Cambridge Monographs on the History of Medicine
EDITORS: CHARLES WEBSTER AND CHARLES ROSENBERG

From medical chemistry to biochemistry

From medical chemistry to biochemistry

THE MAKING OF A BIOMEDICAL DISCIPLINE

Robert E. Kohler

Department of History and Sociology of Science
University of Pennsylvania

CAMBRIDGE UNIVERSITY PRESS

CAMBRIDGE

LONDON   NEW YORK   NEW ROCHELLE
MELBOURNE   SYDNEY

CAMBRIDGE UNIVERSITY PRESS
Cambridge, New York, Melbourne, Madrid, Cape Town, Singapore, São Paulo, Delhi

Cambridge University Press
The Edinburgh Building, Cambridge CB2 8RU, UK

Published in the United States of America by Cambridge University Press, New York

www.cambridge.org
Information on this title: www.cambridge.org/9780521243124

First published 1982
This digitally printed version 2008

A catalogue record for this publication is available from the British Library

Library of Congress Cataloguing in Publication data
Kohler, Robert E.
From medical chemistry to biochemistry.
(Cambridge monographs on the history of
medicine)
Includes bibliographical references.
1. Biological chemistry – History.
2. Biological chemistry – United States – History.
I. Title. II. Series. [DNLM: 1. Biochemistry –
History. QU 11.1 [K79f]
QP511.K63   574.19′2′09   81–10189

ISBN 978-0-521-24312-4 hardback
ISBN 978-0-521-09047-6 paperback

For my colleagues

Contents

Contents

I

Introduction: On discipline history

Histories of the scientific disciplines are not new, but in recent years historians of science have begun to write them in a new way. Older histories were often written by scientists turned historians and were insiders' accounts of the accumulation of more perfect knowledge.[1] They did not inquire why the world of knowledge is divided up as it is, or how it got that way, any more than naturalists before Darwin's generation worried about the origin and extinction of species. There was no particular reason for scientist historians to see how their disciplines were shaped by processes of social and economic adaptation and competition. Disciplines were the framework for descriptive natural histories of knowledge, not for analyses of the evolution and perpetuation of social forms.

Disciplines are political institutions that demarcate areas of academic territory, allocate the privileges and responsibilities of expertise, and structure claims on resources. They are the infrastructure of science, embodied in university departments, professional societies, and informal market relationships between the producers and consumers of knowledge. They are creatures of history and reflect human habits and preferences, not a fixed order of nature. There have as yet been few studies of sciences as institutions, and it is this aspect of the discipline of biochemistry that will concern me here. I will have less to say about biochemistry as a system of ideas than about biochemists' collective efforts to build and maintain their own institutions. The focus will be on how the symbiosis between biochemistry and medicine was established and how it shaped biochemists' practices. I shall show how different styles or programs of biochemistry developed as adaptations to particular institutional contexts.

The special appeal of studying the history of disciplines is derived from their dual functions as guides for intellectual and political behavior. This was pointed out by both Charles Rosenberg and Russell McCormmach.[2] Rosenberg observed that disciplines are where individual and collective values meet:

It is the discipline that ultimately shapes the scholar's vocational identity. The confraternity of his acknowledged peers defines the scholar's aspirations, sets appropriate problems, and provides the intellectual tools with which to address them; finally it is the discipline that rewards intellectual achievement. At the same time his disciplinary identity helps structure the scholar or scientist's relationship to a particular institutional context. His professional life becomes then a compromise defined by the sometimes consistent and sometimes conflicting demands of his discipline and the conditions of his employment.[3]

Disciplinary affiliation, far more than family, party, class, or even educational experience, shapes scientific careers and discourse. Because disciplines regulate intellectual traffic among scientific communities, they are indispensable for understanding innovations that may occur when academic boundaries and trade relations shift. Departments and professional societies mediate between science and the political, cultural, and economic institutions on which science depends for material and political support.

Disciplinary history also has strategic advantages for historians of science. It provides common ground for the "internalist" and "externalist" camps and opens communications with other historical specialties. Rosenberg hoped that the study of disciplines would encourage historians to accept science and medicine as aspects of social and intellectual history and would alert historians of science to the benefits of a broad historical perspective. For McCormmach, discipline history was a way of taking the blinders off the intellectual history of science without losing that distinctive emphasis differentiating the history of science from general history and justifying its existence as a distinct discipline. The intellectual benefits of discipline history are congruent with the strategic needs of historians of science to consolidate their discipline and win greater support from social, economic, and intellectual historians.

It is surprising, in view of its promise, how little discipline history has been done in the past 15 years. Disciplines have been invoked to explain the process of selection among different styles of science; Rosenberg's analysis of American styles of genetics is exemplary.[4] Disciplines have been used to explain the differential reception of particular theories of discoveries.[5] The style of research schools has been analyzed in institutional terms. For example,

Gerald Geison suggested, in his study of the Cambridge School of Physiology, how intellectual programs were shaped by the needs and opportunities of institution building.[6] But such studies by historians are rare. Sociologists of science, on the other hand, have been much concerned with the social basis of discovery and have been drawn to the study of networks of scientists working on common problems. They have not, however, generally been concerned with units as large as disciplines.[7] Moreover, by adopting, rather naively, the language of paradigms and consensus, sociologists have neglected the crucial role of historical experience and institutional context on the development of science.

There are signs of change, however. Several recent dissertations deal with departments and disciplines as political and intellectual entities: John Servos has written on physical chemistry in America; P. Thomas Carroll, on the University of Illinois department of chemistry; John O'Donnell, on American psychology. Dorothy Ross and Margaret Rossiter have laid the groundwork for comparative institutional histories of the social and agricultural sciences.[8] Daniel Kevles's book, *The Physicists*, although it does not attempt a systematic analysis of departments and styles, does reveal how American physicists were integrated into economic and political institutions.[9] Why this new interest in a program that has had its prophets for almost two decades? Perhaps we are feeling the effects of the burgeoning post-1960s academic market for "science and society" courses. For a new generation of historians of science, preserving the schism between "internal" and "external" methodologies has neither intellectual nor occupational benefits. Institutional and disciplinary history are ideal programs for a discipline with a heavy investment in intellectual history, adapting to a market that rewards a concern with the social and political aspects of science.

Some readers of this book may feel that the ideas of political economy – entrepreneurs, markets, constituencies, service roles – are overemphasized and the role of scientific ideas underrated. It may be that in some cases particular discoveries were indispensable resources for discipline building. But I do not believe, as I once did, that particular theories have, in general, a causal role in the creation of disciplinary institutions.[10] Some minimal level of intellectual achievement is, of course, a necessary condition for institution building. But intellectual achievement or the lack of it is not the reason why biochemists failed to build a discipline in nineteenth-century Germany or why they succeeded in America, a provincial backwater if judged by research output. Differences in achievement cannot explain why the timing, location, and character of discipline building differed so markedly in the United States, Britain, and Germany. These patterns have to do with the political and economic support system of science: movements for reform of universities and medical schools, changing hospital practice, expanding markets for scientific professionals, and evolving division of labor among disciplines. The importance of political economy is evident in the two great episodes of discipline building: Germany in the midnineteenth and America in the early twentieth century.

Sociologists Joseph Ben-David and Avraham Zloczower invoked the idea of a decentralized, competitive academic market to explain why so many new biomedical disciplines were created in German universities between 1860 and 1880. They argued that in a decentralized system of state-supported universities competing for students and faculty, specialization was an effective strategy both for ambitious scholars and for university leaders. Organizing a new discipline was a way for smaller universities to attract top faculty, and the competitive market ensured that new specialties would be widely adopted once they were recognized in a few places.[11] Ben-David and Zloczower used a similar market argument to account for the ups and downs of achievement by German physiologists.[1] Their point was that the pace of scientific discovery does not depend on potential opportunities in nature or even on available facilities for research. Intellectual opportunities were exploited and facilities were created only when physiologists believed that achievement would be rewarded with specialized chairs, institutes, and stable budget lines. When every university had its chair of physiology, innovation declined, despite the existence of abundant facilities for research. The success of new disciplines in midnineteenth century Germany had to do with the institutional structure of the academic market and the political support for learning in the Second Empire.

The political economy of science in midnineteenth century German universities was in some ways a hothouse culture, not rooted in the provision of economic services.[13] This was not the case in the second great period of discipline building. In the early twentieth century, new applied science disciplines were created in German technical colleges and especially in American universities and their satellite professional schools. But here too the crucial resources for discipline builders were less intellectual than economic and institutional, arising from new connections between science and agricultural and industrial development, and its sanctioning ideology of professionalism and the "service university." In his 1971 study of agricultural experimental station scientists, for example, Charles Rosenberg developed the idea of the scientist – entrepreneur.[14] He showed how scientist – administrators developed new professional roles that met legislators' and farmers' demands for practical results and also scientists' expectations of freedom to pursue basic research in their disciplines. Institutional contexts were created on the interface of academia and agricultural industry in which scientists could take greater responsibilities for economic growth and development and mobilize public support for science on an unprecedented scale, without compromising their disciplinary goals. Opportunities were created in experiment stations for a whole range of new agricultural disciplines. Other varieties of scientist–entrepreneurs performed similar mediating roles in government bureaus, industrial research laboratories, hospitals, social research commissions, and other institutions that utilized scientific knowledge for producing goods and services. An array of new basic applied sciences were created in schools of engineering, medicine, and social science, which provided skilled professionals for new science-based industries.[15] The establishment of biochemistry as a discipline was part of this historical process.

By World War I most scientific disciplines depended on public financial and political support to maintain their competitive position. A high level of research output and good connections with professional markets were crucial in the competition among disciplines or intradisciplinary styles. Political scientist Yaron Ezrahi offers a very suggestive account of how scientists use prevailing social beliefs and economic or political circumstances as resources for establishing their claims to public support.[16] Ezrahi depicts science as an interest group, not essentially different from any other group:

The unprecedented degree to which science in America is dependent upon external material and political support in order to exist has compelled American scientists to engage actively and continually in competition with other social groups for their share of public resources and political support.... [T]he ability of science to grow and flourish depends no longer merely on the free and successful use of intellectual resources, but also on its adaptability to political action and its capacity to convert its unique resources into effective means of political influence.[17]

Althogh Ezrahi is concerned mainly with the political authority of scientific theories in social policy making, his insights are equally applicable to the social processes that shape disciplines. A central theme of this book is that scientists and their allies use professional ideologies and social reform movements as resources to create disciplinary institutions. Underlying this argument is the belief that one cannot distinguish purely technical aspects of ideas from their role as political strategies in the competition for resources. Decisions about research programs, audiences, and department policies represent investments in a future market for scientific skills. Ideas are judged not only for their truth value but also for their utility in discipline building.

Rosenberg, Ben-David, Ezrahi, and others focus on different periods in the history of science, from the 1860s to the 1960s, and on different parts of the scientific enterprise, from academic ivory towers to the interface with production and the arena of national politics. But they share a conception of scientists as social actors in specific institutional contexts. They all use the language of competition, entrepreneurship, and resource management to understand the changing political map of scientific disciplines.

This conception of a political economy of science provides the central ideas for my analysis of discipline building in biochemistry. My main argument is that biochemists succeeded in establishing independent departments in American medical schools because the medical reform movement there offered opportunities that were not found in Germany or Britain. As medical colleges became postgraduate schools, elementary chemistry was relocated to premedical courses, and an essential service role was created for biochemists in the roster of preclinical disciplines. The belief of American medical reformers that science and scientific methods were crucial to medicine gave biochemists a key role in training physicians. Because of the historic weakness of the biomedical sciences in America, physiologists could not compete for biochemists' turf, as they did in Germany and Britain. American reformers' preference for standardized institutions and separate, specialized departments closed the door to alternative programs espoused by departments of physiology, chemistry, or biology. In Germany and Britain, the lack of systematic reform movements and the presence of powerful claimants to biochemistry in physiology and other disciplines resulted in a more lively competition among disciplinary programs and a more protracted, less successful process of discipline building. This will be the jist of Chapters 1–6.

Disciplines are not homogeneous, consensual communities. They consist of diverse segments, often identified with competing styles or programs. These different programs are adapted to different institutional contexts, and, most important, they prescribe favored relationships with other disciplines. If disciplines are to the political economy of science what nations are to the political economy of production and commerce, then it is no surprise that their domestic affairs may be profoundly influenced by a diverse traffic in ideas and problems with neighboring disciplines. This is especially so for biochemistry, which must adapt to an unusual variety of powerful, sometimes domineering, neighbors.

Prior to 1940 there were at least three distinct styles of biochemistry: clinical, bioorganic and biophysical, and biological. One program took from biology its concern with a broad range of fundamental processes and its tolerance of tentative solutions. Another favored the narrow problems and stringent explanations that chemists prefer. A third prescribed the utilitarian problem solving of clinical science. Each defined a style by pointing to paradigms and constituencies in other disciplines. Analysis of these styles will be the burden of Chapters 7–11.

Briefly, the argument is that biochemists' programmatic conceptions of their discipline were shaped by institutional contexts and relationships, such as channels of recruitment, political alliances, and service roles. In American and many European universities, the biochemists' professional role was teaching medical students and training medical graduates in clinical investigation. Biochemists depended on clinicians for financial and political support, and clinicians depended on them for training and new diagnostic techniques. This symbiotic relationship shaped most biochemists' careers. Problems of clinical diagnosis were dominant intellectual interests for some thirty or forty years. Quite different relationships shaped the careers of those fewer biochemists employed in departments of chemistry, physiology, and biology. Physiologists valued biochemistry as an essential subdivision of their discipline. Consequently, biochemists enjoyed stable support but limited opportunities for discipline building. In contrast, chemists saw biochemistry as an important external market for organic or physical chemists, but not as part of their discipline. Departments of chemistry almost never appointed biochemists to their staffs, but as the principal source of recruits, they profoundly influenced biochemistry. Biochemistry interacted with biology in still different ways. Traditional biologists mistrusted biochemists' reductionist views, and those interested in applying physics and chemistry disdained biochemists as narrow specialists. Very few biologists were recruited to biochemistry, and departments of biology seldom appointed biochemists. Chemical biology flourished in a few independent, self-consciously interdisciplinary institutes, insulated both from medicine and traditional biology. A few market relationships thus shaped the career options of recruits to the discipline.

The connection between institutional contexts and disciplinary styles, what Rosenberg has called the "ecology of knowledge,"[18] can best be seen by looking at university departments. Their mission is to embody and perpetuate disciplines. Programs are often discussed explicitly in connection with appointments to chairs, and these records are often available in university archives, an extremely rich and little-used historical resource. Individuals fashion programs out of their own experience but work them out in building departments. For example, the Cambridge biochemist F. G. Hopkins gradually developed a vision of biochemistry as a broadly biological discipline. His vision was manifested, not in his own research, but in his institute, which included individuals with competencies in microbiology, botany, embryology, and chemistry. It is possible to identify departments that exemplify other disciplinary styles and to relate these styles to the service roles that justified growth and influence. Departmental politics are often revealing of relations among disciplines. Many departments were established by physiologists, chemists and clinicians, and university administrators, who were concerned with the overall division of labor among the biomedical sciences. Innovations were thus stimulated or legitimated by criteria external to biochemistry. As the ecological metaphor implies, department programs were shaped by many actors and a process of adaptation to a complex social and economic environment.

2

Physiological chemistry in Germany, 1840–1900

As biologists have learned to see species as historical creations, not embodiments of some essential reality, so too must historians learn to think of disciplines as human creations, not subdivisions of a fixed natural order. The scope and thrust of biochemistry were, at crucial points in its history, very much up for grabs; at all times, they were subject to some degree of local interpretation. One must think of biochemistry in two complementary ways: as a body of work in the biomedical aspects of chemistry and as a political or institutional rubric that varies with time and locale. I use the term "biochemistry" to refer to the timeless extended family of biochemistries; when referring to specific historical groups, I use the terms they themselves used: physiological or pathological chemistry, medical chemistry, biological chemistry, *and* biochemistry, because that term too identifies a group of historical actors. "Biochemistry" has two meanings here, which is awkward, but inescapable.

Most academic disciplines originated in the rather brief period of active institution building in Germany, from 1840 to 1890. In physiological chemistry, as in most fields of science, Germany took a strong and early lead. Yet physiological chemistry was an anomaly; it was not a story of rapid and successful specialization and growth. Germans led in the production of biochemical research; but there were few institutions of physiological chemistry and these had little growth potential. This weakness became apparent after about 1900 when other countries, notably the United States, took the lead in institution building. This seeming paradox of intellectual success and institutional failure was, I believe, a consequence of the historical relationships of German biochemists with physiologists and chemists.

In most European universities, physiological chemistry evolved as a subdivision of physiology. Its association with physiology was not an inevitable consequence of the nature of that discipline, however. Physiological chemists were attached to physiology in the 1870s after a preceding generation had failed to establish their claim to the emerging specialty of organic chemistry. Only a few found careers in pathology, pharmacology, and hygiene, although chemistry was no less relevant there than in physiology. These patterns have more to do with institutional structures and strategies than with intellectual affinities.

Let us first look more closely at the anomalous pattern of discipline building. In 1905 Cambridge physiologist John Langley and clinician Thomas Clifford Allbutt cited impressive evidence of a biochemistry gap: in 1903, they claimed, 2,500 German workers published over 3,000 papers on chemical aspects of the biomedical sciences, whereas a handful of British workers published 70 papers, mostly of low quality. Although Britain and the United States had only 2 regular academic positions for biochemists, Langley and Allbutt counted 11 in Germany, 8 in Austria, and 15 in five other European countries.[1] Exaggeration of rivals' strengths was a regular part of the "neglect of science" game, of course, and Langley and Allbutt admitted that many of the continental positions were not in physiological chemistry as such. (Most, in fact, were attached to other disciplines.) Nevertheless, perusal of the *Biochemische Zentralblatt* bears out Langley and Allbutt's claim. Biochemical research was flourishing in institutes of chemistry, physiology, pathology, pharmacology, and clinical medicine.

Compared with these other biomedical disciplines, however, physiological chemists had few institutions devoted exclusively to their discipline. In 1906 the medical faculties of all 27 German-speaking universities had *ordinarius* (that is, full) professors of pathological anatomy, physiology, and hygiene, 24 had chairs of pharmacology, but only 9 had *ordinarius* professors of physiological chemistry. Four of these nine were less specialized chairs of "medical chemistry," including general chemistry, and three were combined chairs of pharmacology and physiological chemistry.[2] By 1918 three chairs had disappeared. The prospects for German biochemistry were less rosy than they seemed to be when viewed from across the Channel. In 1926 the Cambridge biochemist F. Gowland Hopkins drew a pointed contrast between the numerous flourishing schools in British and American universities and the marked absence of biochemical institutes in Germany.[3] This disparity was the result of a pattern set in Germany in the midnineteenth century. Physiological chemistry was the *Stiefkind* of the biomedical disciplines.

Taking the establishment of *ordinarius* chairs as an indicator of discipline building, physiology, pathological anatomy, hygiene, and pharmacology (less clearly) all show the same pattern of institutional growth: a few early innovators, then a rush of new chairs, and rapid saturation of the market[4] (see Figure 2.1). The whole cycle took about 30 years, with half to two-thirds of the new chairs being established in only 10 or 15 years.

Physiological chemistry is the single exception to this pattern among the biomedical sciences. Following a brief spate of new chairs in the 1870s, more chairs disappeared than were created until after World War I. Seven universities had no independent institutes of biochemistry until after World War II (see Figure 2.2). The pattern persists if we take a less stringent indicator of discipline growth by including *ausserordentlich* professorships, which were created only for the lifetime of particular individuals (see Figure 2.3). Many were secondary positions in institutes of physiology, pathology, or pharmacology and were subject to the changing priorities of these disciplines.

A still less stringent measure of the recognition of physiological chemistry as a discipline is the total number of specialized personnel, including *Privatdozenten*, the unsalaried instructor–researchers from whose ranks the German professoriat was recruited. Christian Ferber has gathered this data for selected years between 1864 and 1938[5] (see Table 2.1). Again the small size of the academic community of physiological chemists is apparent: one-third the size of physiology, one-half of pharmacology. Physiological chemists had fewer positions than either physical chemists or pharmaceutical chemists. Physiological chemistry had neither the academic prestige of the other biomedical disciplines nor the professional market of the applied chemical specialties. Why?

Joseph Ben-David and Abraham Zloczower have argued that the establishment of specialized disciplines was facilitated by the economic and political structure of the German university system.[6] In a decentralized system of state-supported universities, competing freely for both faculty and students, a strategy of specialization

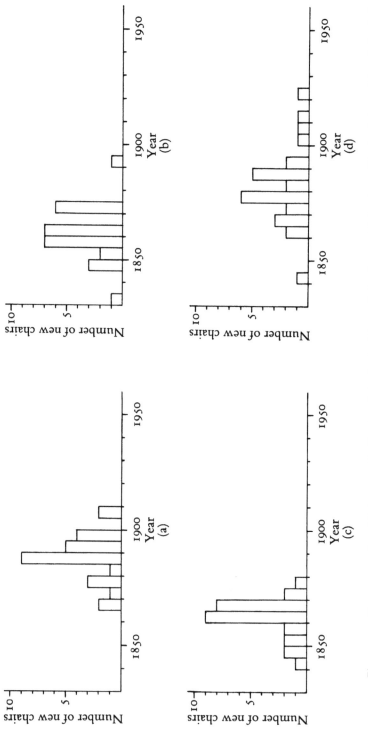

Figure 2.1. Frequency of establishment of *ordinarius* chairs in the biomedical sciences: (a) hygiene; (b) physiology; (c) pathological anatomy; (d) pharmacology.

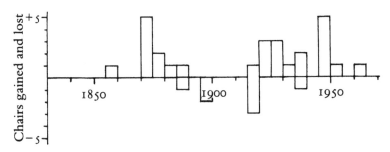

Figure 2.2. Frequency of establishment and disappearance of *ordinarius* chairs in physiological chemistry.

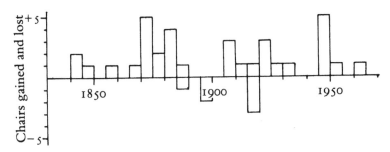

Figure 2.3. Frequency of establishment and disappearance of *ordinarius* chairs and *ausserordentlich* professorships of physiological chemistry.

Table 2.1. *Total number of faculty in the biomedical disciplines*

Discipline	Year								
	1864	1873	1880	1890	1900	1910	1920	1931	1938
Physiological chemistry									
Ordinarius		1	2	3	2	2	2	10	12
Ausserordentlich			4	3	4	5	5	12	10
Privatdozent		1	6	5	8	4	11	10	7
Total		2	12	11	14	11	18	32	29
Physiology									
Ordinarius	15	19	20	20	21	22	25	28	21
Ausserordentlich	3	3	4	6	9	12	15	24	18
Privatdozent	9	1	2	7	20	27	22	23	15
Total	27	23	26	33	50	61	62	75	54
Pharmacolgy									
Ordinarius	7	11	9	14	16	18	20	22	23
Ausserordentlich	3	6	6	4	3	6	4	16	8
Privatdozent	3	5	4	6	6	13	19	17	17
Total	13	22	19	24	25	37	43	55	48

conferred a real competitive advantage. To gain an edge in the competition for the best faculty, a university would invest in a new specialty, such as physiology, which had hitherto been one leg of a chair of anatomy. Specialized chairs and laboratories enabled physiologists to concentrate resources on their special problems without having to satisfy anatomists' expectations. The rate and quality of research, which is the hard currency of the university marketplace, went up. In order to compete, other universities were obliged to follow suit with specialized chairs and institutes. With the promise of instant career rewards, chairs, and laboratories, institutes drew ambitious and talented recruits and stimulated them to still greater exertions. New disciplines thus spread like fashions throughout the system.

Of course there were intrinsic opportunities for discovery in these new specialties. But opportunities are realized only when there is a market for them: when there are institutions to mobilize resources and a social reward system to guarantee steady careers and recognition for discoverers. There is no necessary conjunction between intellectual opportunity and institutional organization, as the case of physiological chemistry reveals. There was no lack of opportunity for discovery in the chemical aspects of the biomedical sciences, witness the outpouring of research observed and envied by Langley and Allbutt. Physiological chemists were certainly no less keen than physiologists to be specialists and masters in their own academic domain. However, their intellectual ambitions were not congruent with the institutional reward system. In this case, institutions impeded the match between ambition and opportunity.

Zloczower has suggested how the competitive market mechanism operated to stifle recognition of physiological chemistry. There were powerful barriers to specialization built into the German system of chairs and institutes. Because institutes had only a single chair, professors were obliged to be generalists and to encompass all aspects of their discipline. Many enjoyed the prestige of possessing encyclopedic learning, and all benefited financially because professors' incomes were largely derived from student fees in the large lecture courses. In an expanding market, specialization was an effective strategy for getting around these barriers. In a static market, however, there were no alternative sources of innovation. Because they were specialized, physiological chemists were considered less eligible for chairs of physiology or chemistry than generalists. Physiologists or chemists who were interested in the border regions between chemistry and the biomedical sciences risked their academic careers by pursuing these opportunities and were rewarded for remaining in chemistry or physiology. As Zloczower points out, by the 1890s the German university system had expanded as far as it could without enlarging the professoriat, and scientific careers were multiplying far more rapidly in hospitals and in technical colleges than in medical faculties.[7]

This explanation is persuasive as far as it goes, but the market mechanism alone does not explain why in one case it promoted specialization and in another suppressed it. Why were specialists in physiology seen as up and coming and physiological chemists seen as *nicht-ordenierbar*? We need to enquire more deeply into the particular historical relations of physiological chemistry with chemistry and other biomedical disciplines.

PHYSIOLOGICAL VERSUS ORGANIC CHEMISTS, 1840–1870

In the early nineteenth century, experimental chemistry was a medical discipline, located in medical faculties or schools of pharmacy. As philosophical faculties were organized, between 1820 and 1850, chemistry was reorganized as a "pure" academic science and transferred from medical to philosophical faculties. Medical faculties were somewhat slower to adopt scientific ideals, and chemists preferred the prestige and status of philosophical faculties. This shift began in the Prussian and north German universities (Berlin, Bonn, Breslau, Leipzig, Greifswald, Jena, Göttingen, and so on), as, after a lag, did construction of teaching laboratories.[8] In the south German universities (Tübingen, Fribourg, Würzburg, Munich, Heidelberg, Marburg, and so on), reform was slower and the association between chemistry and medicine was longer lived. Still further down the gradient of reform, in the Austrian universities, chemistry remained in medical faculties into the twentieth century.[9] Thus for reform-minded ministries, separation of chemistry and medicine was the mark of progress. Chemists shed their reputation as handmaidens of practical medicine and developed bodies of abstract theory, especially in organic chemistry, in emulation of the *rein Wissenschaften*. Medical reformers emphasized the need for strong basic sciences in medical training and insisted that their students be instructed by pure chemists in philosophical faculties.[10] University leaders, state authorities, and organic chemists all embraced the divorce of chemistry and medicine in the name of cultural progress. In contrast, the claims of physiological chemists rested on their traditional role in medical science. This strategy was ill adapted to institutional realities and soon failed.

In the 1840s and 1850s, a number of attempts were made to establish independent chairs of physiological chemistry. Most of these early efforts at discipline building occurred in south German universities: Tübingen (Würtemberg), Fribourg (Baden), and the three Bavarian universities of Erlangen, Munich, and Würzburg. Felix Hoppe-Seyler's institute of physiological chemistry at Strasbourg (in Alsace) was modeled on Tübingen and may be seen as the last of this early group. Except for Leipzig (Saxony), which had an independent chair for a few years, no north German university tried to establish a chair of physiological chemistry.

These early experiments in discipline building may best be seen as an aborted attempt to reform academic chemistry, not as an attempt to create a new discipline of physiological chemistry. Justus Liebig's treatises on animal and agricultural chemistry, which were enormously popular in the 1840s, are usually taken to be the design for a new discipline of physiological chemistry.[11] It is more reasonable to see them as a design for chemistry as a whole, based on Liebig's own experience as a discipline builder. His school of experimental chemistry had developed in the School of Pharmacy at Giessen before being admitted (grudgingly) into the philosophical faculty.[12] Liebig built his program for chemistry on the long-standing association of chemistry with medicine and pharmacy, and his program was in direct competition with theoretical organic chemistry. (It is no accident that Liebig took up physiological and agricultural chemistry after losing the lead in structure theory to the French school of Dumas.) His grandiose theories of nutrition, digestion, and metabolism were designed to provide a theoretical program that was as academically respectable as structure theory was for organic chemistry. Liebig saw chemistry as an applied science, allied to pharmacy, medicine, and agriculture, and he aimed to domesticate this vision to the new philosophical faculties. His strategy was to capitalize on what, in his experience, had been the most reliable institutional support.

In the context of university reform, however, this applied science program was less viable than the broader and more theoretical

programs of general or organic chemistry. The old intimacy between chemistry and medicine was no longer seen as a desirable
alliance. Colleges of agriculture and pharmacy remained segregated
from universities, like technical and business colleges. Liebig's
highly speculative theories aged rapidly after about 1850 and ceased
to be of any use to chemists, whereas organic structure theory
enjoyed one stunning success after another. Liebig gave up teaching.
He went to Munich in 1850 as a popular author, lecturer, and
cultural lion, not as the leader of a research school. After 1850, chairs
of chemistry in all the German states were increasingly occupied by
general chemists, such as Friedrich Wöhler and Robert Bunsen, or
by organic chemists, such as A. W. Hofmann, August Kekule, and
Heinrich Kolbe. Chairs of physiological chemistry were regarded
as second-rate alternatives to chairs of organic chemistry; existing
chairs in medical faculties were reorganized in philosophical faculties. The failure of physiological chemistry to become a discipline in
the period from 1840 to 1860 is the reverse side of the success of
organic chemistry, seen from the loser's point of view.

Despite considerable local variation, there are some common
themes in the rise and demise of physiological chemistry at Tübingen,
Würzburg, Leipzig, Strasbourg, Erlangen, Munich, Fribourg,
and Heidelberg. First, relocation of chemistry from medicine to
science was generally delayed or incomplete. The existence of a
chair of medical chemistry facilitated efforts to establish physiological chemistry. It was no guarantee of success, however; personalities
and local politics were often the decisive factor.

Second, organic and physiological chemistry were often combined in a single chair, thus providing the incumbent with a broader
audience and a stable service role. Where physiological chemistry
was simply an advanced medical specialty separate from organic
chemistry, it had a narrow and vulnerable political base. Where
physiological chemists made a broad claim to chemistry as a whole,
they were vulnerable to criticism for being too ambitious and
specialized and were no match for general and organic chemists. It
was hard to claim neither too much nor too little, and success
occurred in only a few special circumstances.

The first chair of physiological chemistry was established at
Tübingen in 1845 and came closest to realizing the distinctive ideals
of the 1840s' program. It was the only one of the early chairs that
survived into the twentieth century.[13] The first *ausserordentlich* pro-

fessor of physiological chemistry, Julius Schlossberger, had studied with half a dozen of the leading chemists in Germany, including Liebig. He taught all the chemistry courses in the medical faculty, from analytical to organic and physiological chemistry. An active participant in the debates over Liebig's theories, he wrote several popular textbooks on organic and animal chemistry and was promoted to *ordinarius* in 1859, only a year before his untimely death. In 1863, the chair, then occupied by Felix Hoppe-Seyler, was transferred to the philosophical faculty as a second chair in the chemical institute. Hoppe-Seyler was fortunate in having friendly chemical colleagues. Adolf Strecker, who succeeded pharmacist–chemist C. G. Gmelin as professor of chemistry in 1860, was a student of Liebig's and encouraged Hoppe-Seyler's work without trying to divert it to his own chair.[14] Supportive allies and a stable claim to both organic and physiological chemistry were great advantages, and the Tübingen chair enjoyed a century-long succession of first-rate physiological chemists: Hoppe-Seyler (1861–72), Gustav Hüfner (1872–1908), Hans Thierfelder (1908–28), and Franz Knoop (1928–45). All were trained in both organic chemistry and medicine, and none slipped into the narrower role of chemist or physiologist.

The medical faculty at Fribourg also had a firm and long-standing grip on medical chemistry. It was, however, less lucky in its incumbents than was Tübingen. Lambert Heinrich Joseph Anton Konrad Freiherr von Babo inherited a chemical empire as long as his name, embracing inorganic, organic, technical, and pharmaceutical chemistry, minerology, physiological chemistry, and toxicology. Babo fit the stereotype of the academic polymath, spread thin over his domain but guarding every bit with fierce jealousy. Although he had spent a year with Liebig, he taught physiological chemistry only from 1845 to 1851 and prevented others from doing so until 1874, when Johann Latschenberger began to teach physiological chemistry with such success that he was granted a formal *Lehrauftrag* in "physiological chemistry, toxicology, and physicochemical hygiene."[15] Babo retaliated. When his young rival requested space in his laboratory, Babo refused. When Latschenberger petitioned to take over Babo's course in organic chemistry for medical students, Babo refused to allow him even to examine medical candidates in chemistry. Finally, in 1882 Latschenberger demanded his own laboratory and a chair in physiological chemistry. The Karlsruhe Ministry called his bluff and Latschenberger resigned. Babo had alienated his medical colleagues, however, and in 1883 he too was forced to resign and his empire was divided. An organic chemist, Adolph Claus, was appointed to a new chair in the philosophical faculty.[16]

Despite this split, the Fribourg Medical Faculty managed, by a shrewd appointment, to keep the medical course in organic chemistry. Eugen Baumann, who took what was left of Babo's chair, was both an organic and physiological chemist. He was Hoppe-Seyler's first assistant at Strasbourg but habilitated as a chemist in 1876. From 1877 until his appointment at Fribourg, he was head of the chemical *Abteilung* of the Berlin Physiological Institute. Baumann worked mainly in the organic chemistry of natural substances, but he had a lively interest in the chemical processes of metabolism, especially oxidation and biosynthesis.[17] Baumann was in a position to claim both physiological and organic chemistry. This arrangement displeased the chemist Claus, but the medical faculty supported Baumann's claim, believing that medical students should not be instructed by a pure *Organiker*. Working in the same laboratory with Claus, Baumann was often at odds with his irascible colleague. Nevertheless, Fribourg rivaled Tübingen as a center of organic-physiological chemistry until Baumann's untimely death in 1896.[18]

In other universities, the combination of organic and physiological chemistry was politically unstable and short-lived. At Leipzig, for example, physiological chemistry began much as it had at Tübingen as an outgrowth of the chair of chemistry in the medical faculty held by O. B. Kühn. In 1843 Carl Lehmann was named *ausserordentlich* professor of physiological chemistry under Kühn and in 1854 was promoted to *ordinarius*. Lehmann was a discipline builder: he wrote the first recognizably modern textbook, which was far more effective in defining the discipline of physiological chemistry than were Liebig's idiosyncratic works.[19] In Saxony, a medical chair of chemistry seemed increasingly anomalous, however. When Lehmann became professor of chemistry at Jena in 1856, his chair was abolished. When Kühn died in 1863, his chair too was abolished and a new one created in the philosophical faculty for Herman Kolbe, a bright young organic chemist.[20] Physiological chemistry was picked up by Carl Ludwig's growing school of physiology.

Variations on this sequence of events were played out elsewhere. The chair of chemistry at Heidelberg remained in the medical faculty until 1851, when Leopold Gmelin's successor, the organic chemist Robert Bunsen, insisted that it be transferred to the philosophical faculty.[21] Organic and physiological chemistry were split. Bunsen taught the medical course in organic chemistry and created one of the largest and most influential schools of organic chemistry in Germany. In the medical faculty, Gmelin's disciple, Friedrich Delff, taught a narrowed range of clinical chemistry, toxicology, and forensic medicine.[22] Meanwhile, physiological chemistry was picked up by Willy Kühne in the Institute of Physiology. At Erlangen in northern Bavaria, an *ausserordentlich* professorship of organic and physiological chemistry was established by the medical faculty in 1849 for Eugen Gorup-Besanez, a disciple of Liebig. Although Gorup-Besanez taught physiological chemistry until 1872, the combination was increasingly anomalous, and he was succeeded in 1878 by Jacob Vollhard, who founded a vigorous school of organic chemistry.[23] At Würzburg, Johann v. Scherer held a chair of organic chemistry in the medical faculty from 1842 and taught a course based on Liebig's *Animal Chemistry*.[24] Because of the deaths of two professors of chemistry, Scherer also managed to take over the courses in inorganic and organic chemistry for medical students. In 1866 he was given a new institute for medical chemistry, which included basic chemistry.[25] This combination was out of harmony with the trend toward specialization, however, and did not survive Scherer's death in 1869. His institute was stripped of hygiene and transferred to the philosophical faculty, where organic chemists Adolf Strecker and Johannes Wislicenus took charge.[26] Physiological chemistry was incorporated into the chair of physiology, and it did not acquire separate status until 1922.

These cases illustrate how difficult it was for physiological chemists to compete with organic chemists. University leaders were anxious to have a modern organic chemist and found that chairs of medical or physiological chemistry could be easily reshaped to attract an ambitious young *Organiker*. As the 1840s' generation of organic-physiological chemists died or retired, they were replaced by a new generation of organic chemists who took over the lucrative medical courses but did not develop physiological chemistry. The Tübingen model of the 1840s was disrupted by the more rapid development of theoretical organic chemistry in the 1850s and 1860s. There was no shortage of able discipline builders, but younger physiological chemists tended to drift into careers in more stable disciplines. Carl Lehmann turned chemist; others escaped into the biomedical sciences, for example, Max Pettenkoffer at Munich.

Pettenkoffer was appointed *ausserordentlich* professor of medical chemistry at Munich in 1847, but the existence of a chair of chemistry in the philosophical faculty obliged Pettenkoffer to confine himself to medical applications.[27] As he wrote to Liebig, he found his role increasingly irksome:

My duties are to lecture on so-called physiological and pathological chemistry and to perform the familiar and dreary routine analyses of urine, blood, etc., for the clinicians. It is not for the advancement of their own understanding that the clinicians want this help but mainly as extra decoration for their clinical lectures, for the sake of symmetry: a painted window on an artificial building.[28]

In fact, Munich seemed an almost ideal place to develop physiological chemistry. In 1852 Pettenkoffer persuaded Liebig to accept the vacant chair of pure chemistry. Pettenkoffer was promoted to a chair of medical chemistry in 1853, and in 1854 Liebig's long-time collaborator in physiology, Theodor Bischoff, was appointed to the chair of anatomy and physiology. Influential allies were no substitute for a broad and independent base in chemistry, however, and Pettenkoffer found more rewarding outlets for his professional ambitions. He became interested in public health during the cholera scare of 1854, inaugurated courses in sanitary chemistry, and in 1865 had his chair reconstituted as a chair of hygiene. Meanwhile, Liebig lectured to adoring crowds, revised his best-selling books, and enjoyed civic and court society. (When Jacob Vollhard revived organic chemistry in 1863, he started from scratch, equipping the laboratory at his own expense.[29]) Physiological chemistry was picked up by Bischoff's student, Carl Voit, who devoted his career to developing Liebig's theories of metabolism. Voit received an independent chair of physiology in 1863, and a separate chemical *Abteilung* was not established until after his death in 1908.[30]

STRASBOURG

Felix Hoppe-Seyler's famous Strasbourg Institute has been regarded by biochemists and historians as a new initiative in discipline building. It is more accurate to see it as the last of the experiments in discipline building that began in the 1840s and were already outmoded by 1872. Everywhere, physiological chemistry was being divided between organic chemistry and physiology, and the Strasbourg Institute survived only because it was treated like a hothouse flower, protected from the buffets of ministerial economizing and academic politics. Annexed with the rest of Alsace after the Franco-Prussian War, the French University of Strasbourg became a showpiece of German cultural imperialism. The Prussian universities symbolized, for Germans, the superiority of German *Kultur* over French *civilisation*, and the Prussian government wanted Strasbourg to combine the best aspects of all the German universities. It was a demonstration to the French of the superiority of German *Wissenschaft*.[31] Although there was only one chair of physiological chemistry in all Germany, Strasbourg had to have a second, and Hoppe-Seyler was appointed to bring the Tübingen spirit to German Alsace.

The Strasbourg Institute was a response to political needs, not to the market demand for physiological chemistry, and the performance of the Prussian ministers did not match their promises. Hoppe-Seyler had to wait 11 years for a new institute and laboratory; it was the last such institute to be built in imperial Germany.[32] The euphoric enthusiasm of this outpost of German culture made up for the cramped and dilapidated facilities of the old École de Médicine. Albrecht Kossel recalled the intoxication of the early years. When Russell Chittenden arrived from New Haven in 1878, he was impressed by the pace of research but appalled at the crowded and ancient facilities.[33]

The Strasbourg Institute lacked two crucial advantages of the Tübingen Institute: it did not include organic chemistry and it depended increasingly on its service role in hygiene. At Tübingen, Hoppe-Seyler had lectured on organic chemistry, and his successor, Gustav Hüfner, took turns with chemists Strecker and Rudolf Fittig.[34] At Strasbourg, Hoppe-Seyler lectured on physiological chemistry, toxicology, forensic medicine, nutrition, and hygiene.[35] Whereas Hüfner examined students jointly with the chemists, Hoppe-Seyler did so with the physiologists. Hüfner did not approve of this alliance, as he wrote to physiologist Hugo Kronecker: "The physiological chemist must strive to give the physician a general chemical instruction, as I in fact do."[36] At Tübingen, physiological chemistry was the top level of an integrated sequence firmly based in general and organic chemistry. At Strasbourg, it was a top-heavy cluster of minor clinical specialties.

In his inaugural lecture in 1884, Hoppe-Seyler offered an analysis of why physiological chemistry was not getting support as an independent discipline. He pointed to the fact that physiological chemists had come to rely exclusively on clinical medicine, even at Tübingen, whereas organic chemists were developing a broad and lucrative connection to industry. He warned of the vulnerability of a clinical connection, observing that although a few clinicians had become more active in chemical work, the majority were noticeably cooler about physiological chemistry than they had been a decade or two earlier. The therapeutic nihilism of the Vienna school had diminished interest in chemical methods in pathology and bacteriology. Clinicians had come to believe that chemical explanations of metabolism were a very distant prospect and used physiological chemists for strictly routine services.[37]

Hoppe-Seyler was very active in promoting physiological chemistry. He formulated programs for the fledgling discipline, staking out a broad territory of basic chemistry, biology, and biomedical science. He founded and edited the *Zeitschrift für physiologische Chemie* (1877), which combined basic organic chemistry and a concern with biological processes, in the Tübingen style. For 30 years this was the only specialized journal of physiological chemistry. In 1877, Hoppe-Seyler published his popular and influential handbook, a major portion of which was devoted to basic biology. While his active research group churned out experimental work, Hoppe-Seyler formulated synthetic theories of biological function; for example, his theory of the linkage between oxidation and biosynthesis.[38]

Hoppe-Seyler's activities as discipline builder earned him and his institute an international reputation. But he could not remedy the basic institutional weaknesses of his discipline. His research school was excellent, but small. An American visitor, Edwin Faust, reported the following in 1895:

The University buildings here are certainly magnificent. What a pity that a man like Schmiedeberg, with such an institution, should have only eight men working in the Laboratory. . . . I asked Hoppe-Seyler whether there was an *Andrang* to his laboratory for places, and if it were necessary to announce one's intention of working there some time ahead; he smiled sadly, shook his head and said: "Oh, nein, hier ist immer genug Platz," and indeed the place looks quiet.[39]

In his later years, Hoppe-Seyler worried that his institute would not survive him, and in fact, his death in 1895 did raise serious questions as to his successor. Gustav Hüfner was called from Tübingen, but he declined on the grounds that the chair did not include organic chemistry: "the chair at Strasbourg...gives too little ground and foundation under the student, and it does not allow the physiological chemist to shape the whole chemical education of the young doctor."[40] Eugen Baumann was then called from Fribourg, but he too declined for, what one suspects were similar reasons.

Unable to find a successor to Hoppe-Seyler who was both chemist and biologist, the authorities decided to split the chair, giving the bulk of its responsibilities and perquisites to a new chair of hygiene. Physiological chemist Edmund Drechsel wrote in dismay to his American friend, J. J. Abel, of his disastrous blow to their discipline:

It is really sad that there is so little judgment in medical circles and that they have been so blinded by a slogan like "hygiene." This is the most damaging blow of all those that physiological chemistry has suffered in recent times. What people are used to celebrate as the successes of "hygiene" are really nothing but a collection of the achievements of a whole lot of other disciplines such as physiological chemistry and physics, bacteriology, ophthalmology, pathological anatomy, etc., etc.[41]

Franz Hofmeister was called to the chair from Prague, and Drechsel feared he would be left with only "odds and ends" of a *Fach*.[42]

Hofmeister proved to be a most worthy successor to Hoppe-Seyler, however. Edwin Faust reported to Abel that Hofmeister's excellent lectures were attracting an increasing number of students to Strasbourg: "Physiological chemistry is flourishing here at present and it has the appearance that it will continue to do so."[43] In 1902, Paul Ehrlich's first assistant left his well-paid post in the hope of getting a second assistantship at Strasbourg.[44] Hofmeister founded a second journal in 1902 and had a broad and imaginative programmatic vision of the discipline, to which he applied the new term "Biochemie."[45] Strasbourg's continuing influence depended entirely on Hofmeister's personal strengths, however, not on a broad economic and political base. It ceased to exist when Alsace was reannexed by France in 1918, destroyed by the same kind of politics that had brought it into being in 1871.

The 1840s' program was in some respects a viable design for discipline building. The combination of organic and physiological chemistry was intellectually sound. The courses in general and organic chemistry required of all medical students were a firm economic base for specialized teaching and research. Politically, however, the combination was unstable. The increasingly important connections to the synthetic dye industry in the 1860s drew organic chemists away from medicine but did not diminish their desire to keep their hold on the lucrative courses for medical students. In the more "progressive" universities of north Germany, medical faculties generally agreed that their students should be taught by pure organic chemists (at Greifswald, for example).[46] Chemists in the south German universities were under increasing financial and ideological pressure to develop organic chemistry in philosophical faculties, and it seemed inefficient to maintain similar but second-rate chairs of medical or physiological chemistry in medical faculties. Each succession of a chair became a political crisis for the physiological chemists who saw their positions diverted to organic chemistry.

In a few cases medical faculties managed to hold on to a second chair of chemistry, but whether incumbents taught organic or physiological chemistry depended on their personal taste or political clout. There was no structured role for physiological chemistry. Fribourg exemplifies this pattern. When Baumann died in 1896 and again when Claus retired in 1899, the Fribourg philosophical faculty tried to co-opt the chair of medical chemistry. They failed. However, Baumann's successor, Heinrich Kiliani, was not interested in physiological chemistry, and the subject was not offered at all until 1904, when a special *Abteilung* was established by Kiliani for his junior colleague Franz Knoop. Knoop combined the organic chemist's skills with the physiologist's interest in intermediary metabolism and gradually reestablished physiological chemistry. He received a new institute in 1915, after he refused an offer from the Rockefeller Institute in New York, and when Kiliani retired in 1920, Knoop was named professor of physiological chemistry.[47] However, Fribourg and Tübingen were the exceptions to the rule: the 1840s' program was dead by 1870.

CHEMICAL PHYSIOLOGY

In most German universities, physiological chemistry was divided between organic chemistry and physiology. It was taken for granted that chemistry was indispensable to physiology and pathology and should be part of preclinical instruction, though not as a separate

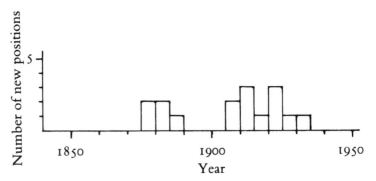

Figure 2.4. Frequency of new *ausserordentlich* physiological chemists in institutes of physiology.

discipline. Physiologists and pathologists provided physiological chemists with modest support and shelter from the tempests of university politics but left them dependent on patrons for whom chemistry was a tool for furthering their own goals. Dependence on physiology was often intellectually stimulating for physiological chemists, but it sharply limited their ability to create independent roles and institutions.

Secondary positions for physiological chemistry in physiological institutes were created in two distinct waves, one in the 1870s and one after 1905 (see Figure 2.4). The first wave was a consequence of the establishment of new physiological institutes in the 1860s and 1870s. This first group included the universities of Berlin, Breslau, Jena, and Leipzig, all of which were in Prussia or north German states. The second wave followed the formal recognition of physiological chemistry as a required part of the state medical examinations in physiology in 1904. The association between physiology and physiological chemistry was determined more by the economics and politics of institution building than by intellectual affinity. The split between physiological and organic chemistry in the 1850s and 1860s was an opportunity that physiologists could exploit to help gain independence from anatomy in the 1860s and 1870s. Their claim to physiological chemistry was supported by state authorities as being financially efficient and intellectually progressive.

Most of the new positions for physiological chemists prior to about 1914 were created by physiologists who were themselves the first to hold an independent chair, and their attitudes were shaped by their roles as discipline builders. Physiological chemistry had both intellectual and strategic importance. Adoption of chemical theories and methods not only opened new intellectual vistas but also served to differentiate physiologists' ideas and skills from those of anatomists. This distinction was crucial at a time when physiologists were breaking loose from anatomy and claiming separate institutes. Because chemical physiology had to do with *processes* in living matter, it was an area in which the contrast with anatomists' structural and morphological concerns was especially sharp. It required skills that the old generation of anatomist–physiologists did not possess and did not care to acquire. Moreover, the connection between physiology and physics and chemistry had a special ideological appeal in midnineteenth-century Germany. It was a banner raised by a new generation of experimentalists and materialists against the old *Naturphilosophie*.[48] It symbolized the ideals of scientific medicine and united the interests of the new physiologists and reform-minded bureaucrats. Intellectual opportunity and political interest coincided.

To assert their independence and importance, physiologists developed an expansive imperialistic program, of which chemical physiology was an integral part. Jan Purkyně's plan for an institute of physiology at Breslau in the 1830s included three sections, or *Abteilungen*, for microscopic, chemical, and experimental or physical physiology.[49] This tripartite program shaped the new institutes of the 1860s and 1870s: histology, chemical or "vegetative" physiology (digestion, assimilation, and metabolism), and physical physiology (nerve–muscle, cardiovascular, sense physiology, etc.). It remained the master plan of the discipline until the 1920s, when a different set of specialties emerged, such as industrial, general, and clinical physiology and physiological psychology. As physiological chemistry was detached from organic chemistry, it was readily assimilated into the growing empire of physiology.

Chemical physiology was crucial to the new ideals of practical laboratory teaching. Chemical physiology lent itself to laboratory instruction on a mass scale: unlike physical physiology, it did not require complex and expensive apparatus or sophisticated knowledge of anatomy and physiology. Chemical work avoided the political problems that arose when students worked with living animals. Isolation of metabolic products from body fluids, experiments with digestive enzymes, and measurements of respiration were the mainstay of elementary laboratory courses. These courses required the services of physiological chemists. Physiologists petitioning for new laboratories and institutes often rested their case on the importance of chemical physiology in teaching.

For all these reasons, physiologists were anxious to encourage chemical physiology but also to resist separatist movements by physiological chemists. Chemistry was vital to physiologists' own claims to separate status as a discipline, to their role as leaders of progressive medical science, and to their ability to pry new facilities out of tight-fisted ministries. Physiologists had to balance their desire to encourage physiological chemists and their fear of losing the field to the experts.

Whether or not semi-independent positions were created for physiological chemists depended on individual attitudes and local circumstances. In some places, physiological chemistry was institutionalized as a formal *Lehrauftrag* or a quasi-independent *Abteilung*, and in others it remained part of the omnibus role of the professor of physiology. In a few rare cases, chemical physiologists occupied chairs of physiology: Willy Kühne (Heidelberg), Albrecht Kossel (Marburg), Gustav Embden (Frankfurt), and Emil Abderhalden (Halle) are the outstanding examples. Generally, however, physiologists who specialized in physiological chemistry ran the risk of making themselves *nicht-ordenierbar*. Physiologists specializing in "vegetative" physiology were not necessarily advocates of specialized roles for physiological chemists. Because their own interest was threatened, they often resisted most strenuously any erosion of their personal territory. Professors who were physical physiologists were often more willing to create *ausserordentlich* roles for physiological chemists; others were simply not interested at all. The absence of a standard institutional pattern thus left physiological chemists at the mercy of personal or political contingencies.

Breslau, Leipzig, and Berlin were the first to establish official positions for chemical physiology, in 1875–8. These universities were among the preeminent institutes of physiology in Germany – breeders of physiologists. All were centers of the new physicochemical ideals, with close ties to the Berlin school of Johannes Müller and Hermann Helmholtz. Emil Du Bois-Reymond was a disciple of Helmholtz's, as was Karl Ludwig, who imported the Berlin ideas to Leipzig. At Breslau, Rudolph Heidenhain continued the tradition of his teacher, Du Bois-Reymond. These physical physiologists were ambitious discipline builders, with an expansive vision of physiology and no proprietary stake in physiological chemistry. At Breslau, Richard Gscheidlen was made *ausserordentlich* professor of chemical physiology in 1875, fulfilling Purkyně's original plan. Gscheidlen and his successors offered a lecture course in physiological chemistry each semester and were more or less independent directors of a chemical *Abteilung*.[50] Karl Ludwig's institute at Leipzig, opened in 1869, had special laboratories for physiological chemistry. Ludwig's plan to get Gustav Hüfner to lead a chemical *Abteilung* was wrecked by local politics; but chemical pathologist Carl Huppert was promoted to *ausserordentlich* professor in 1871, and in 1878 Edmund Drechsel began a lineage of eminent physiological chemists at Leipzig. Ludwig took pains to promote chemical physiology; an assistantship in chemistry was created in 1883, and in 1892 Drechsel's successor, Max Siegfried, was named *Abteilung-Vorsteher*, which, in practice, if not in principle, is an independent chair.[51]

Du Bois-Reymond also used a strategy of specialization to expand physiology at Berlin. His new institute (1877) boasted no fewer than five *Abteilungen*. The chemistry department, led by Eugen Baumann, had the largest portion of laboratory space, and Baumann enjoyed considerable autonomy to develop his specialty, always subject, of course, to the director's vision of a unified, *gesammte Physiologie*. Du Bois-Reymond had no intention of letting physiological chemistry escape as physiology itself had escaped from anatomy:

So great is the pressure toward division of labor in our field that people have already questioned whether the chair of physiology should not be further divided into chemical–physiological, physical–physiological, neuro–physiological, etc., chairs, just as physiology itself previous loosed itself from *Anthropotomie*, *Zootonomy*, and so forth. If this is to be the future of physiology, then we have indeed built unwisely here. For our institute is founded on the belief that above those who teach the individual disciplines stands one who represents the idea of *gesammte Physiologie*.
 The remaining nucleus of physiology is not further divisible because it is like the action of a machine that does not really consist of separable parts. Who would investigate a steam engine by dividing it up among a chemist, to look into the combustion process, a physicist, to study the pressure of the steam in the boiler, a kinamaticist, to study the mechanical linkages,

and a thermodynamicist to deal with the efficiency?...So too in physiology, beginners must be taught the fundamental concepts and ideas of the discipline as parts of a comprehensive, unified whole, in order to have a coherent picture of the animal machine.[52]

By providing specialized roles, political shelter, and material support for physiological chemistry, Du Bois-Reymond forestalled secession. But this relationship depended on individual tact and vision. A later director, Max Rubner, was more possessive and insisted on giving the lectures on chemical physiology himself, with notable lack of success.[53]

The combination of excellent facilities and limited opportunity for promotion and growth made the Berlin *Abteilung* a springboard for first-rate persons on their way to important chairs. Carl Huppert and Edmund Drechsel left Leipzig for chairs at Prague and Bern. Baumann was called to the chair at Fribourg in 1883; his successor, Albrecht Kossel, took the chair of physiology at Marburg in 1895; Hans Thierfelder succeeded Hüfner at Tübingen. The Berlin group was virtually a discipline within a discipline long before it was recognized with an *Ordinariat* in 1928. Especially under Baumann and Kossel, it was one of the most active centers of research and training in physiological chemistry.[54]

Smaller and less prestigious universities could not afford an internal division of roles, and there the disadvantages of dependence were more marked. The checkered history of the chemical *Abteilung* at Jena, established in 1884 by Thierry William Preyer, exemplifies these difficulties. The first incumbent, Friedrich Krukenberg, committed suicide in 1889, allegedly for want of proper support for his *Fach*. His successor, Richard Neumeister, retired in 1897 to medical practice and amateur philosophizing, and his successor made no mark in the discipline.[55] *Privatdozenten* in physiological chemistry at Göttingen, Erlangen, and Fribourg either switched to hygiene or were driven out by competition.[56] Apart from Breslau, Leipzig, and Berlin, only Basel established a formal role for physiological chemistry. There Johann Friedrich Miescher, who had himself done pioneering work on nucleic acids with Hoppe-Seyler, established a second chair in 1886 for Gustav Bunge, who ran a modest, but first-rate, department for 34 years.[57]

The association of physiological chemistry and physiology quickly became an accepted fact. In 1877 Felix Hoppe-Seyler singled out the possessive attitude of physiologists as the main reason why more institutes of physiological chemistry were not being created.[58] Moreover, physiologists ceased to press for an institutionalized division of labor. Besides the one at Jena, no new *Abteilung* for chemical physiology was established between 1880 and 1907. Physiological chemistry was taught in every German university as an integral part of vegetative physiology, but physiologists were no longer interested in creating specialized roles for physiological chemists.

It is not entirely clear why subdivision should have been a less useful strategy for growth in the 1890s than it was in the 1870s. The most likely explanation is that physiologists were no longer encountering competition from the older type of organic-physiological chemists. The spate of new chemical *Abteilungen* in the 1870s may well have been a response to the success of Strasbourg and Tübingen and to contemporary pressures for similar independent institutes for example, at Leipzig. Half a dozen institutes of medical or physiological chemistry were created between 1869 and 1877, although only two of these were in Germany.[59] The determination of such physiologists as Du Bois-Reymond and Eduard Pflüger to preserve the union of physiology and physiological chemistry may reflect their fear that Hoppe-Seyler's and these lesser institutes were a trend.[60] It is suggestive that institutional initiatives in both physiology and physiological chemistry ceased simultaneously in about 1880.

Other possible reasons for the flagging interest in physiological chemistry lie not in physiology as such but in the university system as a whole. Ideological and financial pressures on professors to represent their whole *Fach* certainly impeded the creation of specialized roles. One of the most influential writers on educational policy, Theodor Billroth, deplored the tendency to divide physiology. As the embodiment of *Wissenschaft* and the vehicle of *Kultur* and *Bildung*, the German professor was expected to unite not divide. Pressure on the crowded medical curriculum also discouraged initiatives to establish still more special fields. Billroth was "decidedly opposed" to the practice of requiring faculties to teach small courses in "various branches of medical chemistry under the designations: zoochemistry, physiological and pathological chemistry, chemical toxicology, forensic chemistry."[61] Cut off from chemistry and in an environment hostile to further specialization, physiological chemists had little chance to create independent institutes. Without competition from competing modes, physiologists had little reason to establish new chemical *Abteilungen*.

Recognition of physiological chemistry as an obligatory part of the state medical examination in 1904 created an instant demand for physiological chemists and a renewed spate of institution building. The experience of Friedrich Schulz at Jena is illustrative of the changes brought about by the new regulations. For years Schulz had dragged along with few students; in 1904 he took a semester off for research at Naples. In 1905 he was overwhelmed with students and had to repeat his courses each term to accommodate them.[62] Expanded market demand justified new institutional roles. Carl Voit's successor at Munich saw the establishment of chemical and physical *Abteilungen* as the keystone of reform.[63] Almost invariably, however, physiological chemistry divisions were established as subdivisions of physiology, not as separate chairs. This pattern simply formalized a relationship that had been common practice for 30 years. The hybrid institutes of pharmacology and physiological chemistry at Königsberg, Halle, and Rostock were parted; physiological chemistry was attached to physiology in the new medical faculties created between 1906 and 1914 at Münster, Cologne, and Frankfurt. The history of physiological chemistry in Germany was one of repeated and generally unsuccessful efforts to establish chairs independent of physiology.

VARIANT MODES: PATHOLOGY AND PHARMACOLOGY

Physiological chemistry was also attached to other biomedical disciplines, notably pathology, hygiene, and pharmacology. Although pathologists were somewhat quicker than physiologists to recognize the importance of chemistry, fewer of their institutional experiments survived. Prior to the establishment of physiological institutes, clinics offered better facilities for experimental medical chemistry than did institutes of anatomy. The two earliest journals for physiological chemistry in the 1840s were clinical journals.[64] Because pathological anatomy, bacteriology, and pharmacology remained more dependent on clinical service roles, however, in the long run they were less able than physiology to support roles for physiological chemists.

Between 1871 and 1880, five *ausserordentlich* professorships for physiological chemistry were established in institutes of pathology, at Berlin, Halle, Leipzig, Bern, and Königsberg; joint chairs with pharmacology were created at Rostock and Giessen. The most successful and long-lived of these institutions was the chemical *Abteilung* established by Rudolf Virchow at Berlin. Like Du Bois-Reymond, Virchow was a scion of the mechanistic Berlin school, and his interest in chemical pathology was ideological and strategic as well as intellectual. The key to Virchow's program for pathological anatomy was his belief that the discipline should focus on the physiological processes of disease in order to provide a rational basis for diagnosis and therapeutics. Virchow's tactical problem, like Du Bois-Reymond's, was to define a style and a territory for his discipline that was broader than morbid anatomy, hence not subsumable to it. Pathology had to be indispensable to clinical practice without being dominated by it. A broadly based, subdivided institutional structure that included pathological chemistry served Virchow's aims as discipline builder just as did Du Bois-Reymond's. By 1900 the Berlin Institute consisted of no fewer than six *Abteilungen*, including all of the important research specialties.[65]

Virchow's chemical *Abteilung* was one of the most active and influential centers of physiological chemistry in Germany. Felix Hoppe-Seyler, Willy Kühne, Oskar Liebrich, Ernst Salkowski, and Carl Neuberg were, successively, assistants or department heads. Like its counterpart in physiology, the department of chemical pathology offered limited opportunity for promotion and growth and, hence, served as a feeder for important chairs elsewhere. Kühne became professor of physiology at Heidelberg and Liebrich professor of pharmacology at Berlin. Although Salkowski enjoyed virtual autonomy in running his department, he paid a heavy price for it: he never had a chair of general pathology and did not found a school of physiological or pathological chemistry.[66] The *Abteilung* was intellectually stimulating and financially protected, which made it an excellent context for research but not for discipline building. The Institute of Pathology at Berlin had many admirers but no peers. Several attempts to create a subdivided institute elsewhere thrived for a few years, then failed. In Ernst Wagner's Institute of Pathology at Leipzig, for example, Carl Huppert had an *ausserordentlich* professorship in pathological chemistry in the early 1870s; however, it was subsumed into Ludwig's institute after only one year.[67]

The combination of physiological chemistry and pharmacology grew out of the old discipline of *materia medica*, which had an honored role in the medical curriculum in the era of "heroic" therapeutics.[68] The similarity between pharmacology and physiological chemistry encouraged the establishment of hybrid roles, especially in the smaller medical faculties. Pharmacology, with connections to clinical practice, offered opportunities for career advancement for physiological chemists. For the same reason, however, these hybrid roles tended to be unstable. Halle is a good example. In 1872 Otto Nasse was made *ausserordentlich* professor of physiological and pathological chemistry (in the Institute of Pathology). Confined there to routine clinical chemistry, Nasse accepted a chair of pharmacology and physiological chemistry at Rostock in 1880. Nasse's post at Halle was then merged with a vacant chair of "pharmacology and toxicology" and eventually (1897) became a separate chair of pharmacology.[69] (Physiological chemistry did not revive at Halle until Emil Abderhalden took the chair of physiology in 1911.[70]) A similar pattern unfolded at Königsberg in 1865, when Max Jaffé, a young clinician and physiological chemist, was invited to develop pathological chemistry in Ernst Leyden's Institute of Clinical Medicine. Chemical laboratories were fitted out in the Institute of Pathology, and in 1872 Jaffé was promoted to *ausserordentlich* professor. When the professor of *materia medica* died in 1873, Jaffé was appointed to a combined chair of pharmacology and medical chemistry. Again, however, clinical chemistry offered little opportunity for disciplinary growth, and Jaffé confined his teaching to pharmacology after 1883.[71]

Bacteriology and hygiene likewise provided opportunities for a temporary alliance with physiological chemistry, but these hybrid roles were also unstable. Before the germ theory was widely accepted in the 1880s, physiological chemistry was seen as crucial to understanding the organic "miasmas" that were believed to cause infectious diseases. Physiological chemists were much in demand for water analysis and sanitary surveys and for investigation of the physiology of infection and resistance. As hygiene coalesced as a discipline encompassing bacteriology, physiology, and public health, physiological chemists like Max Pettenkoffer rode the wave of political support into new careers. An *Abteilung* for pathological chemistry and experimental hygiene was established in the Leipzig Institute of Pathology in 1872. The first incumbent, Franz Hofmann, was a disciple of Pettenkoffer and Voit's and like his mentor found nutrition and bacteriology more rewarding than chemistry. In 1878 the *Abteilung* was made an independent institute of hygiene.[72] At

Göttingen, an assistant of Hofmann's, Karl Flügge, took charge of a new institute of medical chemistry and hygiene in 1883, but in 1889 Flügge's successor limited the scope of the Institute to hygiene.[73] Physiological chemistry had no official role at Göttingen until 1918.

A more successful combination of bacteriology and physiological chemistry occurred at Bern, where bacteriologist Edwin Klebs established an assistantship for pathological chemistry (in the Institute of Pathology) in 1872. Klebs's assistant, Marcell Nencki, had studied both chemistry and medicine at Berlin and was an energetic and talented entrepreneur. In 1878 Nencki was promoted to professor and director of a new institute of physiological chemistry, closely connected with pathology. In 1885 he was granted a *Lehrauftrag* in bacteriology, and he did some remarkable pioneering work in bacterial biochemistry. The stability of Nencki's scientific empire depended on his personal presence, however, and when he left Bern in 1891, his institute was divided into chairs of bacteriology, and physiological chemistry plus pharmacology.[74] Edmund Drechsel was called to the latter from Leipzig, and the combination of pharmacology and physiological chemistry continued at Bern until the 1940s.[75] Under Drechsel's successors, however, pharmacology was decidedly the dominant partner.

BIOORGANIC CHEMISTS

Because there were few institutionalized roles and rewards for physiological chemists, biochemical research in Germany was carried on by many different groups in many disciplines for many different reasons. Indeed, most of the original and important biochemical work was done under the rubric of other disciplines. Physiologists and organic chemists in particular dominated the intellectual life of German biochemistry. In the late nineteenth century, such biochemist–physiologists as Willy Kühne, Albrecht Kossel, Ernst Brücke, Friederich Miescher, Gustave Bunge, Leon Asher, and others were at least as influential as the occupants of the few chairs of physiological chemistry. Kühne's laboratory at Heidelberg and Kossel's at Marburg appear to have been more popular and influential than those at Tübingen or Fribourg, at least for foreigners.[76] Because physiological chemistry was attached to physiology, physiologists felt no compunction about pursuing problems in chemical physiology; no institutional division of labor restrained individual predilections. Had physiological chemistry been more developed institutionally, biochemical problems would have been regarded as biochemists' turf, out of bounds for physiologists.

Many of the best German organic chemists also concerned themselves with biochemical problems. From the 1870s to the 1940s, the successive occupants of the Munich Chair, Adolf von Baeyer, Richard Willstätter, and Heinrich Wieland, were leading participants in debates over the chemical mechanisms of fermentation, enzyme action, and biological oxidation. Biochemists adopted Emil Fischer's researches on the structure of sugars and peptides and on the sterochemistry of enzyme reactions as exemplars of their discipline.[77] Fischer's institute at Berlin attracted a stream of German and foreign biochemists. The prominence of organic chemists also reflected the institutional disposition of physiological chemistry. As organic chemists taught the basic courses in the medical curriculum, they had regular opportunities to develop an interest in biomedical problems. Their role also encouraged them to believe that the future of biochemistry depended on regular intervention of organic chemists.

Chemists' theories of biochemical structure and function were credited to a quite extraordinary degree by a discipline that was generally skeptical of speculative theories. In the 1920s, Richard Willstätter's theory that enzymes were small organic molecules absorbed on nonspecific "colloidal" proteins was widely accepted, although the evidence for it could easily have been interpreted otherwise.[78] Other reductionist theories widely believed in the 1920s included Phoebus Levene's "tetranucleotide" theory of nucleic acids; the craze for "colloidal" chemistry, which swept biochemistry in the 1920s; and in the 1930s, the Svedberg's theory of unit proteins and Max Bergmann's theory of simple repeating structures in proteins. One of the hottest events in the 1920s was the clash between Heinrich Wielands and Otto Warburg's theories of biological oxidation, both of which rested on simplistic analogies with simple chemical systems.[79] The credit given to these and other theories reflected an unspoken belief that organic and physical chemists knew the shortcuts to solving complex biological problems. This pattern of deference reflects biochemists' dependent roles in German universities.

The partition of biochemists' domain between chemistry and physiology was an implicit mandate for both hosts to take a proprietary interest in biochemical problems. Because of the career problems that resulted from premature specialization, it was neither the young nor the middling chemists and physiologists who took an active role in biochemistry but the established and accomplished. They alone were sufficiently secure in their careers to take up a line of work that was marginal to the mainstream of their own disciplines. As a result, small, but unusually select and influential groups of physiologists and chemists were attracted to biochemical work.[80] Although the intellectual standards of biochemical work were thus raised to a high level, the leadership of chemists and physiologists did little to strengthen the institutional base of physiological chemistry. Here is the mechanism that produced the familiar pattern of German biochemistry: high intellectual achievement on the margins of the discipline and underdeveloped institutions at the core.

By World War I the official institutes of physiological chemistry were not important centers of biochemical work. These institutes rested on their medical service roles, not their contributions to avant-garde research; few professors were distinguished scholars. The few exceptions, like Franz Knoop and Karl Thomas, were unable to attract able and ambitious students to the discipline. When Franz Knoop sent his students out to study with organic chemists, they were diverted into more profitable careers in organic and industrial chemistry.[81] In 1923 Karl Thomas established a program at Leipzig to retrain clinicians in basic chemistry and biochemistry, in the hope that some would become biochemists; none did. Of 25 fellows, 4 went into pathology, 3 into hygiene, and the rest into clinical research.[82] There were plenty of opportunities for biochemical research in hospitals and biomedical institutes, but no market for professors of biochemistry in German universities.

The most productive and influential German biochemists in the period from 1920 to 1940 worked in research institutes, which did not depend on service roles. Not surprisingly, these institute biochemists resembled the bioorganic chemists and chemical physiologists more than they did their academic confreres. Gustav Embden, a student of Hofmeister's who worked out the crucial steps of the "Embden–Meyerhof" pathway of glucose metabolism, was director of the Institute of Vegetative Physiology at Frankfurt, an endowed research position.[83] Max Bergmann, a leading protein chemist, was director of the Institute for Leather Research in Dresden. Otto Meyerhof, who worked out the chemical physiology of muscle contraction, spent the greater part of his career in Germany as director of the Kaiser Wilhelm Institute of Physiology at Heidelberg.[84] Otto Warburg, perhaps the most admired and emulated biochemist of his generation, directed the Kaiser Wilhelm Institute of Experimental Biology at Berlin.

Warburg combined the biologist's sense of large problems with the chemist's passion for "clean" experimental systems, sophisticated techniques, and simple chemical explanations, befitting a student of Emil Fischer's. His great ambition was to explain the mystery of growth in normal and cancerous cells in terms of metabolism and oxidation. In his early years, he worked on growth and respiration in dividing sea urchin eggs; his colloid-chemical theory of the *Atmungsferment* was one of the leading ideas of the 1920s. In the 1930s, Warburg developed spectro-photometric methods to unravel the enzymes and cofactors of the respiratory chain.[85] His laboratory in Berlin drew crowds of young British and American biochemists eager to learn a style of biochemistry that was more broadly biological and more chemically sophisticated than they had learned in medical school departments.

Research institutes provided opportunities for innovative research but not for discipline building. Warburg received few offers of academic chairs in the 1920s, in part because of prevalent anti-Semitism, but also because his style did not fit the institutional forms of academic physiological chemistry.[86] Warburg had little interest in training a new generation of biochemists. He had few German disciples and used his co-workers as high-grade technicians to crank out research on problems he set, rather than using research to train junior colleagues. American visitors in the 1930s were impressed by Warburg's dynamic personality and intellect but were dismayed by his autocratic methods as director of the institute. Warburg prevented his most brilliant pupil, Hans Krebs, from applying his methods to intermediary metabolism. (This line of work later led Krebs to discover the urea and citric acid cycles.) Warburg directed his workers to freeze out a distinguished visiting biochemist whom Warburg saw as a possible competitor. He maneuvered an American biophysicist, George Wald, out of his laboratory when it became clear that the young man would pursue his own line of research. A bright young American biochemist, Eric Ball, reported that Warburg's laboratory was intellectually isolated and ingrown and no place for an inexperienced man to get a rounded training.[87]

These limitations of Warburg's institute were partly due to Warburg's idiosyncratic character, but they also reflected systematic structural weaknesses in German biochemical institutions: the almost complete absence of a recruitment and reward system; the gulf between a privileged avant-garde and the official academic discipline; and brilliant poaching by physiologists and chemists without much commitment to discipline building. These features of German biochemistry were shaped by the anomalous development of physiological chemistry during the great age of discipline building between 1840 and 1890.

3

Physiology and British biochemists, 1890–1920

In Britain biochemistry developed within departments of physiology, beginning as a specialized subfield, chemical physiology, and gradually achieving independent status as a separate discipline. This was the prevalent German pattern; alternative German modes were virtually absent. There were regional differences, but what is striking is the consistency of British biochemical institutions (see Table 3.1). Lectureships, or assistant professorships, in chemical physiology were first established in the leading medical schools during the period from 1895–1905; the smaller provincial universities of the midlands followed suit from 1909 to 1914, and the larger technological universities in the 1920s.[1]

There were a few exceptions: at Bristol University and Imperial College, biochemistry was attached to chemistry and botany. Chemist Chaim Weizmann was a lecturer and then a reader in biochemistry (really fermentation chemistry) in William Perkins's department of chemistry at Manchester from 1910 to 1915.[2] The most important exception was Liverpool University, where the first chair of biochemistry was established in the School of Public Health. But within a decade it too had reverted to the norm, a chair of chemical physiology. Roles for biochemists were established in a few London hospitals; R. H. A. Plimmer and John A. Gardner taught biochemistry at St. Thomas's and St. George's before World War I. E. C. Dodds made the Courtauld Institute of Pathology at Middlesex Hospital into a leading center of clinical biochemistry in the 1920s.[3] But these were marginal to the mainstream of the discipline. What strikes the historian's eye is the consistent genetic relation between biochemistry and physiology. In no other country was this pattern so evident.

Ultimately, the explanation of this pattern has to do with the general underdevelopment of the biomedical sciences in nineteenth-

Table 3.1. *Establishment of biochemical institutions in British universities*

University	Lectureship in physiology	Dual chair with physiology	Independent chair	Other
University College London	1896	1922		
Cambridge	1896		1914	
Edinburgh	1899		1919	
Liverpool	1907		1902	
Kings College	1905	1928		
Glasgow	1905	1919		
Bristol				1910
Oxford	1909		1920	
Belfast	1909	1922		
Aberdeen	1911		1948	
Cardiff	1912			
Sheffield	1913		1945	
Leeds	1913			
Imperial College				1913
Manchester	1920			
Birmingham	1928			
Durham/Newcastle	1939			
St. Andrews	1938			

century Britain and the selective importation of German models and ideals. Except at Edinburgh, there was no tradition of medical chemistry and no renaissance in organic chemistry in the 1870s. There was nothing in Britain resembling the south German combination of organic and physiological chemistry. When experimental physiology was imported from Germany in the 1870s and 1880s, it was assumed that chemical physiology belonged in physiology. There was no competition from indigenous institutions of organic or medical chemistry as there was in Bavaria and Austria.

Nor was there competition from the more clinical sciences of pathology, pharmacology, and hygiene. Most British medical students learned clinical medicine in hospital apprenticeship programs, where the clinical sciences remained under the control of medical practitioners. Those who took both academic and medical degrees experienced a sharp break between the academic sciences, including physiology, and their practical clinical training. Absence of a centralized system of competitive medical schools and diverse licensing standards precluded the development of specialized biomedical disciplines in Britain. Physiology flourished, but it had no peers. There simply were no viable alternative contexts for developing physiological chemistry besides physiology.

Physiology dominated the medical and biological sciences in late nineteenth-century Britain, more than it did in Europe and far more than in the United States. In the 1860s and 1870s, T. H. Huxley, Michael Foster, and others established physiology as the core of general biology in British schools and universities, thus providing a firm economic base for the discipline in teacher training. Physiology became the highbrow path from academic study into medicine, thus ensuring both able and ambitious recruits and sympathetic and powerful allies among elite British physicians. The location of physiologists in universities, separate from hospital schools, prevented medical service roles from dominating their intellectual style. Physiology was the queen of the biomedical sciences and a dynamic and powerful academic interest in university affairs.[4]

The fountainhead of British physiology was University College London, where William Sharpey was professor from 1832 to 1874. Sharpey himself was primarily an anatomist, did little research, and did not teach experimental methods. However, he did not allow himself to be dominated by surgical anatomists and updated his lectures with reports of the latest German discoveries. He inspired a generation of physiologists who, from 1870 to 1900, established experimental physiology at Cambridge, Oxford, Edinburgh, and Kings (see Table 3.2). The appearance of specialized roles for physiological chemistry followed the same pattern of diffusion as physiology itself. From University College, it spread to Cambridge, Edinburgh, Glasgow, Kings, and Oxford, wherever modern programs of physiology were established.

British physiologists, like their colleagues at Leipzig and Berlin, had an expansionist mentality and saw the development of new specialties as a good strategy for expanding and protecting their territory. In 1914 Charles Sherrington described a department of physiology as comprising three main subdivisions: physical and psychophysical physiology, chemical physiology, and histology. Ideally, Sherrington felt, physical and chemical physiology should have separate chairs. He also noted that opinions varied widely as to the relative importance of these two main branches: he himself regarded physical physiology as having the larger claim on teaching

Table 3.2. *University College London physiologists appointed to leading British chairs*

Physiologist	Years at UCL	Subsequent chair of physiology
Michael Foster	1869–70	Cambridge (1871–1902)
W. Burdon Sanderson	1871–83	Oxford (1883–1905)
Edward A. Schäfer	1884–99	Edinburgh (1899–1933)
Francis Gotch	1882–3	Oxford (1905–13)
W. D. Halliburton	1884–90	Kings (1890–1923)
Benjamin Moore	1895–9	Liverpool (1902–14)[a]
W. A. Osborne	1901–4	Melbourne (1904–38)

[a] Chair in biochemistry.

hours and resources for research, but he acknowledged the case for chemical physiology, primarily because of its importance in laboratory teaching.[5] Institutional expansion of physiology entailed, for Sherrington and others, the creation of specialized roles and chairs. Service roles in medical teaching made chemical physiology a prime area for growth. For this reason, British physiologists were determined opponents of home rule for physiological chemistry and other specialties. Sherrington disapproved of the American habit of creating separate chairs of histology; Walter Fletcher and others lamented the rise of separate departments of pharmacology.[6] Physiologists created roles for physiological chemists and then found themselves in the awkward position of jealous parents, restricting the development of their own offspring.

This pervasive relationship between physiology and biochemistry shaped the experiences of the founding generation of biochemists and determined the distinctive issues of discipline building in Britain. Because chemical physiologists dominated the initial phases of this process, the role of chemists was a crucial issue, and there was a definite point when chemists were seen to predominate in influencing the emerging specialty. The recruitment of chemists was perceived by biochemists as crucial to independence, and physiologists perceived a growing gap between chemical physiologists and biochemists; that is, they began to see physiological chemists as outsiders. The increasing influence of chemists in departments of physiology destabilized the working relationship and necessitated a redefinition of roles. In some cases, a hierarchy of courses and roles in physiological chemistry evolved within physiology and then split off as a daughter department. In other cases, physiologists decided that their responsibility for the emergent discipline had ended and practiced benign neglect. In still other cases, physiologists actively opposed separation of the new specialty. In all cases, however, the root issue was what physiologists and biochemists could rightfully expect of each other. This conflict was the unifying common experience for first-generation biochemists in Britain; particular responses to the generic problem depended on individuals and local circumstances.

Separate roles for physiological chemists evolved gradually out of routine teaching needs in chemical physiology. The role of assistant professor, first established by William Sharpey in 1887, was a response to the expansion of laboratory instruction. Although it was not officially for chemical physiology, the role was often so de facto because laboratory instruction was largely chemical and because most professors were physical physiologists. Gradually it evolved into a junior post for a physiological chemist. University College exemplifies this process.

INTERNAL SPECIALIZATION:
THE UNIVERSITY COLLEGE MODEL

Development of chemical physiology at University College depended at first on the personal predilections of Sharpey's assistants. W. D. Halliburton taught an advanced course in chemical physiology from 1884 to 1890, as did Leonard Hill until 1894, when he substituted a course in psychophysiology. Chemical physiology was reinstated in 1896 by Benjamin Moore and then dropped again by Swale Vincent in 1899. The role stabilized in 1901 when the new professor, Ernest Starling, fitted out a research laboratory for physiological chemistry and put it in the charge of W. A. Osborne, a physiologist who had studied with Hüfner at Tübingen.[7] In 1901 Samuel B. Schryver was appointed to a permanent lectureship in physiological chemistry, and when Osborne left in 1904, he was succeeded by R. H. Adders Plimmer. Both Schryver and Plimmer had been trained as organic chemists at University College and Berlin and, in addition to teaching "chemical physiology," offered courses on advanced topics in biochemistry.[8] An undifferentiated assistant's role thus evolved into specialized positions for physiological chemists, with a stable service role in medical instruction and the rudiments of a disciplinary program.

Physiological chemistry was an important part of Starling's plans for expansion. As he later observed, "the budding off of new subjects made the need of more space for the teaching of the physiological group of subjects still more imperative."[9] This was an effective strategy at a time of dramatic expansion and change at University College. In the 1890s, London University had been only a formal, degree-granting body for the two dozen or so colleges, institutes, and hospitals in London. Academic standards and policies in the biomedical sciences had been largely controlled by conservative practitioners. After nearly two decades of controversy, the London University Act of 1898 enabled the London colleges to incorporate as university faculties, opening the door to rapid reform. Expansion and specialization were the order of the day. It was expected that each discipline would demonstrate its progressive qualities by developing new specialties, and the planning of new buildings was an excellent occasion to formulate ambitious long-term plans. Chemistry was reorganized in 1902, and a new chair of organic chemistry was created in 1905. Ernest Starling took the lead in planning the reorganization of the medical sciences between 1905 and 1907. An anonymous publicist (probably Starling) explained how the new physiology institute, with its integrated subdivisions, was an embodiment of the university idea. When the institute was completed in 1909, it included space for physiological chemistry as a semi-independent department in the Berlin style.[10]

Physiology at Edinburgh, Oxford, and Kings Colleges developed as colonies of University College, and the roles for physiological chemists emerged in much the same way they did in Starling's school. When Edward Schäfer arrived at Edinburgh in 1899, physiology had changed little since the 1870s. Schäfer's predecessor, William Rutherford, had devoted his last decades to his lectures and his vast collection of histology slides. There was no differentiation between elementary and advanced physiology; students simply took the course a second time. Histology was the only recognized specialty; Rutherford's assistant, Thomas Milroy, was interested in chemical physiology but had no specialized role in which to do it. Physiological chemistry was rudimentary, as recalled by Schäfer:

There was also a classroom for Physiological Chemistry with about sixty places, but when these were fully occupied it was almost impossible to enter the room so full was it of fumes and products of combustion. A small amount of Physiological Chemistry conducted in this room and the Histology constituted the whole of the teaching of practical Physiology in the ordinary medical curriculum. In addition there were certain rooms of no great size intended for research work in Experimental and Chemical Physiology. They were, however, very imperfectly fitted and it was difficult for work to be done in them.[11]

Schäfer's improvements followed the example of University College. The old chemistry laboratory was refitted for chemical research, and a lecture hall was converted to a student laboratory in physiological chemistry. Thomas Milroy was appointed "lecturer in advanced physiology and physiological chemistry," and when funds from Andrew Carnegie's Scottish Universities Trust became available in 1901, Schäfer put a chair of physiological chemistry at the top of his shopping list. Scaled down by the university, Schäfer's request was approved, and in 1902 John Malcolm was appointed lecturer in physiological and pathological chemistry. Within three years, Schäfer had staked his claim to histology, experimental physiology, and physiological chemistry, each represented by a special lectureship.[12]

At Oxford, differentiation of chemical physiology began earlier but proceeded at a more leisurely pace. Although John Burdon Sanderson and Francis Gotch were both scions of University College, Oxford was less hospitable to experimental science, and specialization of roles was a less-favored strategy. John S. Haldane may have taught chemical physiology as early as 1887, but his official position as lecturer (later as reader) was not so designated.[13] Physiological chemistry was relegated to a decrepit corrugated iron shed until 1906 when Gotch petitioned for a new annex, pointing to the growing prestige of physiological chemistry and the superior facilities provided by other universities.[14] Walter Ramsden taught chemical physiology from 1897 but was not given a specialized lectureship until 1914 when Gotch was succeeded by Charles Sherrington.[15] (Sherrington may have offered J. S. Haldane a secondary chair in biochemistry because Haldane later boasted that he had refused an Oxford chair because it was designated as "biochemistry."[16]) At Kings College, limited resources, competition from University College, and William Halliburton's personal interest in chemical physiology prevented any early differentiation of roles. The reorganization of London University in 1905 gave Kings access to larger medical audiences and opened up opportunities for specialization. A new laboratory was built for the medical sciences, with laboratories for physical and chemical physiology. In 1905 Otto Rosenheim, an organic chemist in the Department of Pharmacology, was appointed to a lectureship in physiological chemistry.[17]

Further variations on this pattern of subdivision and specialization occurred at Glasgow, Manchester, and the Yorkshire universities. In each case, particular local circumstances shaped the outcome of a process that is recognizably the same in all. At Glasgow, the process of subdivision was facilitated in 1905 when a local shipping magnate gave £8,000* to endow a lectureship in physiological chemistry. Edward P. Cathcart, chemist and physiologist, was appointed to the post.[18] The breakup of Victoria University in 1903 likewise created opportunities for change in the medical sciences at the new universities of Leeds, where a lectureship in physiological chemistry was established in 1913, and at Sheffield, where biochemist–physiologist J. B. Leathes held a joint chair from 1914.[19] At Manchester, where traditional physiology was more entrenched, subdivision did not occur until 1920.[20]

SEPARATE AND UNEQUAL: CAMBRIDGE

At Cambridge, Michael Foster began to develop chemical physiology in much the same way as his mentor at University College. By 1900, however, physiological chemistry began to be perceived as a separate discipline. This distinctive local variant in part reflected Foster's remarkable programmatic vision. Of all the British physiologists, Foster had the broadest vision of physiology as the comprehensive study of biological functions. No one was more assiduous in systematically developing specialized fields. His strategy of internal division of labor is evident less in his programmatic statements than in the diverse interests of his disciples. Especially in the mid-1870s and again in the mid-1890s, Foster seems to have deliberately and systematically guided his students into diverse physiological specialties, including chemical physiology.[21] Believing that physiological processes would ultimately be explained in chemical

---

* During the period discussed in this book, the pound was equivalent to U.S.$5.

terms, Foster sent three of his favorite students, Walter Gaskell, John Langley, and Arthur Sheridan Lea, to learn chemical physiology at Kühne's knee at Heidelberg. He nudged other protégés into chemical problems. When Walter Fletcher decided to take up muscle work in 1898, he asked Foster if he thought there was any promise in the chemical side; Foster, he later recalled, "rolled up his beard with both hands over his mouth and chuckled." The ultimate result of Foster's eloquent silence was the collaboration of Fletcher and F. G. Hopkins on the biochemistry of muscle contraction.[22] Foster encouraged Hopkins to study the chemistry of the developing hen's egg as a way of understanding the processes of morphogenesis. Although Hopkins did not do so himself, he passed the spark of interest to his student Joseph Needham.[23] T. R. Elliott's theory that nerve impulses were transmitted chemically (1904) and John Langley's theory of chemical receptors (1905) also testify to the prevalence of biochemical concepts in Foster's school.[24]

Sheridan Lea was Foster's chief assistant for chemical physiology, and an informal role was transformed by 1895 into a special lectureship in this field. In the mid-1880s, Sheridan Lea did pioneering work on the digestion of proteins and was one of the first in the 1890s to point to the importance of intracellular ferments in growth and metabolism. In his role as assistant professor, Lea lectured on chemical physiology and wrote a chemical appendix to Foster's textbook.[25] At Cambridge, as at London, however, the pursuit of physiological chemistry depended on an individual's aptitude, not on an institutionalized role. When chronic illness forced Lea to retire in 1895, university officials decided that "the immediate needs of the Department" did not warrant continuing his special lectureship in chemical physiology.[26] An histologist took Lea's course in intermediate physiology, and a young graduate, Alfred Eicholz, took over his advanced course in chemical physiology. Trained in comparative anatomy, Eicholz managed to survive for three years by relying on Lea's notes for lectures. He then accepted a post teaching physiology in the new school of agriculture.[27] Some distinguished research in physiological chemistry was still being done at Cambridge. In the Department of Botany, Joseph Reynolds Greene was investigating the nature of intracellular ferments.[28] In physiology, a young medical student, Arthur Croft Hill, had just discovered that digestive enzymes could be made to work in reverse, synthesizing polysaccharides from sugar molecules.[29] But there was no institutionalized role for a physiological chemist at Cambridge.

University authorities agreed with Foster that these and other "recent striking developments" justified at least a readership but, for financial reasons, recommended only that a university lectureship in chemical physiology be created, with no stipend attached. Foster's deputy, John Langley, agreed to contribute £100 from department funds, but only temporarily.[30] After a meeting of the Physiological Society, Foster approached Frederick Gowland Hopkins and offered him the position.

Like Schryver and Plimmer, Hopkins was a chemist by training. The son of a respectable but impoverished petit bourgeois family, Hopkins had been apprenticed to a chemical analyst and subsequently worked for Sir Thomas Stevenson, the leading forensic chemist in London. Encouraged by Stevenson, Hopkins studied medicine and in 1894 qualified at Guy's Hospital. There Hopkins's interest was aroused in problems of nutrition and metabolism by the brilliant and idiosyncratic physician–physiologist F. W. Pavy. He had some contact with the active group of young chemists and physiologists working with Ernest Starling, notably J. B. Leathes and William Bayliss. He collaborated with pathologist Archibald E. Garrod in a study of urinary pigments and, in his spare time, operated a commercial laboratory for clinical chemical analysis. He was the obvious candidate to succeed Stevenson. In contrast to the Cambridge physiologists, Hopkins was a practical clinical chemist, and he felt acutely his lack of collegiate polish and credentials. Encouraged by Foster, Hopkins took the plunge, aged 38, into an uncertain future as an academic biochemist.[31]

The difficulties that Hopkins experienced at Cambridge are legendary. Foster had arranged for Hopkins to supplement his meager stipend by teaching at Emmanuel College. This, Hopkins discovered, entailed teaching gross anatomy, a burden that consumed his time and weighed on his spirits for nearly a decade.[32] Foster's faith in physiological chemistry and his promise of a salaried position could not refurbish the facilities and revitalize the courses that had run down since Lea's day. Hopkins found "no equipment (or sympathy) for the chemical side of work," and heavy teaching responsibilities severely limited research time.[33]

In part, Hopkins's problems were due to the general situation of science at Cambridge. The university was still little more than a degree-granting body; the colleges controlled budgets and academic policy. This decentralized structure impeded the growth of the experimental sciences, which required expensive centralized laboratories. No college wanted to make an investment that would benefit other colleges more than itself, and the university as such had no endowments to maintain laboratories. The colleges controlled all fellowships and had sole access to the emotional and financial loyalties of alumni. They contributed to the university-based sciences only just enough to prevent more radical reform. University officials hoped that new patrons of the sciences would turn up, but they were often disappointed. There were few private patrons of science and competition was fierce.[34] About 1900 the government's board of education began to give grants to aid technical and medical research and training, but powerful university interests feared government interference and Cambridge was the last university to apply for public funds. The medical faculty was bitterly criticized when it finally did so in 1914.[35] Lacking its own endowment, the Medical School was unable to develop new specialties like biochemistry. (Part of the £5000 it sought in 1914 was earmarked for a lectureship in biochemistry.) The frustrations that Hopkins experienced were shared by other discipline builders in genetics, anthropology, and psychology.

There were also specific problems having to do with the relationship between physiology and biochemistry. Foster was aging and took little part in department affairs. Langley lacked Foster's broad vision of physiology and Foster's disinterested concern with specialties other than his own. He was dictatorial and favored neurohistology and neurophysiology, in which he himself was interested.[36] He also lacked Foster's visionary faith in the promise of physiological chemistry and saw every investment in Hopkins's specialty as a diversion of resources that could have gone to more important areas. Competition for limited financial resources exacerbated Langley's growing sense that physiological chemistry was no longer a part of physiology and had no claim upon it.

In 1902, for example, Hopkins declined to take the new chair of biochemistry at Liverpool on the understanding that he would be given a readership.[37] But Langley refused to press the university for an endowed readership in chemical physiology because it seemed to him unlikely that the university could afford it. He proposed instead that the university upgrade Hopkins's lectureship to a readership and double their contribution to Hopkins's salary from £50 to £100.[38] The hard-pressed university officials were only too willing to agree. Hopkins subsequently declined two offers of chairs from American universities and in 1905 discouraged efforts to lure him to University College London.[39]

The key to Langley's policy regarding biochemistry is his conviction that Hopkins wanted (and deserved) an independent position as representative of a discipline separate from physiology, and with a separate budget. That was the gist of Langley's argument to the senate in 1902: problems of chemical physiology had become too technical for physiologists to solve themselves. They were problems for specialists in organic chemistry:

The subject was becoming more and more a special study, the results of which physiologists would be content to accept as they accepted the results of physics. In Germany this had been recognized by the establishment of professorships in the subject with special laboratories.[40]

Langley was unwilling to sacrifice physiology's claims on university resources in order to nurture a specialty that he saw becoming a sub-specialty of chemistry.

Biochemists later ascribed to Langley the belief that biochemistry was already "played out" as a field of research.[41] Perhaps so; the crucial point, however, is that Langley was making a political judgment of the proper relationship between physiological chemistry and physiology. Physiologists might draw upon physiological chemists' work, but in Langley's view, they had no financial or institutional responsibility for supporting it. Whereas Starling and other physiologists nurtured physiological chemistry as a subdivision of physiology, Langley saw it as a competitor for scarce resources. Where Langley's interests were not involved, he supported Hopkins; where there was direct competition for funds, he ruthlessly pursued his own interest. Two episodes illustrate this pattern: the election of the Quick Professor in 1906 and the allocation of the Drapers's bequest for a physiological laboratory in 1910.

The Quick bequest of £30,000 to promote "study and research in the sciences of vegetable and animal biology" was one of the largest at Cambridge and attracted many claimants. Forestry, protozoology, bacteriology, genetics, and biological chemistry all had a record of intellectual achievement and had suffered from chronic financial malnutrition. Langley and Clifford Allbutt, professor of medicine, stated the case for Hopkins:

Physiological or Medical Chemistry has made advances so far-reaching and many-sided that several branches of sciences formerly independent must now look to it as the chief aid to their development. It is indeed almost a commonplace to say that not in a few but in most branches of biology the work of enquiry if not already conducted on chemical lines, can be regarded as a preparation for chemical enquiry. The subject...has been identified in the past with animal physiology and with medicine. Already for a decade or more this identification has been found insufficient and misleading. Chemistry is now supplying fundamental data for the explanation of biological phenomena, and its influence is making in a sense a new biology.[42]

Langley was aware that physiology had no possible claim on the Quick funds. Moreover, a Quick Chair of Biochemistry would have benefited physiology more than any of the other possible dispositions. Hopkins would have provided useful services to physiology (for example, teaching chemical physiology) without being a financial burden on Langley's budget; he would have been an ally, not a poor relation.

Physiologists W. H. Gaskell and Walter Fletcher also backed Hopkins's claim to the Quick Chair, as did biologists Francis Darwin and J. A. Bradbury; F. F. Blackman, plant physiologist and head of the powerful Board of Geology and Biology, gave biochemistry and genetics equal claim.[43] After a year of wrangling, the university agreed upon a plan to endow two chairs, one in "biological (physiological) chemistry" and one in genetics. The Quick trustees had their own idea of what the benefactor would have liked, however, and awarded the prize to protozoology.[44] Hopkins and his friends were dismayed, and Fletcher later complained that the affair had been bungled, allowing "interference of lay opinion outside."[45]

Langley was much less generous when it came to allocating the £22,000 given by the Drapers Company for a new physiology laboratory.[46] Hopkins certainly assumed he would be well provided for. In 1910 he wrote in despair:

I have come to the conclusion that I could not stand my present double activity for many years to come. I should have to make up my mind either to drop science, and settle down to the humdrum of tutorial work and college teaching; or else stick to the laboratory and put up with a small income. Fortunately, I think neither may be necessary in the more or less near future. A Chair and a department of Biochemistry are certainly nearer to becoming realities now than ever they have been before. The Drapers Company have recently given £50,000 [*sic*] which they want spent on buildings, and most likely it will result in a large block in which my department will have self-contained and independent laboratories. I can't absolutely count on it; but it is likely.[47]

In this case there was direct competition between physiology and physiological chemistry, and from the start Langley had intended to cut Hopkins out. He intimated to Vice Chancellor Mason that £22,000 might not suffice for a laboratory "exclusive of a Laboratory for Bio-chemistry."[48] The financial board insisted that biochemistry (and psychology) be included in the plan, however, and the University Association agreed to raise the extra funds by a public appeal. A benefactor for psychology soon came forward, but for biochemistry none. When the new laboratory opened in 1914, Hopkins was left in possession of the old, makeshift physiology laboratories.[49]

As a result of his decade of frustration and neglect, Hopkins came to be regarded as a kind of biochemical saint. His patient suffering exemplified to biochemists their bondage to hostile or indifferent physiologists. Like all myths, this one turns grays to black and white to make a political point. Langley's intent was not to suppress biochemistry, only to put the burden for its support where he felt it belonged, which was not on physiology. He freely acknowledged that Hopkins's facilities were hopelessly inadequate: "whilst I naturally put first the completion of the Physiological Laboratory, I think that the establishment of a separate Department of Bio-chemistry is very pressing."[50] Yet even after 1914 Langley refused to let Hopkins use the fees he earned by teaching physiological chemistry. Hopkins himself was partly responsible for his predicament. He was shy, diffident to a fault, and at a loss in the rough and tumble of university politics. He simply did not stand up to Langley to assert his proper interests.

It was the colleges that first came to Hopkins's rescue. In 1906 Emmanuel College appointed him as a tutor and fellow, although the small stipend entailed extra tutorial work.[51] In 1910 Hopkins was awarded a praelectorship and fellowship at Trinity, the position that had enabled Michael Foster to get a toehold in Cambridge in 1871. It was his friend Walter Fletcher, an adept in university politics, who took the initiative. Fletcher drafted a petition to the Trinity council, mobilized allies, and steered it clear of political snags. He recalled how Cambridge had been the last to recognize Hopkins's achievements: "The situation was painfully ludicrous; it was indeed scandalous, and hostile comment upon it was often heard in London and elsewhere." He pointed out how little things had improved:

Though his remuneration is now adequate, the situation is almost as ludicrous as before – indeed it would be fair to repeat the word scandalous. For the University appears, when judged from outside, to have taken for itself the man in the country most fitted to lead research and teaching in Bio-chemistry, and to have sterilized him by permitting it to be arranged that he shall have no time to do either.[52]

Efforts were once again being made to raise endowment for a chair of biochemistry; meanwhile, Fletcher urged the Trinity council to consider that a fellowship would set Hopkins free to do what Foster had intended when he brought him to Cambridge. Hopkins received the news of the Trinity praelectorship while he was recovering from a nervous breakdown, brought on by years of frustration and overwork.[53]

Hopkins still did not have either a chair or an endowment, of course, and had to carry on in two converted basement rooms with hand-me-down equipment, including an antique centrifuge that shimmied menacingly about the room when run at top speed.[54] Hopkins's situation improved in 1912 when he became co-director of the Nutritional Institute in the School of Agriculture and transferred much of his research to a new facility.[55] But this was another makeshift. When the National Institute for Medical Research opened in 1914, Hopkins's friends advised him that there was a better chance there than at Cambridge of creating a school of biochemistry.[56] Another petition was circulated, and in 1914 a chair of biochemistry was created, without salary or endowment, however.[57] The war put an end to Hopkins's hopes; it was not until 1921 that a large private bequest enabled Hopkins to realize his ambitions for a research school.

The evolution of institutional roles for biochemistry was not much slower at Cambridge than it was at University College. Hopkins's position seemed worse because it was expected that biochemistry would become an independent discipline; because

Langley was less altruistic than Ernest Starling; and because Starling's strategy of internal specialization made less sense in a university that had to rely on unpredictable private benefactions.

A DEVIANT MODE: LIVERPOOL

Liverpool University was the one major institution in which physiological chemistry did not evolve out of physiology. A chair of "biochemistry," the first so named, was established in 1902 in the School of Hygiene and Public Health. It was an exception that proved the rule, however, for in 1914 this chair became, in effect, a secondary chair of chemical physiology. The establishment of the Johnston Chair of Biochemistry was part of the reorganization that occurred when Liverpool broke loose from the federated Victoria University. The movement for educational reform focused on local commercial needs, and as Liverpool's wealth depended on its overseas trade with the tropical colonies, local benefactors favored tropical medicine, hygiene, and public health. Eight of the ten new chairs established between 1902 and 1913 were in these fields; among them, biochemistry.[58]

The guiding hand of this outpouring of civic spirit was Professor of Pathology Rupert William Boyce. An energetic and impetuous Irishman, Boyce already had a record of progressive civic reform. When his colleagues balked at an offer from the Colonial Office to found a chair of tropical medicine in 1898, Boyce offered his own laboratory and in three months raised the necessary funds from local merchants. As city bacteriologist and member of a royal commission on the problems of sewage disposal, Boyce knit together the interests of town and gown. He led the movement for education home rule and was instrumental in founding the School of Public Health.[59]

The first chair of biochemistry in Britain differed both in its conception and its economic base from the usual positions in chemical physiology. Boyce was interested in chemistry for its relevance to bacteriology and hygiene, and his assistant, A. S. Grünbaum, taught a course in "biochemistry" for public health students before 1900.[60] Boyce obtained the endowment for the new chair of biochemistry from his father-in-law, William Johnston, a wealthy ship owner.[61]

The first Johnston Professor, Benjamin Moore, was a scion of University College but not a typical chemical physiologist. An

Irishman like Boyce, Moore had a restless energy and flamboyant temperament. He was trained in industrial chemistry before turning to physiology and had a broad and eclectic range of interests. He spent a year with Wilhelm Ostwald at Leipzig, where he picked up physical chemistry and a taste for Ostwald's militantly reductionist philosophy of science. Moore was a socialist and an ardent advocate of scientific social reform. He speculated on the origins of life, pamphleteered for national health insurance, was active in public health surveys, and during the war pressed for measures to protect munitions workers from TNT poisoning. Brash, opinionated, and vehement, Moore left turbulence in his wake wherever he went.[62]

Moore was not a regular medical professor; he was the director of an endowed research department, which did not depend on service courses in chemical physiology. Moore could afford to be different. His broad-ranging interests included the colloidal chemistry of proteins, enzymes, bacteriology, clinical chemistry, and photosynthesis. His program lived up to the connotations of its name, *bio*chemistry. Moore was also a discipline builder. In 1906, when Langley refused to publish some of his papers in the *Journal of Physiology*, Moore organized the *Biochemical Journal*. At first mainly an outlet for Moore's school, the *Biochemical Journal* became the unofficial professional journal for British biochemists and in 1911 was purchased by the new, nationally based Biochemical Society.[63] Unfettered by a strong connection with physiology, Moore cultivated diverse institutional connections: with the Marine Biological Station at Port Erin, the School of Public Health, and the departments of Pathology and Pharmacology. He lectured at the College of Surgeons and acted as chemical pathologist to the Royal Infirmary.[64] Moore's textbook, *Biochemistry*, was organized around his theory of biological energy transformers and his own work on photosynthesis. It expressed his idiosyncratic program for a new discipline of biochemistry.

Physiology seems to have been the one base Moore did not touch, and there physiological chemistry evolved in the usual way out of medical teaching. When Charles Sherrington introduced laboratory instruction in 1907, following a tour of American medical schools, he emphasized chemical physiology:

After visiting America last year I returned impressed with the progress there ... and especially in their methods of teaching as compared with our own. Their teaching is more practical. The lecture room is used less and the practical laboratory more. This involves more expense but I am convinced turns out their students with on the whole more useful knowledge than ours have, though their teachers may be less learned than ours.

On return I went over my own laboratory to see how far I might put my own house in order in that respect and place ourselves abreast of American teaching. I decided to get leave from our Medical Faculty to replace two lectures per week by two practical classes. In this way the students now instead of seeing *me* analyze milk, foods, expired air, urine, etc. at a lecture table do these things *themselves* in the laboratory. Formerly only certain advanced students did so.[65]

Sherrington had doubted that his students would share his enthusiasm for laboratory work, but enrollment almost doubled in one year, from 52 to 91. So great was the demand that Sherrington was obliged to seek extra resources for chemical work. The university agreed to refit a large room as a laboratory of chemical physiology. In 1909 Sherrington asked for a special lectureship in chemical physiology for his assistant, Herbert Roaf. The lectureship was created but was designated for "clinical physiology," perhaps to avoid competition with Moore.[66]

Sherrington himself lectured on both physical and chemical physiology. When he left for the Waynefleet Chair at Oxford in 1913, however, the Liverpool authorities were unable to find a successor of equal breadth. Sherrington advised them to split the chair, appoint a physical physiologist, and draft Moore to teach chemical physiology:

Our University is in the fortunate position that it possesses already a Chair of Bio-chemistry, Bio–chemistry being practically a synonym for Chemical Physiology. And the Chair of Bio-chemistry is filled by a Professor who previously to his acceptance of the invitation to it had held a Chair of Physiology. It is true that the Chair of Bio-chemistry is at present *de facto* a research Chair. The University should in my opinion endeavour to use this Chair as a provision for Chemical Physiology. To throw upon the Chair of Bio-chemistry the additional burden of a considerable amount of somewhat elementary teaching is perhaps to invade seriously the Chair's amenities and opportunities. But such a change would be greatly to the advantage of the students of Physiology in the University.[67]

Moore apparently approved, and Sherrington's plan was adopted.[68] This was the opening wedge for the physiologists. Six months later Moore resigned to join the new National Institute for Medical Research in London.[69] He was succeeded by Walter Ramsden, a typical chemical physiologist. The medical faculty even petitioned to change the designation of the Johnston Chair to "chemical physiology" but were refused.

Although it kept its distinctive name, Moore's department soon lost its distinctive character. Ramsden's policies reflected his experience at University College and Oxford. He organized "the usual classes in chemical physiology" (as well as courses in clinical chemistry) and spent much time on clinical analyses and autopsy reports for the Royal Infirmary.[70] Ramsden had been considered a promising researcher on the basis of a few highly polished papers on biological colloids. By 1920, however, he had abandoned research, and his lack of energy and poor lecturing style attracted few research students. The Liverpool department thus reverted to almost total dependence on its service roles in physiology and medicine. The reversion of Moore's deviant style to the norm of chemical physiology illustrates how institutional pressures shaped the nascent discipline.

NEW ROLES FOR CHEMISTS

Routine service roles in medical teaching, absence of alternative clienteles, and acceptance of physiologists' traditional claims to physiological chemistry dominated the first phase of discipline building. Chemical physiology was recognized as a subspecialty of physiology, requiring specialized chemical skills. As more chemists were appointed to junior positions in physiology, however, it became more apparent that they constituted a distinct academic species. More departments had to face the issues that divided Hopkins and Langley. Internal specialization of roles entailed a second and more drastic phase in which discipline boundaries were redrawn.

Who were the chemical physiologists who filled the new lectureships? Of the 20 individuals who had specialized academic positions prior to 1914, eight came from physiology, ten from chemistry (two were not identified). Recruits trained in physiology dominated in the early years, but chemists came to the new specialty in greater numbers after about 1905. Of the eight chemical physiologists, five also studied physiological chemistry on the continent, two with Salkowski and one each with Emil Fischer and Hüfner (see Table 3.3). Yet six remained ultimately in physiology. This pattern of careers suggests a transitional generation. A chair of physiology remained a greater attraction for physiologists than a

Table 3.3. *Founding generation of biochemists trained as physiologists*

Biochemist	Physiology training	Physiological–chemical training	First position in physiological chemistry	Ultimate career
E. P. Cathcart	Glasgow	Berlin (pathology)	Glasgow	Physiology (Glasgow)
A. S. Lea	Cambridge		Cambridge	Physiology (Cambridge)
J. B. Leathes	Guy's Hospital	Berne (Drechsel) and Strasbourg	St. Thomas's Hospital	Physiology (Sheffield)
J. Malcolm	Edinburgh		Edinburgh	Physiology (Dunedin)
J. A. Milroy	Edinburgh	Berlin (pathological chemistry)	Belfast	Biochemistry (Belfast)
W. A. Osborne	Belfast	Tübingen	University College	Physiology (Melbourne)
W. Ramsden	Oxford	Berlin, Vienna Zurich (chemistry)	Oxford	Biochemistry (Liverpool)
H. M. Vernon	Oxford	Naples (biology)	Oxford	Physiology (National Institute for Medical Research)

chair in a new, more specialized discipline populated increasingly by chemists.

The ten academic biochemists who came from chemistry had distinctly different career patterns. (see Table 3.4). Six were trained by leading European chemists; two (Cramer and Rosenheim) were German emigrés. Unlike the physiologists, many of the chemists had worked as professional researchers in the medical research institutes of London, and none of this group reverted to chemistry. The chemists' transition to biochemistry was irreversible. Only one, Henry Raper, became a physiologist (and he had been trained in physiology). Five found permanent positions in hospitals or research institutes, and only three (Hopkins, Moore, and Edie) occupied university chairs of biochemistry.

In the larger group of individuals who worked as nonacademic biochemists prior to 1915, chemists outnumbered physiologists by 11 to 3. Two came from the departments of chemistry at Cambridge and University College, and two from Julius B. Cohen's group of organic chemists at Leeds, which deserves a special place in the history of British biochemistry.[71] The research institutions of London were the most important market for professional biochemists before World War I. The Lister Institute was the largest of these institutions. Apart from the permanent staff, Plimmer, Leathes, Robison, Raper, and others spent formative years there.[72] The Wellcome Physiological Research Laboratory, supported by Wellcome Borroughs, Ltd., was an active center of biochemical work when Henry Dale was there. The National Institute for Medical Research, which opened in 1914 under the general direction of Walter Fletcher and the Medical Research Committee, became a productive center of biochemical research after the war.[73] The research institutions provided training and employment for a generation of biochemists before there were large schools, abundant fellowships, and a regular market for biochemists in British universities. They provided a pool of recruits as specialized chairs were created.

The different styles of the early chemical physiologists and the first biochemists demarcate two distinct scientific subcultures. The chemical physiologists were members of an academic elite who specialized, but never severed, their attachment to greater physiology. The biochemists were members of an emerging occupational or professional community located in institutions that developed science for practical reasons, such as industries, hospitals, sanitary

Table 3.4. *Founding generation of biochemists trained as chemists*

Biochemist	Chemistry training	Physiological–chemical training	First position	Ultimate career
W. Cramer	Berlin (Ph.D.)		Edinburgh	Medical Research (Imperial Cancer Fund)
E. S. Edie	Edinburgh	Liverpool	Aberdeen	Biochemistry (Capetown)
J. A. Gardner	Oxford Heidelberg (Ph.D.)		St. George's	Medical chemistry (London hospitals)
F. G. Hopkins	Apprenticeship	Guy's	Cambridge	Biochemistry (Cambridge)
B. Moore	Belfast Leipzig	University College	Liverpool	Biochemistry (Oxford)
R. H. A. Plimmer	University College Geneva, Berlin	Lister	University College	Medical chemistry (St. Thomas)
H. S. Raper	Leeds	Lister, Strasbourg	Leeds	Physiology (Leeds, Manchester)
O. S. Rosenheim	Würzburg	Leeds	Kings	Medical Research (NIMR)
S. B. Schryver	Leipzig	Wellcome	University College	Biochemistry (Imperial College)
W. W. Taylor	Edinburgh		Edinburgh	Biochemistry (Edinburgh)

commissions, and experiment stations. Specialization brought the chemical physiologists few career rewards; the positions they might have occupied were increasingly filled by chemists, whose training and outlook suited them for specialized research roles.

First-generation biochemists were aware of the changes occurring in chemical physiology and believed that the growth and prosperity of their discipline depended on recruiting more chemists. Edward Mellanby, who studied with Hopkins from 1902 to 1907, recalled that although chemists were generally not yet interested in biological problems, the biochemists were acutely aware of the need to entice first-class chemists into the discipline.[74] In fact, chemists had begun to notice the career opportunities in the biological sciences. In 1902 the Royal Institute of Chemistry officially recognized "biological chemistry" as a professional specialty with its own qualifying examination. This certificate was apparently intended mainly for sanitary chemists and brewing chemists, for the examination focused on the biology and chemistry of microorganisms and fermentation.[75]

Hopkins was especially active in recruiting practical chemists like himself to physiology and biochemistry. In 1906, for example, he exhorted the Society of Analysts to fill in the gap left by the declining interest of organic chemists in messy biological problems:

Such work really requires special instincts and the pure chemist has largely lost them. He is but a poor analyst, as the physiological explorer finds on turning to him for help. I feel that this help, so far as the immediate future is concerned, will have to come from the pupils primarily trained in your own laboratories, where the analytical instinct is developed. . . . There are the beginnings just now of a renewed interest in biology on the part of all chemists. May the analyst feel this too.[76]

Hopkins's most powerful programmatic statement, "The dynamic side of biochemistry," (1913) was delivered to the physiological section of the British Association for the Advancement of Science, but Hopkins made it clear that it was really organic chemists whom he hoped to convert to the biochemical faith:

I have been in a position to review the current demand of various institutions, home and colonial, for the service of trained biochemists, and can say that the demand will rapidly prove to be in excess of the supply. It will be a pity if the generation of trained chemists now growing up in this country should not share in the restoration of this balance. You certainly have the right to tell me that I ought. . .to be addressing another section; but it may be long before any member of my cloth will have the opportunity of appealing to that section [chemistry] from the position of advantage that I occupy here [in physiology].[77]

Hopkins hoped that biologists and physiologists would also turn to biochemistry but felt that it was easier to learn new problems than new techniques. The reversion of chemical physiologists suggests that Hopkins's instincts were sound.

Hopkins observed that academic chemists were no longer ignorant of biochemistry although few were really sympathetic:

I do not find any more the rather pitying patronage for an inferior discipline, and certainly not that actual antagonism, which fretted my own youth; but I do find still very widely spread a distrust of the present methods of the Biochemist, a belief that much of the work done by him is amateurish and inexact.[78]

Hopkins acknowledged that much biochemical work was amateurish and inexact but vigorously denied that these faults were inherent in biochemistry. The burden of his address was that the pure chemist had much to learn from studying the step-by-step degradations and syntheses in living cells, each reaction catalyzed by a specific enzyme and the whole organized as efficiently as a chemical machine shop. In the 1920s, chemists were themselves delivering sermons from the pulpits of science on the opportunities in biology and medicine.

In 1921 Hopkins was invited to address the chemical section of the British Association.[79] At the same meeting, Fletcher harangued the physiologists on the benefits that would accrue to organic chemists if they would work in biology and medicine: "Many signs point to the near approach of the time when organic chemists will feel the need of fresh inspiration coming from the intricate laboratory of the living cell."[80] Meanwhile, the president of the chemical section exhorted his audience with the same message.[81] Fletcher later pointed to this meeting as the turning point in chemists' attitude toward biochemistry:

The organic chemists one after another admitted that the best developments in the study of the carbon compounds must lie in observing not so much what transformations could be effected by the forcible means of the laboratory as those which were actually managed in living cells.[82]

He looked forward to a stream of valuable recruits from organic chemistry. The entire presentation bears the unmistakable marks of Fletcher's handiwork. Discounting somewhat Fletcher's report of a "complete change of attitude," it is doubtless true that some chemists had come to see biochemistry as a promising source of jobs for their students.[83]

The migration of chemists into physiology began to strain institutions like the Royal Society, which altered disciplinary categories at a glacial pace. In 1931, for example, Walter Fletcher complained to chemist Robert Robinson that his section of the Royal Society was not taking their fair share of responsibility for appointing bioorganic chemists and that the whole system of recruitment had failed to adjust to new realities:

Chemists at the R. S. appear to me to act often from what seems a narrow and sectional point of view. If a well trained organic chemist does brilliant original work within a field of interest to the biologists, the chemists appear at once to disown him and to throw the whole burden of his support upon the biological side. I can think of many instances of this over several years.

Action of this kind seems to me to be vicious because it . . . must have the effect of tempting a young man to keep in the old ruts and in the well-worn parts of the field, if he wants to get into the R. S., instead of finding new ways for himself. Incidentally, the principle works at present so as to burden quite unfairly the active parts of biology. . . . It would be fair enough that we should bear part of the burden, so to speak, of biochemistry, namely, that part which is effectively chemical physiology; it is grotesque that we should have to include that part of biochemistry which is being developed by the brilliant influx of organic chemists who are now seeing that the study of life processes may teach them more of what chemistry means in the eyes of the Creator. . . .

I see clearly that the progress of medicine is being held up at many points because men with first-class training in chemistry or in physics are kept away from the wonderful opportunities they might have, because of the present organisation of scientific education in the schools and Universities, and in large part also by the faulty organisation of the Royal Society. Clever boys are made to do chemistry and physics because that gives the easiest road to scholarships at Oxford and Cambridge. . . . When they reach either Oxford or Cambridge they are actually allowed to get a First degree in natural science without touching anything outside their own subject. At the R. S., if a chemist studies living matter the chemists appear to throw him over. We are trying hard to get physicists to enter the gold mines of interest and value waiting for them in biology and medicine, but I am afraid that if and as we succeed we shall find that the physicists will throw them over. . . . I can get well-trained organic chemists in almost any quantity by lifting my finger and offering a beggarly stipend. It is very difficult to find any men at all with decent biological knowledge together with a sound training in either chemistry or physics.[84]

Robinson replied that physiologists tended to be too easily impressed by chemists' achievements just because they had to do with biologically interesting substances. The real fault, he asserted, was the failure to recognize biochemistry as a distinct discipline:

On the wider question I am in full agreement but I do not think your criticism of the chemical R. S. committee is quite just. Everything possible should be done to encourage young chemists and physicists to enter the fruitful borderline regions and especially those relating to biology or medicine and so far as the R. S. is concerned it is the limitation to two new Fellows a year which is the fault in organisation. The number of men of first rate caliber who are not yet in the sacred precincts is very considerable and at the present rate of entry some injustice, even to the pure chemist, is inevitable. Consequently every candidate must be considered as a chemist, without prejudice or favour and obviously this operates against borderline men. . . . It is all very difficult but I feel that "biochemistry" or "physiological chemistry" is evolving its own standards and the real solution must be to have it recognized as a distinct subject electing perhaps one new Fellow each year.[85]

Two things are clear: first, organic and biochemists had already entered into a mutually beneficial relationship. Second, the strains of this new relationship were magnified by the persistent dependence of biochemistry on physiology.

THE PAINS OF PARTURITION

The influx of chemists into university departments of physiology resulted in the gradual recognition of biochemistry as an independent discipline. Biochemistry began to split off from physiology just before World War I, and several new chairs were established in the postwar period of reconstruction. In the large medically oriented universities of London and Edinburgh, parturition occurred when biochemists acquired the responsibility for teaching organic chemistry to medical students. This reshuffling of roles caused a conflict of interest between physiologists and chemists. At University College, biochemistry remained associated with physiology, but at Edinburgh, it was detached and linked to chemistry. At Cambridge and Oxford, where the demands of medical teaching were less immediate, the process of fission took a different course. Independent chairs were created by well-connected academic entrepreneurs. In this context, internal competition for service roles was less important than the national politics of science patronage. Competition developed, not between chemistry and physiology, but between biochemistry and other biomedical disciplines.

The internal evolutionary pattern can be seen most clearly at University College, where biochemists gradually expanded into organic chemistry and developed a sequence of elementary, intermediate, and advanced biochemistry courses parallel to the courses in physiology. At that point, physiology and biochemistry parted, like a replica from a template. Intermediate and advanced courses in physiological chemistry were first offered by Plimmer in 1909 as part of the honors B.Sc. course in physiology.[86] Plimmer hoped these courses would attract recruits from chemistry. In practice, however, few intending physiologists saw biochemistry as an attractive career. The key to tapping a large audience of potential recruits was the course in organic and applied chemistry required of all medical students, taught by E. C. C. Baly in the Department of Chemistry.

The place of organic chemistry in the medical curriculum had long been the subject of debate in the medical faculty, and Baly's departure in 1910 reopened the question of who should teach chemistry to medical students.[87] Ernest Starling proposed that a readership in biochemistry be established in physiology; chemists J. Norman Collie and William Ramsay approved. Starling then proposed that the new reader take charge of organic and clinical chemistry. Ramsay and Baly countered with the suggestion that elementary, organic, and medical chemistry be taught by a "teacher of chemistry," nominated by the medical faculty but appointed in chemistry. This motion was approved. However, Ramsay, Baly, and Starling then proceeded to divide the responsibility for organic and medical chemistry between Baly's successor and Plimmer, thus leaving the original dispositions unchanged.[88] The physiologists wanted organic and medical chemistry but not elementary chemistry (which had not yet been made a prerequisite for entry to the bachelor of medicine course). The chemists wanted to keep organic chemistry and were able to do so because they taught elementary chemistry.

This ad hoc arrangement was continued from year to year until 1917 when the chemists were so swamped with war-related work that they agreed to let Plimmer take full charge. Plimmer groaned under the extra burden of organic chemistry on top of chemical physiology and advanced biochemistry.[89] But control of this vertically integrated sequence of service courses was the basis for developing biochemistry as a distinct discipline. Plimmer did not reap the fruits of his labors (he left University College in 1919), but Jack Drummond, his successor, did. An organic chemist specializing in nutrition, Drummond had ambitions to be a discipline builder:

> I am greatly looking forward to working with Starling and Bayliss and have great hopes of getting a school of Biochemistry going there. There is also the attraction of academic circles. My only pessimistic moments are when I think of the penniless condition of the College to which I am going.[90]

Drummond's ambitions were realized sooner than he expected.

In the spring of 1920, a delegation from the Rockefeller Foundation discovered the new clinical units established by the Board of Education at University College Hospital. Impressed by the similarity of these units with their own plans for full-time academic clinical chairs, Richard Pearce persuaded the foundation board to give $5 million for new facilities and staff in the biomedical sciences. The plans included $250,000 for a new biochemistry laboratory attached to the University College Hospital. Starling proposed that biochemistry be set up as a semi-independent department alongside physiology, with a professor, an associate professor, and two assistants.[91]

Biochemistry at University College was shaped by this new connection to clinical medicine. The renascence of physiology after 1904 had been made possible by segregating it from the dominating clinicians. (University College Hospital had been incorporated separately for just that purpose.) By 1920, however, medical reformers aimed to reestablish a more equal partnership between the biomedical and clinical sciences. Physiologists and biochemists applauded this trend. Starling, who had just resigned to take a post at St. Thomas's Hospital, decided to remain at University College to lead the reorganization. H. H. Dale wrote Pearce that the most serious deficiency in physiology at University College was the absence of clinical connections. Starling agreed that the success of the clinicial units required close contact with the biomedical sciences.[92] A new readership was established in pathological chemistry to connect with T. R. Elliott's clinical unit. Unable to find a suitable biochemist, Drummond drafted Charles Harington, a young chemist in George Barger's department, and sent him to study clinical chemistry with D. D. Van Slyke at the Rockefeller Institute.[93] The medical curriculum was reorganized: general chemistry was made a premedical requirement, and organic chemistry was expanded. At A. V. Hill's suggestion, Drummond organized a full lecture course in advanced biochemistry and the M. B. degree examination was revised accordingly. When Drummond was promoted to professor in 1923, biochemistry became an independent department, but one closely allied with physiology.[94]

A similar process of fission occurred at Edinburgh, only in chemistry rather than physiology. The key figure there was James Walker, a physical chemist of thoroughly modern views and with a strong interest in medical teaching.[95] As professor in the medical faculty at Dundee from 1897 to 1908, he had reorganized the teaching of chemistry to integrate basic theory and clinical application. At Edinburgh, chemistry had long been connected with medicine (the medical chair was the only chair of chemistry until 1893). This tradition and Walker's experience shaped his plans after he succeeded to the chair in 1908. Walker's master plan, drawn up in 1914, included accommodation for "possible future developments...in the field of medical chemistry." Money was appropriated for a new laboratory, but wartime shortages put a halt to all construction. Not to be balked in his plans, Walker proposed, in 1917, that part of the building fund be used to endow a new chair of medical chemistry, to teach an integrated sequence of courses from basics to clinical applications:

The ideal to be aimed at is a Department of Medical Chemistry, which should be in close association with the Departments of Physiology, Pharmacology, Pathology and Bacteriology, and in which the medical student should be taught not only his First Professional Chemistry, but the chemistry he requires in his later studies. If all this teaching were done in one department under one head, coordination and continuity could be absolutely secured, and the student would not have the unfortunate idea that after he had passed his First Professional Examination he was done with chemistry for ever, and that the Physiological Chemistry that he met with in his second year...was something quite different from his First

Year's Chemistry instead of being a continuation and application of the same.[96]

The university senate approved, and in 1919 George Barger was appointed to the chair of "chemistry in relation to medicine."[97]

Edward Schäfer was bitterly opposed to Walker's evident designs on chemical physiology. He too had submitted a master plan in 1914, which had as its centerpiece a new chair and institute of chemical physiology. For him too physiological chemistry was a strategic area for expansion and had outgrown the existing lectureship: "Unless an independent chair is established, it is impossible to attract or keep the best man, who will not consent permanently to occupy a subordinate position."[98] Although Schäfer's plan was approved, Walker's clever maneuver had established the chemists' claim to biochemistry as a fait accompli. Schäfer could not block Barger's claim to the large courses in general and organic chemistry, but he did make sure that Barger would not take over W. W. Taylor's course in chemical physiology and initiate a new course in clinical chemistry, as Walker had planned.[99] In 1920 Schäfer renamed Taylor's lectureship "biochemistry" and refused to budge. Richard Pearce, on tour for the Rockefeller Foundation in 1923, described the stalemate:

Each department, especially physiology, feels it should be complete in itself, and there is no tendency to use space in common for work of the same character. Large classes and a reverence for a traditional curriculum have made the situation as to space almost intolerable. Also there has been curious expansion – dependent again on ideas of water-tight departments. Schäfer, determined to hold on to Histology, has built a laboratory for his subject... used only three months of the year, while bacteriology is crying for space.... To crown all one finds Barger, one of the greatest of biochemists, teaching inorganic and organic chemistry, because Schäfer insists on teaching biochemistry in his department of physiology. It is only fair to say that the Principal and the Faculty recognize their fault, but fearing Schäfer, are waiting for his retirement, probably within two years, before making a change.[100]

Schäfer did retire in 1925, and Barger began to teach biochemistry to students in bacteriology and chemistry, not, however, to physiologists; the biochemistry lectureship remained part of physiology.[101] As Schäfer had predicted, however, it failed to attract first-rate biochemists and remained a minor service role.

The relation between biochemists and physiologists in other British universities turned on similar issues of territorial rights. In some smaller universities, biochemistry remained attached to physiology. In some cases, limited resources necessitated hybrid roles, as in the smaller German universities; in others, physiologists deliberately blocked separation. When Otto Rosenheim left Kings in 1920, the readership in biochemistry remained vacant for seven years, even when organic chemistry was transferred from chemistry to physiology in 1922. William Halliburton was preoccupied by his compulsive labors as editor and compiler, and when he broke down mentally and physically in 1922, there was no one to exploit the opportunity for discipline building.[102] At Glasgow, it was a story of co-option, not neglect. In 1919 William Gardiner endowed a separate chair of physiological chemistry, and Edward Cathcart, then Grieve Lecturer, was appointed professor. Cathcart proceeded to turn the Gardiner Chair of Biochemistry into a second chair of physiology. He had become interested during the war in fatigue, industrial physiology, and basal metabolism and turned his back on his earlier chemical work.[103] Like J. S. Haldane, he became a strong advocate of holistic physiology, a program having little room for biochemistry. In a lecture entitled "Dynamic biochemistry," which was a deliberate echo of Hopkins's 1913 address, Cathcart railed against biochemists who saw organisms as chemical factories and reveled in the minutiae of cellular chemistry:

The whole mechanistic outlook is to me anathema. . . . Our methods may be muddy, may be amateurish, may be childish, but we at least do not shut our eyes to the fact that we are dealing with a living organism, and that it is no use pottering about with isolated fragments.[104]

Appointed Regius Professor of Physiology in 1928, Cathcart continued to dominate his successors in the Gardiner Chair of Biochemistry until he retired in 1946.[105]

Most physiologists were more sympathetic to biochemistry than was Cathcart. For example, the second chair of physiology established at Manchester in 1923, despite its title, was intended by A. V. Hill to be a chair of chemical physiology or biochemistry.[106] The first occupant of the chair was Henry S. Raper, who combined the skills and outlook of chemist and physiologist. It was Raper who took up Cathcart's challenge in 1930 and made the case for a chemical physiology of the cell.[107] Yet even sympathetic physiologists were a mixed blessing to biochemists. Sheltered institutional niches limited opportunities for discipline building. Hybrid chairs of physiology and biochemistry provided prestige and intellectual opportunities, but they often reverted to pure physiology. This pattern was especially marked in the smaller English universities. At Leeds, for example, physiology was subdivided in 1919 into two hybrid chairs of "physiology and biochemistry," and "experimental physiology and pharmacology," occupied by Henry Raper and A. Lovatt-Evans. Within months, Lovatt-Evans resigned; his chair was reduced to a lectureship, and Raper was left in sole charge of physiology. When Raper himself left, Leeds had no biochemist at all: a lecturer was appointed in 1926, but he had only a marginal role. There was no chair until 1946.[108] A similar pattern occurred at Sheffield, where J. B. Leathes took the chair of physiology in 1914. Leathes enjoyed the benefits of a chair of physiology, but he had no incentive or opportunity to develop biochemistry. When he retired in 1933, his chair and even the lectureship in chemical physiology reverted to physiology. Biochemistry did not begin to revive until 1938, when Hans Krebs was given a research position in pharmacology.[109]

CONCLUSION

The institutional problems that many British biochemists experienced had their roots in the historical evolution of "chemical physiology." Physiologists and, later, organic chemists recognized the marginal benefits of a strong biochemistry, but neither was willing to support it at the expense of their own central interests. During times of expansion, biochemistry was a good cause for obtaining resources that would not otherwise have been accessible. In lean times, when hard trade-offs had to be made, support was not forthcoming. Dependence on physiology hampered efforts to create separate departments. Physiologists either lacked incentives to nurture biochemistry or thought it too important to let go. University leaders found it easy to cut corners by forming hybrid departments. The lack of an independent reward system made academic careers in biochemistry less attractive than careers in medicine or physiology. In the recurrent spasms of expansion and reform, biochemistry gradually evolved into a quasi-independent discipline; but there was nothing like the sustained, nationwide reform movement that swept biochemistry into being in the United States. In 1925 there were only four independent chairs in Britain; in the United States, there was one in almost every medical school. Despite constant laments from Fletcher and others of the shortage of home-grown biochemists, this shortage continued until after World War II.

The intellectual style of biochemistry in most British universities also reflected its historical evolution as chemical physiology. It was largely limited to animal and human physiology, especially those areas accessible to chemical investigation: vitamins and nutrition, metabolism, and hormones. As physiologists adapted their priorities to growing opportunities in clinical research, biochemists likewise concentrated on problems of human physiology and pathology. This relatively narrow range of subject matter reflected the limits imposed on biochemists by their service roles in physiology and medicine.

There were exceptions: a distinctive style of "general biochemistry" flourished at Cambridge, so much so that Hopkins's style has seemed more representative of British biochemistry than the more numerous and typical schools of chemical physiology. However, Hopkins's school and similar institutions were endowed institutes, not tied to service roles in medical physiology. The situation was similar to that in Germany, where a few independent institutes like Otto Warburg's overshadowed the official academic institutes of physiological chemistry. A distinctive political economy supported a distinctive disciplinary style.

4

General biochemistry: the Cambridge School

"General biochemistry" differed from "chemical physiology" in both scope and emphasis. It was a broadly biological program, taking as its domain all forms of life: microbes, plants, invertebrates, and higher animals. It was concerned ultimately with fundamental processes – growth, development, energy transformation, and biochemical control – rather than special problems of human physiology and pathology. General biochemists looked to more varied constituencies: zoologists, botanists, microbiologists, as well as physiologists and pathologists. This broad conception of biochemistry was both an intellectual design and a political strategy for discipline building. Breadth and diverse audiences legitimated independence from physiology and provided access to wider institutional support systems.

General biochemistry required a broader base of support than that provided by service roles in physiology and medicine. Consequently, it was limited prior to 1945 to a few institutions: F. G. Hopkins's school, Rudolf Peters's at Oxford (an offshoot of Cambridge), David Keilin's group at the Molteno Institute, and a few small research units. Endowment and favored connections to external patrons of basic research freed these groups from dependence on a single source of support and recruits, namely medical teaching. An undergraduate degree program in biochemistry gave Hopkins an unusually large and diverse pool of recruits. The broader programmatic missions of government councils and private foundations found expression in the researches they supported. Just as chemical physiology was congruent with its limited basis in medical physiology, independence from service roles facilitated more general, avant-garde research.

Hopkins's intellectual vision of general biochemistry can be traced back to at least 1910, although it was not realized institutionally until the 1920s, when Hopkins finally got the financial means to do so. The basic themes of Hopkins's program apparently evolved gradually between 1906 and 1913 out of his reading in the literature of protein metabolism rather than out of his own research.[1] The idea that all forms of life are unified at the level of metabolism is implicit in his celebrated 1913 lecture to the British Association for the Advancement of Science. In 1918 Hopkins stated that he had planned to teach general biochemistry when he received his chair in 1914 and was prevented from doing so only by the war and lack of suitable equipment for work with a range of biological materials.[2] After some fumbling attempts to translate his program into specific research, in 1919 Hopkins stumbled onto glutathione, a widely distributed, reversibly oxidizable small molecule, which he believed was involved in cellular respiration.[3] Biological oxidation became the core of an increasingly diverse research program, developed by Hopkins's disciples but inspired and integrated by Hopkins's remarkable vision of a broad, internally specialized discipline.

There is an intriguing problem here: Hopkins was only one of many biochemists who read the literature and saw the promise of intermediary metabolism for discipline building, yet Hopkins was the only one (except for Benjamin Moore) who formulated a systematic disciplinary program. There is little in Hopkins's previous achievements to explain his creative vision. (He was best known, before 1914, for his isolation of a new amino acid, tryptophane.) The key, I believe, is the institutional context in which Hopkins worked. Hopkins owed a great deal to the ideals implicit in the structure of Michael Foster's school and, ironically, to Langley's benign neglect.

The key to Hopkins's genius as the architect of a discipline was his awareness of the strategic uses of ideas. This awareness was sharpened, I believe, by the problems that confronted and frustrated him daily for over a decade. Hopkins needed a program that would make him independent of physiology. General biochemistry was simply too big to be swallowed or contained by physiology. It was big enough to justify separate institutions, with special claims on university resources, and broad enough to attract a variety of powerful allies. Hopkins and Langley both wanted an independent chair for biochemistry. Langley's brief for Hopkins's claim to the Quick Chair in 1906, depicting biochemistry as a discipline underlying all biological sciences, could have served as a text for

Hopkins himself ten years later.[4] This assumption by both parties that biochemistry should be separate set Cambridge apart from other universities, where biochemists looked forward to a semi-independent role *within* physiology. There is a specific match between the unique institutional situation at Cambridge and Hopkins's unique role as discipline builder.

The subdivided structure of the Physiological Institute provided Hopkins with a ready model for a subdivided institute of general biochemistry. Hopkins need not have been consciously imitating Foster's strategy. He worked in an institution that embodied Foster's programmatic vision: it was an immediately available resource, ideally suited to his strategic needs. We may begin to see why, of the many biochemists who were interested in metabolism and frustrated by physiologists, it was Hopkins alone who combined ideas and strategy in a powerful disciplinary program.

Hopkins was unusually explicit about the strategic value of particular research problems. In 1914 he pointed to the importance of internal unity and varied constituencies:

The recognition of Biochemistry as a specialized departmental subject is mainly justified . . . by the fact that in the study of metabolism it provides a common ground and a common technique for biologists whose special interests and ultimate activities may greatly vary.[5]

To counter physiologists' complaints that biochemists were too narrowly specialized to be a separate discipline, Hopkins observed that physiology was only one constituency of a greater biochemistry:

In leaving an Institute supposed to deal with the whole of animal physiology for one equipped for more embracing studies of the chemistry of living organisms as a whole, the biochemist would be far from narrowing his interests. If his intellectual frontiers would shrink on one side, they would extend in the other and, for him, more logical directions. The Institute I have in mind would steal something from the activities (usually, however, minor activities) of various existing physiological institutes, but would justify the theft by a highly profitable combination and coordination of stolen materials.[6]

In the 1870s Michael Foster freed physiology from anatomy by appropriating parts of biology; fifty years later, Hopkins used his mentor's strategy to free biochemists from their constricting role as chemical physiologists.

Financial independence was no less essential than a viable program for discipline building. Hopkins's professorship was not endowed, and he had no access to research funds until 1921, when a large gift from the estate of Sir William Dunn finally enabled him to realize his ambitions. Walter Fletcher was once again Hopkins's guardian angel, this time in his role as secretary of the Medical Research Council.

THE MRC AND THE DUNN BEQUEST

The establishment of the Medical Research Committee (MRC) in 1913 (it became a council in 1919) was one outcome of a decade-long agitation by scientific interests for government sponsorship of scientific and medical research. Backed by influential allies in the British government, Arthur Balfour, Richard Burdon Haldane, and H. A. L. Fisher, the science lobby exploited mounting fears of German economic and military power. They pointed to the German government's active support of universities that trained scientists and engineers and of industries that put them to work on research and development. They argued that the British state must likewise take an active role in training scientists and physicians and encouraging the application of science to national development.[7]

The Medical Research Committee was created by the National Insurance Act of 1911; it gave the secretary an open-ended mandate to sponsor medical research, an annual appropriation of £50,000 for a program of grants in aid, and a central laboratory, the National Institute of Medical Research. It was protected from vested bureaucratic interests by its position under the Privy Council. The first secretary of the MRC was Walter Fletcher. Fletcher's plans were disrupted almost immediately by the outbreak of war, and he was soon preoccupied with organizing medical manpower and facilities for national service. In the long run, however, war service greatly strengthened the position of the MRC.

Scientists' war service was the most effective demonstration of the benefits that science and medicine could bring to the national welfare, and scientists lost no opportunity to drive the point home. The MRC became a central institution in medicine and biomedical science, with a proven record of achievement and a network of powerful connections with physicians, academics, and politicians. In 1914 Fletcher was a respected scientist and university administrator; in 1919 he was a scientist–statesman with a national reputation. As secretary of the MRC, he was in a strategic position to influence the postwar reconstruction of medical and scientific institutions. He had the respect of the medical profession and was widely sought for advice on the disposition of funds, as he was, for example, by the Dunn trustees. His opinions on the organization of biomedical science carried the weight of practical achievement as well as academic expertise.[8]

Fletcher quickly revealed an extraordinary flair for administration. He was intelligent and aggressive, a keen judge of men and ideas, and his quick sense of humor extended to his own human foibles:

His ardent courage and his frankness made him a vigorous critic, sometimes too trenchant in his denouncement of others, and often too outspoken in giving unsought advice. But his heart held neither malice nor bitterness, and he was always eager to make amends.[9]

Trained as a laboratory scientist and thrust into the role of a civil servant, Fletcher combined the ideals of basic research and practical service. The mission of the MRC was to promote clinical research and improve clinical practice; but the principle means of doing so, in Fletcher's view, was by better utilizing basic knowledge of physiology, biochemistry, and pathology. Fletcher was much concerned with developing roles and institutions that could make basic knowledge accessible to clinical practice. However, he was also concerned with developing the biomedical disciplines, and he used his influence with potential patrons to gain support for areas of basic research that would complement MRC projects. Fletcher had a remarkable sense of the national system of biomedical sciences as a whole and of his responsibility to shape and manage this system. His efforts on behalf of Hopkins exemplify his role as scientist–manager.

Biochemistry was an important part of Fletcher's plans for the MRC, and his close relationship with Hopkins continued after Fletcher left the laboratory bench for the council table. Hopkins was one of the original members of the committee, and one of his first tasks was to survey the needs and resources of biochemistry, with an eye to the disposition of government grants. He turned to his student, Edward Mellanby, for assistance:

My job is to research after researchers. The new Committee is going to be no joke. Indeed I want to ask you the biggest favor I ever asked of you. . . . I want you to try and appraise the current work in physiology, pathology and pharmacology. . . . If by the end of the first week in October you could prepare some sort of document pointing out the main lines on which chemical research is likely to help practical medicine you would be doing much for me and for chemical research. . . . What I am asking is really rather a big thing, but I feel that the matter is important. What we do during the next year may determine the fate of that £60,000 [sic] for a long time to come. To make a strong case, I want a young and alert mind to help my rusty one and it is to you alone that I can turn.[10]

Fletcher frequently called upon Hopkins to locate biochemists for MRC projects or to organize committees on urgent biochemical problems. Hopkins was one of the first to recognize the importance of vitamins in nutrition, and in 1915 Fletcher sought his help in making knowledge of vitamins available to the public.[11] When the food shortage became acute in 1917, Fletcher asked Hopkins to head a committee of the MRC to organize nutritional research and to see to it that physicians were made aware of biochemists' knowledge of essential food factors. Hopkins's committee played an important role in the public acceptance of the new idea of vitamins.[12]

The biochemistry of infectious diseases was a second problem that brought Fletcher and Hopkins together. Hopkins had been interested in bacterial metabolism for some years before trench warfare reinstated infectious diseases as major health problems. He responded eagerly to Fletcher's proposal that he initiate research on pathogenic bacteria.[13]

Their wartime experiences reinforced Hopkins's and Fletcher's conviction that the shortage of biochemists was a serious long-range problem for British biomedical science. In 1917, for example, Fletcher asked Hopkins to suggest a biochemist to join a team in France investigating trench nephritis. Hopkins could think of no one who was suitably trained: "I have always felt in my bones that some day or other one would come up against the paucity of trained biochemists in this country as something of a disaster. I feel it now. . . . It is really painful."[14] In 1919 an opportunity arose for Fletcher to help Hopkins remedy the shortage of biochemists. In the fall of 1918, Charles D. Seligman, trustee of the William Dunn estate, contacted Cambridge biologist William Bate Hardy for advice regarding a possible large gift to biomedical science. (Hardy was biological secretary to the Royal Society and chairman of the MRC Food Committee.) Hardy directed Seligman to Fletcher, who quickly gained the confidence of the Dunn trustees.[15]

The war and postwar enthusiasm for rationalizing and strengthening national institutions affected the perceptions of philanthropists as well as government officials. The traditional ideal of ameliorative charity gave way to the idea of "preventive" philanthropy. Rather than alleviate the sufferings of victims of social ills, the idea was to support institutions and individuals who could prevent the causes of social ills.[16] Medical and scientific research and professional experts became the favored beneficiaries of the new "scientific" philanthropy. Decimation of British youth in the trenches and the postwar fashion for social engineering put a premium on training a new generation of scientific and medical experts. Cambridge and other universities, of course, were quick to encourage this policy.

The history of the Dunn benefactions exemplifies this change. The estate of over £1 million was left to charity in 1900. For almost the next 20 years, the trustees had been doling it out in small doses to the needy: £70,000 to 52 hospitals, £6500 to 15 nursing homes, £20,000 to 23 orphanages, £105,000 to YMCAs, the Salvation Army, and so on. In 1918, however, Seligman initiated a sharp change of policy. A few large gifts were made to biomedical research and education: a readership in pathology at Guy's Hospital (£25,000), the Dunn Institute of Biochemistry at Cambridge (£210,000), the Dunn Institute of Pathology at Oxford (£103,000) and a clinical research unit at the London Hospital (£10,000).[17] Between 1919 and 1925, £464,000 were invested in biomedical science, all with the advice of Walter Fletcher.

Biochemistry was only one of many claimants to patronage, of course, and it was not at all clear at first that Hopkins would receive any part of the Dunn largesse. The advice that Hardy and Fletcher offered Seligman in November 1918 reflected their somewhat different institutional interests. Hardy gave priority to three schemes: biochemistry, ethnology and applied psychology, and parasitology. All three were new disciplines, for which the Cambridge biologists had tried and failed to raise endowments before the war. Although Hardy did not mention Hopkins by name, it is clear from the way he made his case for biochemistry that he had Hopkins in mind.[18] In contrast, Fletcher's initial proposals to Seligman reflected some of the projects he had in mind for the MRC and NIMR: a national laboratory for biological standards, clinical units in the London hospitals, and a national institute for human nutrition.[19] Fletcher's proposals focused on specific medical problems and on institutions for performing research; Hardy gave priority to developing academic disciplines and institutions for training researchers.

The proposals by Hardy and Fletcher reflect different views of the appropriate match between private patrons and public needs. Fletcher did not think biochemistry or universities were less important than Hardy did; only that national laboratories were more appropriate objects for large private benefactors. The relationships among private patrons, government, and university science were in a state of flux in 1919. Legislation making the MRC a permanent council and defining its scope was being negotiated. Fletcher's chief objective was to secure the Dunn estate for medicine and wait for the situation to clear.

By August 1919, Fletcher's advice to Seligman had changed significantly: Fletcher now emphasized university departments over national research institutes and training as well as research. It was clear by then that practical medical research at the National Institute for Medical Research would have ample public support. Fletcher knew that the council would be able to channel substantial sums of money into university research by means of an extramural program of grants to individuals. It was clear to Fletcher that the chief need was to expand quickly the training of biomedical and clinical scientists to staff the growing departments and clinical units and to spend the new research funds. As the MRC was legally prohibited from giving gifts of endowment, Fletcher saw private benefactors, like the Dunn estate, as filling this vital role. Fletcher's first priority became to obtain endowment for an institute of biochemistry at Cambridge.[20]

When Fletcher informed Hopkins that his long-cherished hope for an institute might be realized, Hopkins poured out his problems to his old friend:

In all honesty it is a justifiable desire to want to train some biochemists as soon as possible. In two months I have had inquiries for workers and have none to suggest. Burroughs and Wellcome, unless Hartley consents to go with them, which is uncertain, propose to take Raistrick away. O'Brien tells me they can find nobody else good enough. I long to develop the special part II course in General Biochemistry which would train the kind of people wanted. I sketched it out in my mind 10 years ago when H. A. Roberts put the subject at the head of the desiderata here, and collections from the "friends of the university" were supposed to be under way. (If you remember there were *some* few earmarked sums got together which disappeared into Langley's scheme.) But the years are slipping away. Quite honestly I can only think now of getting things ready for my successor, if I am to have one. *That* much I should like to do.[21]

Hopkins's laboratory had been drained of students during the war. Academic salaries were eroded by inflation, and universities were experiencing stiff competition from chemical industries invigorated by the war. Petty academic squabbles prevented Hopkins from expanding into more adequate facilities. A postwar malaise, felt especially by young scientists, was sapping the intellectual vigor of university science. Sydney Cole, who ran the big medical course, was threatening to leave Hopkins in the lurch. A brilliant young biochemist whom Hopkins had pegged for invertebrate work had decided to travel. Opportunities in medical practice opened up by the war were attracting medical students away from careers in science.[22]

With Fletcher behind the scenes marshaling support from other influential advisors, preaching Hopkins's cause, and blocking competing schemes, the Dunn trustees agreed to endow an institute for Hopkins and to do it on a handsome scale. Fletcher hastily wrote Hopkins and Hardy to prepare a detailed plan for spending twice the sum of money they had previously discussed. Their plan called for £165,000, including £60,000 for a new laboratory and an equal sum for a research fund – an extremely large amount for the time. The trustees approved, and in 1924 the new Dunn Institute was opened with fanfare in the press and an address by Arthur Balfour, both arranged (and largely written) by Fletcher.[23]

HOPKINS'S SCHOOL

The Dunn bequest had an immediate impact on Hopkins's group. In February 1921, the sight of his laboratory humming with activity gave Fletcher a twinge of regret at having left the bench for the desk.[24] Again thanks to Fletcher's intercession, Hopkins was given permission to use the interest from the research endowment fund in 1922, and the number of workers in his group soared from 10 in 1920 to 59 in 1925.[25] (see Figure 4.1). Hopkins's school produced nearly half the papers published in the *Biochemical Journal* in the mid-1920s. Biochemists trained in Hopkins's school were favored candidates for the new positions opening up in hospitals and clinical units. Fletcher played an important role in developing the market.

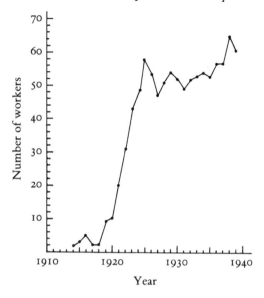

Figure 4.1. Number of workers in the Dunn Institute of Biochemistry at Cambridge, 1914–39.

In 1922, for example, he urged Seligman to create a clinical research unit at the London Hospital to make the best use of the biochemists being produced by Hopkins:

The proper equipment of these laboratories, especially on the biochemical side, would supplement in a really valuable way the work you have done at Cambridge. The Dunn Institute there, under Hopkins, will quite certainly turn out every year a regular small stream of well trained men coming on to medical work in London. Pinton and Marrack, in charge of these London laboratories now, are old pupils of Hopkins and have his spirit, and at this immense clinical centre the best men from Cambridge (and presently Oxford too) will be able for the first time to work in a full scientific way in the hospital wards. The Dunn Laboratories at Whitechapel will be a real battleground for men trained in a primary way at the Dunn Institute at Cambridge.[26]

Fletcher was thus able to stimulate both the supply of biochemists and the demand.

As funds for equipment and workers became available from the Dunn bequest, Hopkins began to realize his long-thwarted ambition for a general biochemistry. He systematically appointed junior staff to develop specialized subfields in microbiology, plant physiology, and developmental biology. Many he trained himself, as

Foster had done 50 years before. J. B. S. Haldane, Hopkins's first reader, had very diverse research interests and moved gradually into genetics, eventually into a chair of genetics at University College.[27] Muriel Wheldale Onslow, who had worked with geneticist William Bateson on the inheritance of flower pigments, was appointed lecturer in 1927. She taught an advanced course in plant biochemistry and carried out pioneering research on the biochemical genetics of plant pigments until her untimely death in 1932.[28] Wheldale's successor in plant biochemistry was Robin Hill, who developed a line of work in the biophysical chemistry of plant proteins and photosynthesis. In the 1930s, Hill worked closely with David Keilin on plant cytochromes and the bioenergetics of isolated chloroplasts. Described as a "shy genius type," Hill was equally master of plant morphology, physiology, and organic and physical chemistry.[29] Malcolm Dixon, who was appointed lecturer in 1928, made enzymes his specialty. Enzymology was crucial to Hopkins's core interest in intermediary metabolism and biological oxidation, and Dixon was eventually made director of a special subdepartment in the Dunn Institute. In the late 1930s, Dixon's group of over a dozen workers was the leading school of enzymology in Britain.[30]

One of the hallmarks of Hopkins's school was its concern with the biological organization of chemical reactions in cells and tissues. The germ of this line of thought was Hopkins's vision of the living cell as an intricately organized enzymological machine shop in which colloidal structures in the cell segregated and coordinated the processes of molecular assembly and disassembly.[31] In the 1920s, Rudolph Peters and Judah Quastel developed this conception along more concrete biological lines, investigating the microstructures that existed in the cell.[32] At the level of tissues, Dorothy Needham was carrying out her work on the biochemical mechanisms of muscle contraction.[33] Other Hopkins disciples extended biochemical ideas to the level of organisms and species. In the 1930s, Ernest Baldwin systematically developed Hopkins's nascent ideas of comparative biochemistry and pioneered the study of organic evolution at the molecular level.[34]

The unifying theme of Hopkins's school was its concern with biological form and function. This biological outlook shaped the department's teaching. Hopkins lectured to his advanced classes on the biochemistry of bacteria, fungi, plants, and marine invertebrates.[35] The Part II course in the biochemistry tripos, the first undergraduate program in Britain, was organized in a most unusual, even quixotic, way. The routine biochemistry usually presented as dry chemical taxonomy was instead worked into student investigations of three type organisms: hen's egg, barley seed, and mammalian liver. (The resemblance to Huxley and Foster's use of type organisms to teach general biology is striking and not coincidental.) Systematic chemistry was sacrificed in order to accustom students to thinking in terms of biological systems. In the second term, 30 out of 40 hours were devoted to enzymes, biological oxidation, muscle action, and microbial physiology. Only 10 hours were given to nutrition and metabolism, the mainstays of orthodox courses in biochemistry. The third term was devoted wholly to chemical morphology, plant biochemistry, and comparative biochemistry.[36] This unique course was a daring realization of Hopkins's vision of general biochemistry.

Not everyone in Hopkins's group was happy with the emphasis on biology. In 1935, for example, Norman Pirie argued that the course should give a longer and more systematic treatment of organic and physical chemistry, intermediary metabolism, and industrial applications of biochemistry. In short, it should be more like the usual courses in other universities.[37] (Pirie was a physical chemist interested in the physical properties of proteins and viruses.) A second proposal was made by Eric Holmes, a doctor of medicine who had worked in pharmacology, to increase the time given to animal metabolism and clinical biochemistry.[38] Both these proposals were countered by the biological caucus, Marjory Stephenson, Robin Hill, and Dorothy Needham, who argued in favor of keeping a strong emphasis on biological process and function.[39] After some discussion, it was decided not to make any real change in the Part II course.[40]

Physiological and medical chemistry did not disappear altogether from the Cambridge scene, but after 1922 they were minor service roles. Sydney Cole, Hopkins's chief assistant from 1898, continued, as a special lecturer, to teach the large course in chemical physiology to students of physiology and medicine.[41] Eric Holmes and one or two others did research on clinical subjects, with grants from the Medical Research Council; but these were peripheral to Hopkins's program.[42] Hopkins no longer had to depend financially and politically on service roles in physiology and medicine.

Nutrition was one of the chief areas in which biochemistry overlapped with physiology and medicine. Although Hopkins was most widely known for his pioneering work on essential amino acids, he abandoned nutritional research after the war; he apparently felt unable to compete with the Lister Institute and other research institutes with large programs in nutrition.[43] (The large-scale animal feeding experiments needed for nutritional work were very expensive, and Hopkins had no inkling in 1918 of his future opulence.) Fletcher pressed Hopkins to continue research on vitamins. In 1928 he squeezed the last £6000 out of the Dunn estate for a Dunn Nutritional Laboratory at Cambridge, hoping that Hopkins would take a more active role in its activities.[44] Hopkins did not do so, despite exasperated pleas from Fletcher:

I told Hopkins that, having somehow bagged the credit for inventing vitamins, he spends all his time collecting gold medals on the strength of it, and yet in the past ten years has neither done, nor got others to do, a hand's turn of work in the subject. His place bristles with clever young Jews and talkative women, who are frightfully learned about protein molecules and oxidation-reduction potentials and all that. But they all seem to run away from biology. The vitamin story is clamouring for analysis....Yet not a soul at Cambridge will look at it.[45]

Ironically, many of Hopkins's postdoctoral fellows came to work with him in nutrition; but Hopkins's real interest was general biochemistry, and he shied away from medical applications.

Two other Cambridge specialties also reflect Hopkins's vision: Marjory Stephenson's work on bacterial physiology and Joseph Needham's on chemical embryology. The chemistry of microbes captured Hopkins's imagination before the war and had a central part in Hopkins and Fletcher's postwar plans.[46] Marjory Stephenson came to work on vitamins in 1919, but at Hopkins's urging, she turned her talents to bacterial biochemistry. She studied bacteriology and began to lecture in the advanced course in 1925. Whereas most biochemists regarded microbes as convenient sources of enzymes, Stephenson was interested in the physiology of microbes as biochemical systems, responding constantly to their chemical environment.[47] The influence of Hopkins's grand scheme is evident. Stephenson selected her research problems less with an eye to medical application (despite pressure from Fletcher, who was paying the bills) than with an eye to basic biological processes. She carried

out fundamental researches on dehydrogenation enzymes and an-
aerobic respiration in microbes from river sludge. She was the first
to systematically explore the remarkable phenomenon of enzyme
adaptation, in which microbes manufacture and secrete different
enzymes as different nutriments are available in their growth medi-
um.[48] Although she herself did not pursue this problem after 1940,
she laid the foundation for the later work of Jacques Monod and
other biologists.

Chemical microbiology, like enzymology, gradually became a
quasi-independent subdepartment of the Dunn Institute. From
1929 Stephenson worked as a full-time "external" MRC staff member at Cambridge. In 1946 she was appointed reader in chemical
microbiology and, just before her death, her disciple, Ernest F.
Gale, was named director of a MRC research unit.[49] In 1948 a visitor
described Cambridge as "deservedly the Mecca of microbiologists
all over the world."[50]

Hopkins also lost no time in developing his interest in the biochemistry of growth and morphogenesis. In the early 1920s, two of
his best students, Michael Perkins and Joseph Needham, began to
work with developing embryos. Perkins died at a young age in
1927, but by the mid-1930s, Needham was the leading advocate of
biochemical embryology.[51] Hopkins's interest in the biochemistry of development was apparently kindled by Michael Foster.
Needham heard Hopkins tell how, over breakfast in 1898, Foster
had urged him to explore the chemical changes that occurred in the
developing embryo. He in turn passed the spark to Perkins and
Needham: "Hopkins was most enthusiastic about the developing
egg as the seat of dramatic syntheses and gave the warmest encouragement to the pursuit of research along the borderline of biochemistry, embryology, and experimental morphology."[52] Needham's
interest in how chemical processes shaped the form of developing
tissues is yet another indicator of Hopkins's influence:

Chemical work on the adult body may be perhaps carried on with a blind
eye to the organization within which its reactions are proceeding. But a
system where the organic form is continually changing with time renders
the comparison between morphological form and biochemical properties
absolutely inevitable.[53]

Needham investigated the distribution of enzymes in developing
tissues and the role of chemical "organizers" in causing differential

rates of metabolism.[54] Needham's strength was his broad knowledge of both biochemistry and biology and his willingness to
theorize boldly.[55] He could do so in the context of Hopkins's
school.

Between 1935 and 1937, Needham attempted to organize an
interdisciplinary institute of "physico-chemical morphology" within
the Dunn Institute. Proposed members included Needham, Ernest
Baldwin, zoologist C. H. Waddington, philosopher J. H. Woodger,
mathematician Dorothy Wrinch, and physical chemist John Desmond
Bernal. His plan provided for research on growth and regeneration,
organizers, biochemical genetics, physical chemistry of chromo-
somes and nucleic acid, x-ray crystallography of proteins, and
comparative metabolism.[56] Needham approached Warren Weaver
of the Rockefeller Foundation, who was developing an ambitious
program in the application of physics and chemistry to biology.[57]
Weaver was impressed by Needham and liked his proposal; but
Needham was never able to marshal sufficient support from the
university. Not surprisingly, his notions of a "theoretical biology"
did not win him friends among orthodox chemists, who considered
him "sloppy," or among zoologists, who would have none of his
wild chemical notions.[58] Such criticism did not trouble Weaver.
What did, however, was the lack of support from university officials who did not like Needham's radical politics or his untidy
discipline. They made it clear that Hopkins would get no support
for Needham's institute.[59]

The principal impediment, however, was Hopkins himself. He
was 75 years old in 1935 and was slowing down. In 1936, for
example, he dodged an appointment with Rockefeller scout W. E.
Tisdale on the grounds that his impending retirement made any
future enterprises in his department unreal to him.[60] Each year
Hopkins announced his retirement – for the next year. He did not
actually step down until 1943. Until it was known who Hopkins's
successor would be and whether he would continue to support
Needham's unusual line of work, Weaver would not risk more than
small yearly grants. Both felt that a mutually beneficial relation had
been thwarted.

Hopkins had never found it easy to administer a large and diverse
group. Only a few years after receiving the Dunn bequest, he began
to run annual deficits, which scandalized the university, puzzled the
Dunn trustees, and finally exasperated his friend Fletcher, who had

been keeping a watchful eye on his handiwork. Fletcher bailed Hopkins out, securing him extra money from the Dunn estate, soothing his nervous anxiety, and, at the same time, exhorting him to curb the size of his school and give other places a chance.[61] It was Hopkins's way to encourage his junior staff to take the initiative in developing new areas of research, and as he aged, this virtue became a vice. In the 1930s, he was not alert to his protegés' needs for material support. Dorothy Needham carried on her first-rate work on a third-rate salary; Joseph Needham felt that Hopkins failed to advance his disciples professionally, for example, in the Royal Society. Hopkins allowed Robin Hill to subsist from year to year on grants, and Marjory Stephenson was constantly having to beg for small sums and to cope with major disruptions caused by changes in single individuals' plans.[62] In part these were normal problems of a large and extremely diverse group, supported by a plethora of grants and fellowships and held together by "Hoppy's" gentle charisma.

Hopkins's genius was his knack for bringing forth the best in people, for turning geese into swans, as Needham put it, by applying the hormone of encouragement:

He was a great giver and receiver of moral support – if he gave freely of it to all his collaborators and colleagues, he also needed it, for he frequently passed through periods of depression. And this was one of his secrets, that he was open to receive it from the most junior of his research workers, so that they did not feel he was encouraging them like some *deus ex machina*, but as one of themselves; in other words, he fully understood and practiced the great doctrine of leadership *from within* and not from above....He had the knack of surrounding himself with people of striking personality...But nothing ever put "Hoppy" in the shade. No one could fail to recognise in the little figure, rubbing its eyes in a characteristic gesture during a conference, loitering with its overcoat unbuttoned in the hall, proceeding with a ruminative walk past the colleges, the authentic gold of intellectual inspiration.[63]

No other biochemical institution came close to Cambridge in its diversity of research specialties and its broad biological vision of biochemistry as a discipline.

These qualities did not long outlast Hopkins's presence. David Keilin, who was trained as a biologist and could well have sustained Hopkins's program, firmly declined the Cambridge chair in 1937.[64] A. C. Chibnall, who succeeded Hopkins in 1943, had much narrower interests in plant proteins and found the strain of administering a large school intolerable. In 1949 he resigned. Hans Krebs, who had a broad biological conception of biochemistry, was unacceptable to the Cambridge powers; Chibnall vetoed Needham and Dixon.[65] In the 1950s, Cambridge reverted to a more orthodox medical style. Meanwhile, the Oxford school under Rudolf Peters and his successor, Hans Krebs, carried on the Hopkins tradition.

OFFSHOOTS: THE OXFORD SCHOOL

The Oxford department resembled Hopkins's in its origin, economic basis, and intellectual style. It too was liberated from dependence on medical service roles by a large gift of endowment. Benjamin Moore infused Oxford with some of the old Liverpool spirit during his brief tenure as Whitely Professor, and Peters was a self-conscious missionary of the Cambridge style.

Change began in a conservative way. The moving spirit behind the establishment of the Whitely Chair in 1920 was Charles Sherrington, and the Liverpool connection was crucial, financially and programmatically. The donor of the chair, Edward Whitely, was the son of a former mayor of Liverpool and a former student and friend of Benjamin Moore's.[66] It was Whitely who nominated Moore as first professor, and Sherrington provided him with laboratory space and £400 from his own budget for research and teaching expenses.[67] Moore was responsible for the course in chemical physiology, and biochemistry was part of the doctor of medicine examination in physiology. It was precisely the arrangement that Sherrington had proposed for Liverpool in 1913: a quasi-independent chair of biochemistry within physiology.

It is not clear that Moore would have been content with that role, however: in his 1920 textbook (patched together out of his earlier programmatic pieces), he announced that Oxford would promote "dynamic" biochemistry, presumably meaning his own eclectic and idiosyncratic interests in bioenergetics and photosynthesis.[68] What Moore would have done with this program we cannot know, for he died suddenly in 1922. Rudolf Peters had several advantages that Moore did not: a more coherent and realistic program, acquired at Hopkins's knee and, in 1923, independent financial means. In that year, the Rockefeller Foundation made a large grant for a new laboratory and research endowment.

The aims of the Rockefeller Foundation in medical research and education were shaped by the same social forces that shaped the MRC. Before World War I, the foundation had been active in public health campaigns against hookworm and yellow fever, programs that reflected prevailing progressive ideology and ideas of preventive philanthropy. After the war, however, foundation leaders were looking for broader and less directly interventionist missions. Medical education and biomedical and clinical research appealed to a new generation of managers as vehicles for their larger social mission, without the explicit moral thrust of earlier programs. Wycliffe Rose led the General Education and International Education Boards into vast programs of support for research in medical schools and universities, to the tune of hundreds of millions of dollars. Rockefeller Foundation leaders like Richard Pearce, who traveled the European circuit, shed older programs and took the lead in fashionable areas of scientific and medical research.

Internationalist ideals and deference to European leadership in science made Britain and Germany favored areas for Rockefeller largesse. Pearce and others were thoroughly committed to the ideal of scientific medicine and believed that clinical science required steady infusions from the basic biomedical sciences. Moreover, foundation policy was to invest in the people and institutions with established records of success: "Make the peaks higher" and let emulation and competition do the rest.[69] Pearce's aim was to round out the biomedical sciences at Oxford and Cambridge. The Dunn trustees had endowed pathology at Oxford and biochemistry at Cambridge; Pearce proposed that the foundation endow pathology at Cambridge and biochemistry at Oxford.[70]

The leading role in negotiations with the foundation was taken by Archibald E. Garrod, chemical pathologist, Regius Professor of Medicine, and an enthusiastic supporter of biochemistry since his early days with Hopkins at Guy's. Peters was ambitious to build a school that would shine as brightly as his alma mater and advised Garrod that £144,000 would build a laboratory and support 5 staff and 20 research workers.[71] Having learned from bitter experience not to put the stakes too high, Garrod helped Peters to trim his sails, charmed Pearce, and undertook to raise the required matching funds from the university and private donors.[72] The new laboratory opened its doors in 1926.

Peters shared Hopkins's biological conception of his discipline and, by 1930, had developed a distinctive program in "coordinative biochemistry," which focused on how cellular microstructures coordinated metabolism and oxidation. Peters adapted and renewed Hopkins's vision of the machine shop cell as Hopkins had adapted and updated Foster's conception of "living protoplasm," by incorporating into it modern ideas from cell biology. This programmatic vision was much more evident in Peters's personal research, however, than in the structure of his department. He was less successful than Hopkins was as an institution builder.

Independent means did not entirely free Peters from reliance on his powerful allies and patrons in the biomedical sciences, especially Sherrington. Peters was much younger and less experienced than Moore and lacked Hopkins's professional authority. He was in no position to put a dramatically new program into effect, and Oxford in the 1920s and 1930s mixed elements of the Cambridge style and of chemical physiology. Peters's main service role was teaching medical students, and without a separate bachelor of science program in biochemistry, students in physiology were his sole source of recruits. Although it was a separate administrative unit, Peters's program was closely tied to physiology.[73] Peters was not the magnet for grants and research fellows that Hopkins was, and he had no more than three permanent staff until after World War II. Consequently, there was less opportunity for specialized subdivisions. Ernest Walker developed chemical microbiology, and an MRC unit in that specialty was established in 1946 under Donald D. Woods, a Stephenson protegé.[74] But the Oxford school was overshadowed by Cambridge until Hans Krebs took the chair in 1953.

CONCLUSION

Hopkins was a Moses figure: he saw clearly what could be done and had the spiritual authority to inspire others to do it. He himself, however, remained a captive of his training and his times: he was an analyst, preaching chemical biology but practicing physiological chemistry. His work on glutathion was less innovative than that of many of his young disciples. In the 1930s, Hopkins was still lecturing his puzzled classes on the evils of the protoplasm theory, although his audience had no notion of what all the fuss was about.[75] In contrast, Peters took for granted the conception that Hopkins had labored to conceive and he had the training to put it into practice in his own research. But he lacked the saintly authority that had enabled Hopkins to attract resources; his disciplinary program was realized less in the institution he built.

Moore, Hopkins and his group, David Keilin, Hans Krebs, and a few others constituted a small avant-garde in British biochemistry. Chemical physiology was the norm, and it was not until after World War II that aspects of Hopkins's program began to take root in many departments. General biochemistry developed as part of an unusual pattern of institution building, involving a visionary entrepreneur and connections with external patrons, a rare combination. Meanwhile, chemical physiology thrived on routine service roles in medical instruction and research. Historical precedents and institutional support systems strongly influenced intellectual styles. As the ideas of general biochemistry became more familiar and accessible, however, particular institutional contexts were no longer as strongly determining of scientific style as they were at first. A new generation of biochemists routinized Hopkins's vision, and wider availability of government patronage diluted the structural importance of service roles in traditional departments. Although Cambridge and Oxford lost their special character, other departments came to resemble what had once been the avant-garde.

5

European ideals and American realities, 1870–1900

Because Germany was so advanced in developing scientific disciplines, German influence was inevitably a major force in the development of the biomedical sciences in Austria, Russia, Japan, Scandinavia, and the United States. Some German laboratories had more foreign than German students. Walter Jones's description of the polyglot character of Kossel's institute at Marburg is typical:

> On the day of my arrival I met a young Russian named [Phoebus] Levene who has worked for several years in New York....Levene introduced me to two of his Russian friends, that is I believe he introduced me to them for it was done in the Russian language and I cannot be certain. These three Russians, a Frenchman, an Englishman, an Irish professor from Belfast named Thompson, the two assistants, another German and myself are the present workers in the Physiological Research Laboratory. It often happens that several of us go out together to dinner and you would be amused to hear the four languages.[1]

Some universities organized special courses in English, and foreign students were regarded as an important vehicle of German cultural imperialism.

Apart from Russia, the United States was probably the most avid consumer of German *Wissenschaft*. It has been estimated that about 15,000 American doctors studied in German (or Austrian) universities prior to 1914, or about one-third of the upper elite of American physicians.[2] The importance of German contacts in agricultural chemistry and in the establishment of American agricultural experiment stations has also been documented.[3] Careers of individual scientists offer abundant evidence of the stimulating effect of German experiences and ideals. The role of Johns Hopkins University and Medical School has long captured the imagination of chroniclers and historians of the German connection.[4] Medical and scientific reformers between 1870 and 1900 harped constantly on the contrast between American and German achievement and saw themselves as creating Leipzigs and Heidelbergs on American soil.

Such claims and perceptions were, of course, strategies to mobilize resources for science in a society that was intensely nationalistic, competitive, and ambivalent about European culture.[5] It was in the interests of reformers first to dramatize the gap between German and American science and then to exaggerate the effectiveness of German exemplars in the new American universities. Historians have recently begun to recognize the importance of distinctively American forms and initiatives. The land-grant colleges, with their populist ideals and emphasis on the basic applied sciences, were as effective an agent of university reform as highbrow German models.[6] Scientific schools, which combined the cultural values of the liberal arts college with the utilitarian thrust and professional clientele of land-grant colleges, were crucial in the transition to university status for many old elite colleges.[7] Daniel Gilman's plans for Johns Hopkins were probably shaped at least as much by his experiences at the Sheffield Scientific School and the University of California as by European models.[8] Ira Remsen's school of chemistry at Johns Hopkins more closely resembled a traditional American college, with its emphasis on character and mental discipline, than it did a German research school.[9] Enthusiasm for things German enlivened traditional careers in college teaching as well as avant-garde research.[10] German cultural ideals were flexible and adaptable designs for reshaping local American institutions.

The ability of German universities to spawn new disciplines depended on the whole system of German society: the uniform, high-quality system of *Gymnasia*; the crucial role of *Wissenschaft* in Germans' national identity; the monopoly of bureaucratic, paternalistic governments over university budgets and policies; and the hierarchical, elitist character of German society, with a weak entrepreneurial middle class and strong university-trained elites. American colleges and medical schools developed in a society without a national system of high schools; where higher learning was not a part of nationalist sentiment; where the federal government was chronically weakened by states' rights politics and antipathy to a professional civil service; and where the potential audience for higher education was a diverse, democratic, entrepreneurial middle class. Joseph Ben-David has argued that the distinctive features of American universities were created when German standards of achievement were introduced into a utilitarian and egalitarian cultural system. The department, with its substructure of equal, specialized chairs; the graduate school, which routinized what in Germany was an informal apprenticeship in research for a small elite; the diversified university, with its collegiate core and varied professional schools; the proliferation of basic applied sciences within academia: these remarkable institutional innovations were adaptations of elitest German practices to a democratic mass society.[11] Star-struck American pilgrims to German universities saw only what their previous experiences prepared them to see. They took home only what they could actually use to build scientific institutions at home. German ideals of achievement acted as a leaven in the diverse American system of liberal arts, scientific, and medical colleges.

This argument is convincing, so far as it goes; but it is only a rough guide to understanding how the mechanics of cultural diffusion worked in practice. Americans went to Germany to study particular disciplines. Their aim on returning was to create departments and graduate programs in their disciplines, not departments or graduate schools in general. To understand how cultural adaptation and innovation worked, we must look at this process in the context of individual disciplines. Depending on when they went abroad and where, Americans observed their disciplines in particular phases of development and in the form of particular local styles. We must therefore ask what intellectual resources were available to scientist–entrepreneurs in their European experiences and how they selectively borrowed disciplinary styles to fit American institutional contexts. We must inquire as to the specific opportunities and limitations of colleges, scientific schools, and medical colleges. What service roles, audiences, and disciplinary alliances did discipline builders marshal to support their work in the style to which they had become accustomed during their German *Wanderjahre*?

American biochemical institutions between 1875 and 1900 strongly resembled German institutions; indeed, one recognizes almost every one of the varied styles described in Chapter 1. Wilbur Olin Atwater, Samuel W. Johnson, and other physiologists and agricultural chemists were direct descendants of Justus Liebig. (As in Germany, however, few of this school became biochemists; most made their mark as chemists or nutritionists.) At the Sheffield Scientific School, Johnson's student, Russell H. Chittenden, combined physiology and physiological chemistry in the style of his mentor, Willy Kühne. At the University of Michigan Medical School, Victor C. Vaughan combined physiological chemistry with hygiene, much as Pettenkoffer had at Munich. Jacques Loeb's school of general physiology at the University of Chicago included chemical physiology, and several of his students became influential biochemists. Finally, physiological chemistry was included in John J. Abel's Department of Pharmacology at Johns Hopkins Medical School, where it eventually developed as a separate discipline. The question is, did these familiar styles reflect trans-Atlantic borrowing or parallel adaptation to similar institutional environments? The answer is, both.

The German influence is evident in nearly every case. Chittenden borrowed his research style and his program from Kühne's institute; trained as a chemist, he came to regard himself as a physiologist. Loeb was German and embodied – even caricatured – the ideals of German academic science. Abel was an ardent Germanophile (at one time he considered emigrating); he spent seven years studying in Germany and had an M. D. degree from Strasbourg. All three had active, continuing connections with German colleagues. Vaughan alone of the four founders never studied in Europe, but he made a point of visiting the European centers of hygiene before setting up his department. It is striking that not one of the four founders of biochemistry in America was first and foremost a biological chemist but bootlegged biochemical work into a more established discipline. They experienced the same constraints of audience and limited resources as did their German counterparts. The universities of Michigan, Chicago, and Johns Hopkins were consciously founded on German models, and structural similarities help to explain why similar disciplinary styles emerged there. Opportunities were far more limited in the United States, of course, owing to the general lack of development of medical schools, especially in physiology. But contexts that did offer opportunities for biochemists gave a selective advantage to one or another German styles.

These were highbrow options, of course. On a lower professional level, agricultural and medical chemistry were the principal career options for biological chemists prior to 1900. Nearly one-third of the tiny band who later founded the American Society of Biological Chemists were employed in agricultural colleges in the 1890s. But neither agricultural nor medical chemistry offered much opportunity for specialization in biological chemistry. Chemists were hired by medical and agricultural colleges to teach general chemistry. Such courses did include some biological chemistry, but generally very little. Agricultural and medical students had little time or inclination to pursue specialized work. Advanced courses usually concentrated on such practical applications as toxicology, clinical analysis, fertilizer and soil analysis, or animal nutrition rather than theoretical biochemistry. Whereas university departments of chemistry were beginning to develop basic specialties in organic, physical, or occasionally biological chemistry, chemistry in agricultural and medical colleges remained a unified discipline, the common denominator of a variety of applied science specialties serving specialized professional audiences. Physiological chemists had higher academic status than agricultural or medical chemists, but they were vastly outnumbered and their specialized credentials were not always an asset in a generalist's market. Chittenden, Vaughan, Loeb, Atwater, and Abel are the atypical individuals who were able to maintain specialized roles on the basis of routine service roles.

CHEMICAL PHYSIOLOGY: R. H. CHITTENDEN AT YALE

The Sheffield Scientific School was established by S. W. Johnson to train technical chemists in the 1850s, and by 1880 it had become a superior college of engineering and experimental science. Chittenden began to teach physiological chemistry in 1874 and in 1882 was appointed to the first chair of physiological chemistry in America, from which he dominated the discipline for three decades (retiring in 1921).

Chittenden's success as a discipline builder depended on a supportive institutional context, a viable intellectual program, and a dependable clientele. The Sheffield School offered all three, and Chittenden demonstrated remarkable entrepreneurial skill in making the most of these resources. The combination of practical and academic values embodied in the Sheffield School was nicely congruent with the ambiguous status of physiological chemistry: a basic applied science, with disciplinary aspirations, but rooted in premedical training. Sheffield was kept at arm's length by Yale College, where some science (mainly natural history) was taught for its cultural, not its practical, value in research or application. Although collegians considered Sheffield's three-year Ph.B degree inferior to the B.A. degree, Sheffield was never a purely technical school. Almost from the start it adopted the ideal of a liberal education in the sciences, analogous to (and eventually competitive with) the classical liberal arts course in Yale College.[12] Moreover, the Scientific School catered increasingly to students who wanted an appropriate general education before receiving technical training in one or another of the professions. A three-year course, "Biology Preparatory to Medicine," was inaugurated in 1870. Consisting at first of basic chemistry and biology, modern languages, and a smattering of history and political economy, the course was expanded in 1874 to include physiology and a laboratory course in physiological chemistry.[13] These courses were meant to prepare students for medicine by presenting physiology and physiological chemistry as basic academic disciplines. This combination of ideals actually was more closely akin to the style of a German university than either the purist ideals of Yale College or the utilitarian ideals of the Yale Medical School. It was an appropriate context for a basic applied discipline like physiological chemistry.

Chittenden had no programmatic vision of this discipline when, as an advanced student, he was called upon to take charge of the laboratory course in physiological chemistry. He was a chemist, innocent of any knowledge of physiology; he saw physiological chemistry simply as a kind of chemical anatomy useful to, but distinct from, physiology. Experience expanded his vision; he perceived that the combination of chemistry and physiology offered intellectual opportunities, and his prospects for a career were made more concrete by Johnson's promise of a permanent position at the Sheffield School.[14] In 1878 Chittenden was packed off to Germany for postgraduate study, which was the customary prologue to academic promotion at that time. During a year of study at Heidelberg with Willy Kühne, his nascent conception of physiological chemistry took shape.

Chittenden had actually arranged to study with Hoppe-Seyler, but, as he later recalled, he was repelled by the run-down condition of the institute at Strasbourg and the absence of everything he had expected of a German university. So within a few days he departed for Heidelberg, without so much as a letter of introduction.[15] Fortunately, Kühne had read and admired Chittenden's first publication and gave him a warm reception. Wittingly or unwittingly, Chittenden's abrupt change of plans was a strategic decision. Kühne's program was closer to what Chittenden had known at the Sheffield

School and was more appropriate to his future plans there. Hoppe-Seyler's institute combined physiological and pathological chemistry and had strong links to clinical medicine. The Sheffield School had no connection with clinical medicine and offered physiology as a basic biomedical science, as Kühne did. Chittenden went to Germany to imbibe chemical physiology, and he found what he wanted at Heidelberg. He soon discovered to his surprise and delight that he was a much better chemist than any of the European students there. Kühne also quickly appreciated his skill and made him his first assistant, ahead of more experienced students.[16]

Chittenden returned to Yale as a convert to Kühne's conception of physiological chemistry. Their extensive correspondence documents a continuous close relationship. Kühne regarded Chittenden as one of his favorite disciples and, in the 1880s, initiated a cooperative research project, by trans-Atlantic mail, on the degradation of proteins, which was to become the basis of Chittenden's reputation and his life's work.[17] The combination of rigorous practical training in chemistry with strong connections to physiology and nutrition became the hallmark of the Yale School. Fifty years later, another scion of Kühne's line, Karl Thomas, told Chittenden's successor, Lafayette B. Mendel, that of all the American departments of biochemistry he had seen, the Yale department was the closest to his own at Leipzig: "Proper pure chemistry is done; but without ever losing sight of physiology."[18] Chittenden himself taught physiology and was active in the American Physiological Society. His school embodied the dominant style of German physiological chemistry. This was not a case of random or slavish imitation of a German model, however. Kühne's style of chemical physiology was as appropriate to the institutional context at New Haven as it was at Heidelberg.

Although Chittenden did teach service courses for medical students, his principle audience consisted of premedical students who desired both collegiate and medical degrees. This was the political–economic basis of his growing program. It is surprising at first sight that a premedical program could survive at all when, for example, the medical course at Yale consisted of two ungraded years and when few schools required even a high school diploma for admission. Even in the 1880s, however, there was a sizable minority of medical students who came to medical school with a liberal arts education. By 1880, 20% of the entering class of Northwestern

Medical College had B.A. degrees and another 10% got the B.A. before graduating.[19] This is probably representative of the better medical colleges. The great majority of physicians had no pretentions to liberal collegiate culture, of course; but collegiate credentials and collegiate style were a real advantage to those who aimed to practice in urban middle class communities and teach in the better medical colleges. Chittenden catered to this elite preprofessional clientele with remarkable success.

In the 1880s and 1890s, a growing number of students took the premedical biology course, and Chittenden outgrew his makeshift quarters. When Yale College erected a chemistry laboratory in 1886, biology expanded into the vacated first floor of Sheffield Hall. In 1889 the entire Sheffield mansion was refitted for biological work, the Laboratory of Physiological Chemistry occupying the first floor. More and more students in Yale College were crossing the cultural frontier at Hillhouse Avenue to take the biological course. In 1888 Yale College officially recognized the Sheffield biology course as an elective course for the B.A. degree. By 1892, 35 to 40 Sheffield students were enrolled in the biology course, 20 to 40 Yale College juniors were in physiology, and 20 to 25 Yale seniors were taking physiological chemistry.[20] Chittenden estimated in 1886 that the biology course was sending ten graduates per year into medicine. After 1888, ten Yale College students per year went through Sheffield to medicine.[21] Graduates of the Sheffield biology course were especially popular with the new Johns Hopkins Medical School, the first school to require a B.A. degree for admission. Of the 370 Hopkins graduates from 1893 to 1905, 74 (20%) were graduates of the Sheffield biology course. William Welch and W. H. Howell both testified to the superior training of Sheffield graduates.[22]

Despite the structural differences between the German and American medical courses, Chittenden's situation was functionally quite similar to Kühne's. German students studied physiology and physiological chemistry as academic subjects in a single degree program; Sheffield students simply took their scientific and medical studies in different places and got two degrees. Chittenden's European experience served him well: Kühne's disciplinary program was well suited to the political economy of the Sheffield Scientific School. As a result, physiological chemistry flourished in New Haven a full decade before there was an academic market for professional physi-

Table 5.1. *Careers of selected graduates of the Sheffield biology course*

Years	Physiological chemistry	Research	Medical education	Biological education
1872–9	0	1	8	5
1880–7	1	0	11	1
1888–95	6	3	36	6
1896–1903	13	10	9	6

Source: R. H. Chittenden to A. T. Hadley, 17 January 1906, Hadley Papers, box 17 f.322.

ological chemists. No other scientific school managed so successfully to combine academic and professional ideals. Chittenden's premedical course had no equal, and because collegiate work was not required by medical schools, one strong institution could virtually dominate the limited market.

When demand for physiological chemists did expand after 1900, Chittenden's program was the major, almost the only, source of supply. More students stayed on for a year or two of graduate study to prepare for specialized teaching or research careers in physiological chemistry. A two-year graduate program in public health was organized around courses in physiological chemistry and bacteriology. Sheffield graduates took positions in agricultural experiment stations, boards of health, government laboratories, medical research institutes, sanatoriums, and medical schools. A selected list of Sheffield graduates who went on to teaching or research, compiled by Chittenden in 1906, gives a rough measure of these trends (see Table 5.1).[23]

CHEMISTRY AND HYGIENE: V. C. VAUGHAN

In the 1880s and 1890s, medical colleges were far less viable contexts for physiological chemistry than the Sheffield Scientific School. Even the best were primitive by German standards, especially in the preclinical sciences. A three-year course was still the rule in the 1880s, and anatomy occupied most of the time devoted to the preclinical sciences.[24] Not until the four-year course was introduced in the 1890s was there room in the curriculum for experimental physiology, general pathology, or physiological chemistry. The preclinical sciences were taught by teacher–practitioners, not salaried professional teachers. Even the best medical colleges did not require a high school diploma and most of the freshman medical year had to be devoted to elementary physics, biology, and chemistry. Preclinical disciplines occupied the narrow space between the elementary and the clinical sciences. Only in rare cases was it possible for physiological chemists to organize advanced courses and define specialized roles.

One such case was the University of Michigan Medical College, where a specialized position in physiological chemistry was established in 1875.[25] Victor C. Vaughan's long reign, from 1879 to 1921, overlapped Chittenden's almost exactly. Like Chittenden's, Vaughan's role evolved within a successful school of applied chemistry, only in a medical context. Under President Henry C. Tappen, an ardent admirer of the Prussian universities, a strong Department of Chemistry was established at Ann Arbor, serving mainly the large and successful medical college.[26] The Department of Chemistry was a medical department, initiated by the medical faculty and expanded in the face of indifference on the part of the faculty of letters and science. In 1878, 374 students took chemistry, of which 346 (93%) were students of medicine, dentistry, or pharmacy. This large and steady market encouraged the development of specialized roles in clinical chemistry. A position in organic and applied chemistry was created for Albert B. Prescott in 1865, in the Liebig style. In 1875 physician–chemist Preston B. Rose was promoted to assistant professor of organic and physiological chemistry.[27]

The audience for physiological chemistry at Michigan was quite different from Chittenden's premedical students at Yale. Medical students were interested in chemistry only for its practical use in toxicology and urinalysis. (Stories abound of the rough and ready way that medical students expressed their impatience with teachers who tried to waste their time with fine points of physiological chemistry.) Rose's course consisted largely of basic analytical chemistry plus urinalysis and was extremely popular. (In 1871/72, 143 of 350 medical students took his advanced elective in urinalysis.)

Victor Vaughan was one year from a Ph.D. degree in chemistry under Prescott when, in 1875, he was thrown by chance into Rose's role of medical chemist. Shortly after Rose was promoted, he was accused by the laboratory director of embezzling laboratory fees. After a bitter confrontation, Rose was dismissed, and Vaughan was drafted to teach Rose's courses in physiological chemistry and "urology." His students were skeptical of the young chemist; but Vaughan had hurriedly learned everything there was to know about kidney function and urine and was soon promoted to lecturer and then assistant professor of medical chemistry. He earned an M.D. degree in 1878 and, in 1883, was named professor of physiological and pathological chemistry, therapeutics, and *materia medica*.[28] His varied titles suggest the scope and clinical emphasis of medical chemistry in the 1870s. Physiological chemistry as Chittenden practiced it was only a small part of Vaughan's formal duties.

Meanwhile, Vaughan was being drawn away from physiological chemistry into hygiene and public health. His interest in hygiene grew out of an investigation of a contaminated water supply in 1880. In 1881 Vaughan initiated a course in sanitary chemistry in the School of Political Science and soon found himself doing bacteriological analyses of water samples from Michigan towns. In 1883 he was appointed president of the Michigan State Board of Health.[29] In 1884 he opened a makeshift hygienic laboratory and, in 1885, began to lecture on the subject. Two years later the board of health, aided by a reluctant board of regents, squeezed $40,000 for a hygienic laboratory from the state legislature, and Vaughan was appointed to a chair of hygiene.[30] He made Frederick Novy, an organic chemist with Prescott, his assistant professor and sent him to study with Robert Koch. They assembled a collection of bacteriological apparatus in Berlin and Paris and initiated an active research program on the chemistry of bacterial metabolism and toxins.[31]

Vaughan was also active in the cause of medical reform at Ann Arbor and in the profession. In 1891 he refused the chair of hygiene at Bellevue Hospital in New York and was appointed dean of the medical school, a position he held for 30 years.[32] Under his leadership, Michigan became one of the leading centers of the nascent biomedical sciences in the United States.

One science that did not benefit from Vaughan's activities was physiological chemistry. Novy took charge of the department in 1891, but when Novy was appointed to a chair of bacteriology in 1892, physiological chemistry ceased to exist as a separate department. It was taught by Vaughan and Novy until 1921 as a minor service role within bacteriology and hygiene. No junior staff was appointed, and the poor state of biochemistry at Michigan became a professional scandal.[33] When Vaughan finally retired in 1921, a separate department was organized by an outsider, Howard B. Lewis.[34]

If Chittenden's school represents the north-German style of chemical physiology, Vaughan and Novy's represents the variant style of Pettenkoffer's school at Munich. The resemblance is striking and is a revealing instance of how institutions limit and shape individual ambitions and disciplines. Pettenkoffer and Vaughan specialized in physiological chemistry at a time and in places where they were officially limited to teaching "urology." Large teaching medical schools, emphasizing clinical practice, limited intellectual opportunities in physiological chemistry. Vaughan and Novy found that the applications of physiological chemistry to other biomedical disciplines offered greater scope to their ambitions than toxicology and "urology." Medical chemistry was too narrow a base to support an academic discipline of physiological chemistry. Talented individuals sought opportunities where service roles were more congruent with high intellectual goals.

BIOCHEMISTRY AND PHARMACOLOGY: J. J. ABEL

If the University of Michigan Medical School was the American Munich, the Johns Hopkins Medical School was the American Strasbourg. It opened in 1893 as a showpiece of American elite academic culture; like Strasbourg, "The Hopkins" displayed all of the most up-to-date features of the best German universities. The biomedical disciplines were all well represented, including the minor ones of pharmacology and physiological chemistry. Because four years of collegiate study were required for admission, including both inorganic and organic chemistry, medical or physiological chemistry could be taught as an intermediate biomedical discipline rather than as an elementary service course.[35]

As at Strasbourg, however, ambitions outran financial resources, and physiological chemistry became attached to pharmacology, a makeshift that lasted over a decade. William Welch and the other founders of the school had planned to open with a separate chair and department of physiological chemistry. Welch hoped that Chittenden could be tempted to accept the chair, although he feared that the cost of such a star would strain their limited resources. When Chittenden declined, Welch decided that a chair of physiological chemistry was a luxury that the school could forgo for the present.[36] At the eleventh hour, he asked J. J. Abel to add physiological chemistry to his responsibilities in pharmacology, as an emergency measure. Diffident of his chemical skills, Abel accepted, "so as to give us time to look about and also to give us some idea of our available resources for a good special man in this line."[37]

Abel had at one time intended to be a physiological or medical chemist, and his career illustrates the flexible options open to biomedical scientists in the "heroic" period. Abel's first love was physiology, which he studied with Henry Sewall at Michigan (B.A., 1883), Henry Newall Martin at Johns Hopkins (1883/4), and Carl Ludwig at Leipzig (1884–6). Recognizing the difficulties of making a career in pure physiology in American medical schools, Abel determined to get an M.D. degree and aim for a professorship of internal medicine, in the style exemplified by William Osler. The role of clinical consultant, he felt, would enable him to support a career of research in physiology, pathology, and pharmacology.[38] Abel proceeded to study clinical medicine at Strasbourg, where he got his M.D. degree in 1888.

It is clear that in 1888 clinical medicine was a more secure base for an academic career in the biomedical sciences than the disciplines as such. It also appears that chemistry offered more opportunity for biomedical research than did physiology and better protection from the pressures and temptations of clinical practice. As expert analysts, medical chemists possessed indispensable service roles and had the closest connections with university science. They could, if they wished, pursue problems in physiology, pathology, or pharmacology and profited from the almost mystical faith of progressive clinicians in chemical diagnosis and therapeutics.

Abel's interest in physiological chemistry and pharmacology was aroused during his years at Strasbourg by Hoppe-Seyler and Schmiedeberg, and in 1889 in Vienna, he determined to become a medical chemist. He wrote to his wife of his plans:

If I prepare for Physiological Chemistry I am sure to get a place in a medical school. That branch is appreciated much more than "die gesammte Physiologie.". . . Once at Clark University or anywhere else with a salary sufficient to save a little out of, I could run over every summer for a couple of months like other house clinicians and practice myself in diagnosing, and in treatment (say in London) and within a very few years be able to bring everything to bear on that best of positions, the clinical teacher's, and consultant for diagnosis. I believe from what I have seen that that is the best position to hold among doctors, most of whom bear you no ill-will for your $10.00 fee as long as they can keep the patient for treatment, an arrangement which would suit me only too well. The other way of beginning, as a Percussion and Auscultation teacher, or what not, I mean such positions as Doland here holds in Philadelphia, are all given to the home men. Doland began at 16 and has already been an M.D. for seven years and it is that sort of protégé that is always on hand for that sort of thing I fear. Now my way if we can do it will also get us there, jut as it has gotten...Osler there.[39]

Abel was diffident of his abilities as a physiological chemist but acknowledged that he would have to teach both normal and patho-logical chemistry when he returned. European chairs were organized that way, and Abel intended to live up to that ideal. To prepare himself, he planned to study clinical chemistry with Marcel Nencki at Bern. His aim was to learn enough chemistry so that, as an internist, he would not have to depend on professional chemists.[40]

Like Schmiedeberg and Hoppe-Seyler, Marcel Nencki favored close connections between chemistry and clinical medicine. As a young medical graduate, he too had taught himself chemistry. Abel found at Bern a broad program of medical chemistry well suited to the better American medical colleges. He wrote his wife Mary of his delight with Nencki's program:

I am trying hard to do the whole chemical side of medicine, understanding by that, Physiological and Pathological Chemistry, resting on a basis of *sound organic chemistry*....I hope to be able to [do] the best sort of work in *disease* by the chemical study of normal and abnormal stoffwechsel, etc., etc.[41]

Abel was hoping to land a job in medical chemistry at home and was corresponding with his old teacher, Victor C. Vaughan. Abel hoped ultimately to have a chair of clinical medicine; but when Vaughan offered him a chair of *materia medica*, he accepted with alacrity.[42] At Ann Arbor, he began research on Vaughan's favorite problem, the toxic degradation products of protein metabolism. In 1892 he spent a summer at Bern, working with Nencki's successor, Edmund Drechsel, who held a joint chair of pharmacology and physiological chemistry.[43] When Abel accepted Welch's offer, Drechsel was struck by the resemblance with his own situation: "Wie sonderbar denn wir beide uns in ähnlichen Zwangslagen befinden. Sie müssen als Pharmakologe noch physiologischen Chemie lesen, und ich als physiologische Chemiker noch Pharmakologie."[44] This was not so strange a coincidence, given Abel's European experience and the ideological and structural similarities between Johns Hopkins and smaller European universities like Strasbourg and Bern.

Abel still felt his lack of systematic training in chemistry and had no imperialistic designs on physiological chemistry.[45] Indeed, he himself taught it for only one year and then assigned the chore to junior assistants. Both he and Welch tried to find an experienced man for the job, but their lack of success suggests that they did not really know what they wanted. T. B. Aldrich, with a doctorate in chemistry from Jena, was promoted to associate in 1896 but was fired two years later. An offer was then made to Chittenden's star student, L. B. Mendel, who declined. So too did Edwin Faust, a pharmacologist–biochemist protégé of Abel, then studying with Hofmeister and Schmiedeberg. Otto Folin, A. P. Mathews, and several other young chemists were considered and rejected by Abel, despite Welch's prodding to get someone hired.[46] Finally, Aldrich's young assistant chemist, Walter Jones, was packed off to Germany for a year of advanced training with Albrecht Kossel. On his return, he took charge of physiological chemistry, and when a separate department was finally established in 1907, Jones was promoted to professor.[47]

Walter Jones had had no training in physiology prior to 1898, and the style of his department, like Chittenden's, was shaped in part by his formative year in Germany. Jones's school was an American variant of Kossel's: a union of organic chemistry and physiology, with the emphasis on chemistry. Jones's success in making the Marburg plant grow in Baltimore's soil also depended on local institutional goals. Welch, Abel, chemist Ira Remsen, and others who designed the new medical curriculum believed that medical students should be instructed in pure organic chemistry by organic chemists in the German fashion.[48] (Remsen had himself done so before the new school was built.) Moreover, physiology was already a well-established department at Johns Hopkins, and there was a well-defined division of labor with physiological chemistry. It would have made little sense for Abel or Jones to develop physiology, even if they had wanted to do so.

Jones had no training in biology or medicine and no desire to acquire any. He devoted his career to the chemistry of nucleic acids, an interest he acquired from Kossel. Phoebus Levene, who shared a bench with Jones at Marburg in 1899, recalled how even then Jones had shown little interest in biological processes:

> Jones was given the concrete problem of making derivatives of thymin. The work was progressing successfully and was destined to shape his principal interest in nucleic acids. My own problem was rather fantastic for I conceived the idea that vitellin must contain the chemical nucleus of nucleic acids since the nucleus developed during the growth of the embryo in the yolk. The problem being fantastic, and originating with myself, it naturally progressed poorly. Kossel was of much help to Jones and little to me. Jones became a devoted admirer of Kossel. I was more impressed by Hofmeister, who... was certain that he held the key to the solution of the structure of the Protein molecule.[49]

Jones found at Marburg a disciplinary style that suited him personally and was congruent with his role at Johns Hopkins. His course at Johns Hopkins emphasized bioorganic chemistry. In selecting his assistants and junior staff, Jones preferred organic chemists: training in physiological chemistry was desirable, but they were chemists first and foremost.[50] With few students outside of medicine and overshadowed by Abel, Jones had little need or opportunity to expand his disciplinary vision.

Chittenden, Vaughan, and Abel were the only three American biochemists with international reputations prior to 1900. The institutional basis for similar roles did exist elsewhere: premedical science courses existed at the universities of California, Pennsylvania, and Johns Hopkins and undoubtedly other places.[51] But they did not produce their Chittendens. Some medical school chemists went abroad to study physiological chemistry in the hope of improving their professional roles. But they had neither the vision nor institutional resources of an Abel or Vaughan. The demand for collegiate premedical training was limited, and the success of one or two programs was more likely to discourage than to stimulate competition. The lack of demand by medical students for physiological chemistry made it difficult to sustain specialized roles, except where unusually talented entrepreneurs or favorable local conditions made it possible. There was little in the American medical system that could be systematically mobilized to build a discipline, and talented men drifted away into chemistry, medicine, pharmacology, or hygiene.

PHYSIOLOGY IN AMERICA

Physiology was a much less important resource for American biochemists than it was for Europeans; it was an underdeveloped

field. In medical colleges it was taught by part-time practitioner–teachers long after it had been taken over by professional
physiologists in Europe. The more pressing need for basic biology
and clinical practice left little room for physiology in the medical
curriculum. Anatomists and clinicians saw physiology as an adjunct to anatomy and clinical medicine, and the battle for academic
status that German physiologists had won by 1870 was still being
waged in American medical schools in the 1890s.[52] Twenty years
later, European visitors noticed the strong clinical bent of American
physiology and the absence of anything like the tradition of Huxley
and Foster. Walter Fletcher and Wilmot Herringham, on tour in
1921, noted this bias:

The work is focused strongly upon its medical application. . . . This, in
itself, is excellent, but it brings dangers of narrowness of outlook and
neglect of fundamental principles. At most of the Universities, physiology is regarded as a subject special to medical students, and is not given
independent rank in the university curriculum as a great primary branch of
knowledge, worth pursuing for its own sake. This seems indefensible on
any grounds.[53]

They were struck that Harvard, for example, had no university
department of physiology and ascribed the small size of the profession to the absence of such schools.

Opportunities for physiologists in American colleges and universities were limited by the long-standing hegemony of zoology and
botany. Entrenched in college curricula, zoology and botany gave
access to the best recruits and jobs as well as the best facilities for
experimental research in the 1890s and 1900s. In Britain, general
biology developed out of physiology; in America, general physiology remained a minor part of biology. Some zoologists were sympathetic with physiology but were not inclined to give up their
position of leadership. Charles O. Whitman put it in a nutshell in 1896:

The zoologists since Darwin's time have almost monopolized experimental biology. Among the physiologists in this country, I doubt half a dozen
could be named, who have taken any active interest in this direction. It is
strange that Physiology, which is so largely an experimental science,
should be the last to come forward in general biology. The reason is not far
to seek. Physiology has found its raison d'etre in medicine, and has limited
its field to man and higher vertebrates. This ought not to be, and physiologists are beginning to see their mistake.[54]

Whitman's plans for a department of biological sciences at the University of Chicago included physiology, along with anatomy, botany, zoology, paleontology, and anthropology, as one branch of a grand united empire of biology.[55] Whitman felt about physiology as physiologists did about biochemistry; it was too vital a part of biology to be allowed to develop separately yet not important enough to vie with botany and zoology.

When President Harper pressed Whitman to give more space and attention to physiology, Whitman replied with a spirited defense of zoology:

Is it not certain that the plans and needs of Zoology are far greater than those of any other department? Which departments take the lead in marine work and in Experimental Biology? Physiology and Anatomy (I mean the Anatomy designed for medicine) both fall far behind either Zoology or Botany. Where do you expect to get the biology needed by the general students of the University? It is now supplied mainly by Zoology, and this must in the nature of the case continue to be so.[56]

The facts supported Whitman's claims. In 1894/95, 329 students enrolled in zoology; 181 in physiology. There were ten jobs for zoologists in biology teaching for every one in physiology. At the Woods Hole Laboratory, zoology attracted the most workers: despite efforts by Whitman and Jacques Loeb to promote physiology, only 8 of 199 workers chose that field. Whitman had hired Jacques Loeb in the hopes that he would develop general physiology at Chicago; but the limits of his altruism were clear.

The chronic ill-health of the American Physiological Society, founded in 1887, was symptomatic of the fragile condition of the discipline. Attendance at annual meetings dropped to a handful in the mid-1890s, and it was uncertain for some years whether the society would survive. The *American Journal of Physiology*, founded in 1898, was in constant danger of collapse, owing to lack of subscribers.[57] In medical colleges, physiologists were confined by entrenched clinicians; in liberal arts colleges, by entrenced natural historians. Physiologists were hard pressed to maintain their own discipline, much less to act as patrons to biological chemists. The historical fact that physiologists and biochemists were fighting simultaneous battles for independent status made it impossible for physiologists to co-opt biochemistry. Survival was still the game in the 1890s.

There is some evidence, in fact, of a reversal of roles: of physiologists using physiological chemistry as a resource for discipline building. Chittenden's school was probably the most prosperous and influential school of physiology in America in the 1890s. Seven of the 32 articles in the first volume of the *American Journal of Physiology* came from Chittenden's laboratory. It was Chittenden who, as president from 1894 to 1904, saw the society through its darkest years. Chemical physiology remained a much more important part of the discipline in America than in Europe. The Canadian physiologist John Tait, visiting in 1921, was struck by the contrast:

This trip gave a good opportunity of seeing how things are handled across the border, and it is a surprise to see how munificent accommodation and equipment are provided there. One soon came, however, to sense a difference between British and American physiology. British is operative and experimental, American is largely chemical in outlook. American university teachers who are not physiologists seem just to assume that physiology is a chemical branch of science, to such an extent is physiology there bound up with chemistry.[58]

What Tait and Fletcher saw in 1921 were the lingering effects of decades of underdevelopment in the 1880s and 1890s. By the time physiologists could afford to have expansive ambitions, biochemists had established separate institutions. American physiologists lacked the prestige and power of their European counterparts, and American biochemists were far more successful in establishing their independent claims.

There is one exception to this rule: Jacques Loeb did have a significant role in the history of American biochemistry, though not the central role he might have had. Loeb was the most vocal advocate and most visible exemplar of "general physiology" in America, perhaps in the world. His belief in the importance of physics and chemistry in biology was rooted in his passionate and militantly materialist philosophy, which looked to positive science as an escape from the evils and follies of social and political customs. In search of a scientific ethic, Loeb had turned to medicine and biology, then to the comparative physiology of the brain, to the physics and chemistry of tropisms and behavior in lower animals, and finally to the pure physical chemistry of proteins. In each phase of his remarkable career, Loeb did battle with "vitalism" and championed the ideals of a reductionist experimental biology based on physical chemistry.[59]

For a time, during his years at the universities of Chicago (1896–1902) and California (1902–10), Loeb led the movement to liberate biology and physiology from the domination of conservative zoologists and clinicians. He was constantly fulminating against the enemies of experimental biology:

It has been the curse of medical instruction, especially in this country, that physiology has been taught not with an emphasis upon the fundamental conceptions and laws of this science but with an emphasis upon certain applications of very petty and trivial details which the practitioner considers as important. For instance, it is a common fact that a medical student will know and consider some trivial manipulation in the analysis of urine as a great physiological discovery, while he has no conception of and does not care to know the main laws of metabolism. The outcome is that we have a class of physicians and clinical teachers who are the worst enemies of medical progress.[60]

Loeb was inspired with the idea that scientific physiology was about to emerge from medicine just as chemistry had been liberated half a century before: "Physiology is in a period of transition to a new and more comprehensive science, namely, Experimental Biology, and it has been the special aim of my work and my department to accelerate this transition as much as possible."[61] For all his disdain of popularity, Loeb had a gift for attracting attention, and works such as *The Dynamics of Living Matter* (1907) were widely read and attracted many young people into biology. Loeb's charismatic appeal is captured in the character of Max Gottlieb in Sinclair Lewis's *Arrowsmith*.[62]

Loeb had real opportunities to put his program of general physiology into practice. Whitman brought him to Chicago in 1892 to build a school.[63] Development of the medical course gave Loeb the audience and service role on which to build chemical biology. In 1898 a separate course in physiological chemistry was organized, mainly for medical students.[64] Loeb's budget included lines for assistant professorships in pharmacology and physiological chemistry. However, Loeb soon found that teaching physiology to medical students was not to his taste, and he began to look around for a position limited to research and graduate instruction.[65] In 1902 he departed for the University of California where, he was promised, he would be insulated from medical demands. There too, however, medical students were the main audience for physiological chemistry. Opposition from conservative medical factions in

1909 again caused Loeb to look elsewhere, and in 1910 he moved to a full-time research position in the Rockefeller Institution, where Loeb's group produced important and influential work; but he had, in effect, given up his ambition to create a discipline of general physiology in America.

For all his quixotic charisma, Loeb was not an institution builder. He lacked the aptitude and the patience, and his high ideals and quick temper made him a poor politician. Loeb never adapted to the American role of academic entrepreneur, a role that Vaughan and Chittenden played so well. Loeb remained the individualistic scholar, disdaining academic politicians like Chittenden. He advised Abel in 1904:

Make your journal a journal for the workers...and not a place where the political boss who exploits science for commercial or other selfish interests has full swing. This has already happened with the *American Journal of Physiology*. A man like Chittenden should not be asked to participate or if he has already been asked he should not be allowed to exercise any influence. Instead of men like Chittenden ask men like Taylor, Gies or Loevenhart, i.e., the actual and honest workers...to give their name to the journal.[66]

Loeb was quick to weary of his own efforts to establish general physiology. When attacked, his impulse was to retire and explode in the privacy of his circle of friends. When a group of clinicians at the University of California staged a counterrevolution, Loeb refused to sit down with them, because they "literally nauseated" him.[67] He grew increasingly pessimistic about the prospects for realizing his vision of general physiology in a university context, as he wrote Simon Flexner in 1910:

I do not think that the Medical Schools in this country are ready for the new departure; the Experimental Biology in the Zoological departments will be one sided and remain so. The only place in America where such a new departure could be made for the cause of Medicine would be the Rockefeller Institute or an institution with similar tendencies. The medical Public at large does not yet fully see the bearing of the new science of Experimental Biology...on Medicine.[68]

Such prophecies tend to be self-fulfilling. Loeb's style of general physiology remained an eddy in the mainstream of American physiology.

Biological chemistry was an essential part of Loeb's program. He himself was drawn to the chemistry of cellular metabolism and oxidation as the basic chemical mechanism underlying growth, development, and behavior.[69] However, he never did create specialized positions for biological chemists in his departments. (A. P. Mathews taught a specialized course on the effects of chemicals on organisms but not a general course.) Loeb had no professional interest in biochemistry as a separate department of knowledge, tending to see it as the proper province of biology. He was slightly disdainful of professional biochemists, no doubt regarding them as too-loyal handmaidens of medicine. Consequently, general physiology was not an important resource for building the discipline of biochemistry.

THE BEGINNINGS OF MEDICAL REFORM

After 1900 physiology and physiological chemistry developed rapidly within medical schools in a more equal partnership with clinical medicine. Preclinical chairs ceased to be used as stepping stones to more prestigious chairs of medicine and surgery. Leading medical colleges began to replace practitioner–teachers with salaried teacher–researchers and to expect their preclinical faculty to have academic as well as medical credentials and to engage regularly in research. Physiologists and pathologists began to put German ideals into practice. In 1881 Henry Sewall was the first professor of physiology at Michigan to have a doctorate and research experience in Germany. He was succeeded by William Henry Howell, another scion of Henry Newall Martin's school at Johns Hopkins, and Warren Lombard, a student of Harvard's Henry Pickering Bowditch. Among Bowditch's younger staff were William T. Porter (M.D., 1885), a veteran of six years in European laboratories, and Walter B. Cannon (M.D., 1900). At Pennsylvania, surgeon–anatomist Harrison Allen was replaced in 1885 by a full-time professor of physiology, Edward Tyson Reichert, a doctor of medicine with research experience in Berlin, Leipzig, and Geneva. At Columbia, T. Mitchell Prudden (M.D. Yale, 1875) taught himself bacteriology and was made professor of pathology in 1891; John G. Curtis gave up a rich consulting practice to take the chair of physiology in 1883. Curtis was succeeded in 1904 by Frederick S. Lee, who was trained at Johns Hopkins (Ph.D., 1885) and Leipzig. Richard Olding Beard, professor of physiology at Minnesota, practiced part-time until 1900 and did no research, but in 1908 he appointed a young

Ph.D. physiologist from Starling's school to build up a research school. In the 1880s and 1890s, physicians with a taste for research made full-time careers teaching physiology or chemistry. In the late 1890s, they appointed a new generation of young Turks, trained at Leipzig, Harvard, and Johns Hopkins, and gave them carte blanche to render their mentors obsolete.[70]

Methods of teaching also began to change in the 1890s. Lectures were enlivened with demonstrations, and demonstrations gave way to laboratory exercises. At Western Reserve Medical College, laboratory work in histology and physiology was required in 1888, in bacteriology in 1894, and in pharmacology in 1898.[71] The earliest physiology laboratories, like William James's at Harvard, had offered the opportunity for experimental work to a few advanced students, in the European manner. In the 1890s, chemical physiology and then physical physiology were introduced as required laboratory courses for all medical students. By 1900 many American medical schools were providing better routine training in the laboratory than European schools. Europeans began to come to America to see how it was done – Charles Sherrington, for example.[72] Clinicians saw laboratory instruction in the preclinical sciences as a step toward more practical teaching in the clinics and wards. Diagnosticians hoped that laboratory work would develop practical skills of observation and scientific reasoning. For the preclinical teachers, experimental teaching was a way of promoting the idea of scientists as creators not just dispensers of knowledge.

Although the pioneers of laboratory instruction saw themselves as imitating European practice, in fact they were doing something distinctly new. German universities provided excellent laboratory instruction to the select few; American medical schools made it available to all. European ideals, put into practice in a more democratic and less hierarchical society, resulted in institutions with much greater potential for growth, recruitment, and participation. In the 1890s, laboratory construction became a regular burden on the budgets of medical colleges, and annual demands for more space and modern equipment became a regular part of the lives of deans and university presidents. The role of the teacher–researcher was recognized as the ideal for the preclinical sciences, and laboratory experience was considered a necessity for modern medical teaching. Facilities for research were viewed as a necessity of life in a modern medical college, and the number of colleges with such ambitions was growing. By 1900 schools that had held a comfortable lead on the basis of excellent teaching by the best local practitioners were feeling the pressure of academic competition in the laboratory sciences.

Increasing use of time-consuming laboratory courses put new pressures on the traditional medical curriculum. In the 1890s, the school year was expanded from six or seven months to nine or ten. By the mid-1890s, a four-year course was the rule in better medical colleges.[73] The longer course gave room for more specialized disciplines and a more rational division of labor. Omnibus natural science courses differentiated into chemistry and physics. A laboratory course in chemistry was a common sign of an improving spirit in the 1880s and 1890s, and the chair of chemistry was often the first to become a salaried chair. Clinicians offered more specialized courses, reflecting the increasing acceptance by the medical profession of specialty practice.[74] Formerly squeezed between elementary science and clinical medicine, the intermediate sciences expanded to nearly half the medical curriculum. Branches that had been part of clinical medicine were expanded as laboratory disciplines, such as general pathology, pharmacology, and therapeutics. Longer and more expensive courses justified greater investment in teachers with more specialized academic credentials, and they in turn pressed for more hours in the curriculum, more adequate facilities, and more time for research. The spiral of rising expectations began to turn.

Financially, the four-year course was a boon to medical colleges. Increased income from fees enabled colleges to pay salaries for full-time preclinical teachers and to build and maintain the new laboratories needed for the practical courses. A fourth year did not discourage many students, and enrollments rose steadily in the 1890s. In 1898 the president of Northwestern University welcomed the medical faculty's petition for salaried chairs of anatomy and pathology, noting that extra salaries "still leave sufficient income to meet the interest on the building and something beside." Since 1890, enrollment had doubled, receipts had tripled, and the value of the plant had increased from $2 to $5 million.[75] The University of Pennsylvania Medical School ran a healthy surplus in the 1890s, turning one-third of it over to the University Endowment Fund. There was only one full-time professor in the preclinical fields, and he relied on cheap student assistants.[76] In the absence of a well-developed national market for biomedical scientists, wages and expectations were relatively low. Demands for research money were modest. Clinical teaching in community hospitals involved no expense for salaries or laboratory facilities. The 1890s were golden years for the old-time medical college: it was the first flush of reform, accomplished cheaply with promising local talent rather than expensive Europeans with grand reputations and high expectations. (Europeans often demanded large salaries and showed little sympathy with democratic educational ideals.) It was a time of visible improvement at bargain prices.

It is useful, however, to distinguish between *improvement* and *reform*. The internal improvements of the 1890s introduced new ideals of scientific medicine and modest opportunities for professional development. They did not fundamentally change the political and economic structure of the traditional medical college.

Medical colleges were still local institutions, serving local medical communities. Most were organized and controlled by physicians to provide cities and their hinterlands with general practitioners and to provide themselves with professional contacts, hospital facilities, and disciples. Rivalries between competing medical factions were often intense. Legally, almost all medical colleges were "proprietary," that is, organized as profit-making institutions with no or merely symbolic association with local universities. Apart from the small minority of diploma mills, most medical colleges looked to professional self-interest as the source of public service ideals. In mid-nineteenth-century America, this was a quite acceptable and effective strategy of community development, especially in small Midwestern and Western towns. However, as perceptions of disinterested public service changed in the 1890s, it was precisely this mixing of profit motive and public interest that medical reformers found most distasteful and most vulnerable to attack.[77]

The financial support system of proprietary medical schools also began to weaken in the late 1890s. Financially, medical colleges depended entirely on student fees, plus occasional (but increasing) donations from the faculty. Large enrollments meant prosperity and improvement, and competition for students was keen. Improvements that attracted greater numbers of students were acceptable; but improvements that limited the pool of qualified applicants were not; for example, raising formal entrance requirements to include a high school diploma or college residence. Medical colleges could afford to have academic pretensions but not academic standards. This was the dividing line between improvement and reform. The basic structure and market relations of the proprietary medical college put a ceiling on what improvements were possible without radical change in the whole system.

The increasingly academic style of the medical course encouraged a closer relationship between medical colleges and universities. The 1890s witnessed a rash of formal affiliations: the St. Louis Medical College and Washington University affiliated in 1891; Columbia and the College of Physicians and Surgeons, in 1894; Rush Medical College and the University of Chicago in 1898; Toland Medical College and the University of California in the same year; and so on. In virtually every case, however, affiliation was more or less a formality, not an organic union. Control of curriculum and appointments remained in the hands of practitioner–teachers. Universities carefully avoided any financial commitments. Affiliation gave real benefits to both parties without the risks of organic union. An attached professional school gave colleges the status of a "university," a valuable plant and equipment, and a dedicated and nonsalaried faculty, all with minimal financial and legal responsibilities. Medical colleges gained the prestige of a university name and connection and the chance to cooperate with or to borrow scientific faculty, without relinquishing control over clinical staff appointments and educational policy. Having university professors teach chemistry and physics enabled medical colleges to compete in scientific "quality" without having to lay out vast sums for a salaried staff.

The limitations of such token reforms are also evident, of course. Medical schools were still proprietary institutions, resting on a limited and vulnerable financial base. The local medical community was still more influential in the selection of staff than a national market and national professional standards. Having a few token researchers in the preclinical disciplines was a far cry from systematic discipline building. In sum: the improvements of the 1890s were German university frosting on an American college cake.

A curious mixture of high ideals and old practices was characteristic of the 1890s. At Columbia, the medical faculty announced in 1894 that the preclinical and clinical disciplines were "essentially a department of physical science theoretical and applied"[78]; yet the high school requirement was not enforced until 1898. Improved courses met counterpressures. The four-year course introduced at Michigan in 1890 included a required laboratory course in physiology, but competition for space in the curriculum became so intense that this course was made optional in 1892 and was not restored as a requirement until 1904. In 1901/02, only 53 of 282 eligible students took laboratory course work.[79]

Although research promise was a criterion in hiring, one gets the impression that high-level accomplishment was not really expected. The emphasis was still on teaching. Reputations in the 1890s were made not by research but by teaching or writing textbooks to replace translations of German texts. Victor Vaughan's career is exemplary. Simon Flexner complained to William Welch in 1902 that bacteriologist Alexander Abbott was the only one of the preclinical professors who was doing real research at Pennsylvania: "What outlook is there for a group of workers? Chemistry can yield nothing, anatomy is doomed to sterility, and physiology is, I fear, not very promising."[80] Yet George Piersol, John Marshall, and Edward Reichert, whom Flexner scorned, had been the young Turks of the 1890s. Flexner had hoped to found a research school but left in 1902 to direct the Rockefeller Institute. Research was not yet a routine part of academic careers.

CONCLUSION

German ideals of research and scientific medicine were widely current in the 1890s; but the market for Ph.D.s in the biomedical sciences was limited by old institutions and traditional practices. When the directors of the Rockefeller Institute decided in 1901 to sponsor the training of researchers rather than building facilities to employ them, J. G. Adami worried that too many men might be attracted to research, glutting the limited market in medical colleges.[81] This was perhaps an accurate reading of the market in 1901, although certainly not a prescient forecast. Prior to the reforms of the 1900s, it was generally taken for granted that there would never be room in the system for more than a handful of research schools like Harvard, Chicago, or Johns Hopkins. The limits of improvement had almost been reached within the old institutional structure, and further change would require structural reorganization of the whole system. The luxuries of a few could not become the necessities for all without systematic reform of the system of proprietary schools and the market for biomedical scientists.

Every generation is "transitional" by definition, but the heroic generation of the 1890s combined, to a marked degree, the different qualities of old and new. Many of this generation were trained as physicians or had practiced before becoming professors; they believed in the ideal of research but did little research themselves. It was this generation who initiated improvements and led the movement for radical reform of medical schools. They appointed the new generation of Ph.D. physiologists and biochemists from nascent graduate schools. They were the prophets of the new generation of teacher–researchers but did not themselves benefit directly from the reforms they set in motion. The mixture of old and new was especially evident in medical chemistry. The improvements of the 1890s did not result in the establishment of new chairs of physiological chemistry. As long as medical colleges were obliged to provide general chemistry, medical chemists had little chance to specialize in physiological chemistry. Yet the potential for discipline building was there, more systematically than in any other institution. But not until improvement gave way to radical reform were biochemists able to exploit this structural opportunity.

6

The reform of medical education in America

The "heroic" period of medical reform in America was dominated by individuals who cultivated German ideals in a hostile environment. Strategies were improvised; success depended on special local circumstances. After 1900 medical reform was increasingly a collective enterprise, led by national organizations and carried out systematically on a regional or national scale. The Association of American Medical Colleges organized the first survey of colleges in 1900, and the Council on Medical Education of the American Medical Association organized for reform in 1904. The celebrated Flexner Report of 1910 was backed by the Carnegie Foundation, and Flexner pursued his reform ideals as an officer of the Rockefeller General Education Board. Strategies were orchestrated and standardized, and reform spread rapidly from leading schools to every medical college. Institutions that did not meet the new standards were allowed to perish. The number of medical schools reached a peak of about 160 between 1900 and 1906 and then plummeted to about 80 in the 1920s[1] (see Table 6.1). Medical institutions were radically restructured to support new ideals and roles. A national market in the biomedical sciences was created in which competition for the best faculty and well-trained students accelerated the transition from the old system to the new. Not since the reform of German universities half a century before had there been opportunities on such a scale for the creation or re-creation of biomedical disciplines.

The main features of the transformation of the old-time medical college into the university medical school are easily summarized. Most important was the change in the political economy of medical education, as proprietary colleges became university schools. Most of the new laboratories in the 1890s were built on borrowed money not endowment. Student fees more than sufficed to pay interest on

Table 6.1. *Medical college student enrollment*

Year	Number of colleges	Number of students	Number of graduates	Number of graduates with a B.A.	Percentage of graduates with a B.A.
1850	52				
1860	65				
1870	75				
1880	100	11,826	3,241		
1890	133	15,404	4,454		
1900	160	25,171	5,214		
1904	160	28,142	5,747		
1906	162	—	—		
1910	131	21,526	4,490	680	15.3
1915	96	14,891	3,536	858	24.3
1920	85	13,798	3,047	1,321	43.5
1922	81	15,635	2,529	1,455	57.5
1924	79	17,728	3,562	2,020	56.7
1926	79	18,840	3,962	2,388	60.3
1928	80	20,545	4,262	2,708	63.5
1930	76	21,597	4,565	3,211	70.0
1932	76	22,135	4,936	3,525	71.4

the mortgages and the salaries of a few preclinical professors, but paying off debts and further expanding department staffs required the larger and more stable resources that only universities were able to mobilize. University leaders had the social authority and connections to raise the millions necessary to build and endow laboratories and teaching hospitals. Endowment enabled medical schools to give a smaller number of better qualified students a more intensive and much more expensive training. Single chairs expanded into departments having large full-time faculty, technical and office staff, and a regular budget for research. Independent medical colleges became operating divisions of universities, dependent on university funds to meet annual operating deficits. Economic dependence entailed accommodation to academic values, and the role of teacher–researcher became the norm, first in the preclinical sciences and then in the clinical specialties. Medical faculties adopted university criteria of hiring and promotion, including achievement in research. The old conflict between practical and academic values did not disappear, of course: if anything, it grew more intense as

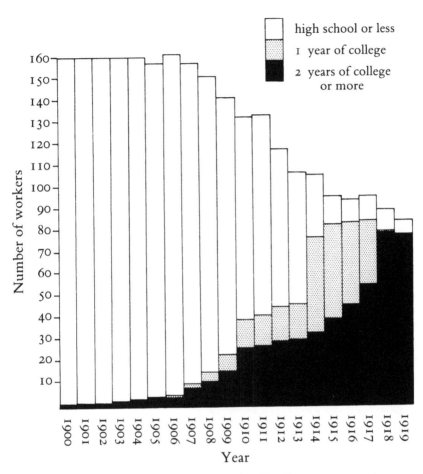

Figure 6.1. Number of medical schools with college entrance requirements.

relations between the two groups became closer. The point is that it was a negotiable issue in 1910; in 1890 it was not.

As proprietary colleges became university schools, they moved up in the educational system from the level of colleges to that of graduate schools. The key indicator here is the requirement of one or two college years for admission to medical school. In 1898 almost no medical college required even a high school diploma. Only Johns Hopkins required a bachelor's degree (and in practice admitted students with three years of college). By 1915 most schools required two years of college work, including basic physics, biology, and general and even organic chemistry[2] (see Figure 6.1). One in four students entering medical school had B.A. degrees, and some two dozen universities offered a six-year combined B.A.–M.D. degree program.

The imposition of collegiate admission requirements had dramatic and far-reaching effects. It disrupted an established market relation with secondary schools and created a new symbiotic market relation with colleges. Reduction of the pool of qualified medical students created a financial crisis for proprietary colleges that depended on student fees. The number of medical students plummeted from 28,000 in 1904 to a low of just about half that number in 1920 (see Table 6.1). Although the average number of students per school fell only slightly and never fell below the figure for 1900, schools that took the lead in raising requirements experienced sharp reductions in enrollment. Financial crises accelerated the pace of change, driving medical colleges into the arms of universities and driving college leaders to accommodate their academic ideals to professional goals. The remedy for financial crisis was still higher academic standards and a closer financial relationship with universities.

The improvements of the 1890s affected only the internal operations of medical colleges, not their market relations. But when reformers began to tinker with the market, they shook the foundations of the whole system. Then one change led to more radical change, and the process did not cease until a new system of medical education had emerged. By 1930 seven out of ten medical graduates had B.A. degrees. In no other country did aspiring physicians spend so much time in school, especially in the premedical and biomedical sciences.

The ultimate aim of the medical reform movement was improved clinical practice. Professors of medicine and surgery supported reform in the expectation of more practical teaching in hospital laboratories and wards. For practicing physicians, reform of medical schools was a strategy for upgrading their professional role from a superior type of technician to community leaders. Medical graduates were expected to acquire the public service values associated with a liberal arts education. As hospitals became middle-class institutions, more physicians were expected to display cultural values of the educated middle class. Hence the sudden change among the American Medical Association (AMA) rank and file from indifference toward educational reform to active leadership circa 1902 to 1906.

It was the biomedical sciences, however, that benefited most from reform, especially at first. The biomedical sciences were the least developed area of medicine in the old proprietary schools and thus the obvious target for reform. Biomedical scientists were an effective pressure group. Politically, it was much easier to put physiology or biochemistry on a university basis than medicine or surgery. Reorganization of physiology or chemistry stripped physicians of only marginal roles; giving chairs of medicine or surgery to full-time teacher–researchers struck at the core of the established system. The biomedical sciences were generally accepted as a necessary preparation for clinical practice (the question was how much, not whether or not), and these disciplines were swept in with the tide of reform.

Conflict between the biomedical and clinical sciences became more overt as clinicians' eyes were opened to the long-term implications of having strong independent departments of physiology, pharmacology, and biochemistry. The "full time" issue, which dominated the reform movement after about 1910, was extremely controversial and divisive. Reorganization of hospitals as operating divisions of universities aroused bitter conflicts between rival medical cliques and threatened physicians' power in their inner sanctum. The later phase of reform was full of *Sturm und Drang*. The gap between the biomedical and clinical disciplines was widest in the decade or so between 1900, when clinical medicine still dominated, and about 1910, when the partnership was reestablished on a more equal basis.

Most histories of medical education have focused either on the heroic or the organized phases of reform, dwelling on the influence of German ideals and Johns Hopkins or on the Flexner Report and the public campaigns of the AMA.[3] These are important aspects of the reform movement, of course, but they are not the whole story. Exactly how high ideals were translated into actual reforms and a broad political movement is still unclear. Most schools could not realistically hope to compete with Johns Hopkins. Competition was local or regional: in New York, Columbia, Cornell, and New York University; in the Midwest, Michigan, the University of Chicago, and Northwestern; in the West, the University of California and Stanford. Local competition for students and faculty shaped reformers' expectations of what was possible, not the impossible standard of the most elite school. Moreover, Abraham Flexner and AMA leaders did not originate reform; they only routinized it. Pressure from the organized lobbies was most effective as a cause of reform in smaller schools after 1910. It is in the preceding decade, however, that reformers actually worked out the strategies for creating new institutional structures and relationships.

In this period, pressure for higher admission requirements came from medical colleges and universities, rather than from state licensing boards or the AMA. The practice of the leading medical schools was well in advance of "official" minimum standards. In 1911 licensing boards in just 8 states required two premedical college years, and only 22 required a high school diploma; but 28 medical schools in 23 states required two years of college for admission. The AMA's Council on Medical Education did not push agressively for higher entrance requirements. In 1905 it set a high school diploma or "its equivalent" (a camel-sized loophole) as standard and recommended that medical schools add a fifth year to teach the basic sciences, rather than require them as premedical courses. In 1910 the council cautiously recommended that a year of college science be required "as soon as conditions warrant."[4] In 1912 it avoided the issue altogether as being too controversial, and in 1914 it came out in favor of reducing the current practice of requiring two college years.[5] Arthur Bevan of the Association of American Medical Colleges (AAMC) rejoiced when the number of schools requiring one year of physics, chemistry, and biology doubled, to nearly 80: "This means, of course, its general adoption. The next thing that must be secured is the compulsory hospital year."[6] Bevan clearly did not anticipate longer collegiate requirements. Two years later, the AMA council ratified the two-year requirement but urged that two years be pruned at the high school level.[7]

The AAMC was an imperfect instrument for reform. It consisted largely of proprietary schools that wanted to keep requirements low and could outvote the more ambitious minority. In 1900 the chairman of the survey committee, E. Fletcher Ingals of Rush Medical College, proposed that a "Federation of American University Schools" composed of the eight or ten leading schools would be a more effective lobby.[8] Secession failed, however, and the reform wing of the AAMC had to build slowly, overcoming internal opposition and the reluctance of some leading schools to join; Pennsylvania was one of the eight or ten still holding out in 1911.[9] In 1914 general feeling in the AAMC was against a college requirement, and secession was again considered by the elite schools.[10]

In short, public and professional agencies ratified the existing practices of a growing minority of medical schools. They were not innovators, but systematizers. So too were the more radical Carnegie Foundation and the General Education Board, which entered the reform campaign after 1910.

It was individual medical colleges that set the pace of reform in the crucial years from 1900 to 1910. The engine of change must be sought at the grass roots, in the activities of local reform groups in a dozen or so large, traditional schools and the half dozen or so new ones. What "heroic" pioneers dreamed of and reformers routinized was created by men who were less concerned with abstract ideals or systematic policy than with resolving problems created by previous improvements. We want to know what particular groups in medical colleges and universities were promoting reform and what groups were opposed to it. What were the internal and external pressures for change, and how were specific strategies of reform shaped by the institutional goals and the market for medical scientists and practitioners? How were the ideals of scientific medicine deployed for political purposes?

THE REFORM COALITION

The reorganization of medical schools was typically accomplished by a coalition of biomedical professors, medical deans, and university presidents. These groups shared a common interest in higher academic standards and organic union of medical school and university. For professors in the biomedical sciences, higher premedical requirements meant students who were better prepared to study anatomy, physiology, or pathology as sciences for their own sake. University control of medical school policy brought them freedom from control by clinicians and practitioners and rewards for contributions to the advancement of knowledge in their disciplines. Professors of anatomy, physiology, and biochemistry looked to the basic university sciences for inspiration and political support.

Medical deans often played a key role in mediating the union of university and medical school. In the earlier years, deans were often preclinical professors: for example, Victor C. Vaughan or John Marshall, professor of chemistry at Pennsylvania. At first they had little power. So long as medical faculties controlled their own administrative and financial affairs, the dean's role was ambassadorial rather than executive. As the only salaried teachers, chemists were often selected for this role, despite their low medical status. In the years when organic union was being consummated, however, the deans' strategic position gave them considerable power of initiative. Because they could speak for both the university and medical school interests, they were a powerful force for the ideals of academic, scientific medicine.

Clinicians as a group neither initiated nor obstructed change. There were a few militant conservatives in every faculty, yet most clinicians recognized the benefits of a university connection. In the early stages of reform, clinicians supported improvements in the preclinical sciences as a prologue to better clinical teaching. Improvement did not threaten their role as physician–teachers as it did later when practitioners were challenged by a new generation of academic clinicians. By then, however, it was too late to turn back. As the clinical branches became the target of reform, more progressive clinical professors took an active role. Samuel S. Lambert was appointed dean at Yale in 1910 to execute the university's decision to reorganize the medical school. David Edsall played a similar role at Pennsylvania, George Dock at Washington University, and others. These academic clinicians were trained in biomedical research and strongly believed that progress in clinical medicine depended on close connections with the biomedical sciences. They greatly influenced the style of the biomedical sciences after 1915.

The university president was perhaps the key figure in the reorganization of medical schools. This was the generation of presidents that brought the modern university into being: William Raney Harper (Chicago), Edmund James (Illinois), Charles W. Eliot (Harvard), Benjamin Ihde Wheeler (California), David Starr Jordan (Stanford), George Vincent (Minnesota), Charles Van Hise (Wisconsin), Nicholas Murray Butler (Columbia), and Arthur T. Hadley (Yale) all took an active personal hand in transforming the affiliated medical college into a university professional school. This generation of presidents transformed the old-time college from a purely cultural institution tied to aging elites and a shrinking market to a mass institution serving as the major entry to a broad range of professional and commercial careers. They expanded the ideal of a liberal arts education to include preprofessional studies in pure and applied sciences and broadened the ideal of a profession to include the cultural and service ideals of the liberal arts college. The reform presidents brought the quasi-autonomous scientific and professional schools that had evolved around the margins of the liberal arts college under central control and presided over the proliferation of new science-based professions. Their interest was clear. The more social roles became the domain of trained and accredited experts, the more were universities indispensable social institutions. The university, with its collegiate core and affiliated professional schools, became the carrier of middle-class democratic culture and values.[11]

It was not obvious even in 1900 that colleges would preserve and enlarge their place in the educational system. Professional schools offered courses in the natural sciences in direct competition with colleges. Some medical colleges proposed to add a fifth year to the medical course for the basic sciences, cutting out the liberal arts colleges altogether. High school reformers envisioned the high school as the central institution of mass higher education, the "people's college," laying claim to the first year or two of college courses.[12] Graduates of Central High School in Philadelphia, Boston English, and other urban high schools were often better prepared in basic science than students with a year or two in a second-ranked college.[13] Some medical reformers looked to improved high schools, not colleges, for better prepared students. College leaders had good reason to fear being "ground between the upper and nether millstone; the technical school above and the high school below."[14]

University presidents sought to preserve the role of the college by academizing professional training and emphasizing science in colleges. Charles W. Eliot was instrumental in orienting high schools toward college admission. He was one of the first to press for medical school reform, and his elective curriculum was designed in part to provide premedical science training. His one great objective was to ensure a central role for Harvard College in the educational marketplace. Many of Abraham Flexner's ideas of medical reform reflected previous experience in college reform. He insisted on the need to rationalize and couple secondary, collegiate, and professional levels and felt that premedical courses were an ideal vehicle for instilling a more serious purpose into collegiate studies.[15] Reform presidents learned the knack of making occupations into learned professions and using academic disciplines as the basis for practical professional careers. The idea was to make "cultural studies" more professional and technical training more liberal. Annual reports of university presidents between 1890 and 1910 are replete with variations on this theme, justifying the instrusion of premedical and other professional courses into the college curriculum.

Yale's Arthur Hadley and others were less than enthusiastic about this trend, but they realized that co-option was the best way of ensuring that preprofessional subjects would be taught in colleges of arts and sciences.[16] The reform of medical schools was crucial to this strategy, especially collegiate entrance requirements. The economic and political basis of Eliot's interest in medical reform was revealed in 1909 when the medical faculty voted to admit students with only two years of college if they had sufficient science. Eliot reacted swiftly to stop any backsliding:

We do not deny that good doctors may be made out of material coming straight from the secondary schools, or from two years of college work, more than half of which is filled with Natural Sciences and Modern Languages....But we have announced time and time again that we are going to use in our professional schools, as far as possible, only the finished product of the American college. The Faculty of Arts and Sciences...has a very decided interest in maintaining the general principle to which the University is committed. It is decidedly to the interest of Harvard College that its students should not be invited to leave at the end of the Sophomore year.[17]

The B.A. degree requirement stood.

University presidents were especially eager to secure a role in training physicians. Medicine had already displaced divinity as the largest and most prestigious of the learned professions. A connection with medicine ensured that colleges would have alumni among an increasingly powerful and well-to-do social elite. University presidents also recognized that a strong program in medical science advertised a university's devotion to the ideal of public service:

As the influence of any educational institution is in proportion to its reputation, and as that reputation depends upon advertising of various kinds any legitimate method of increasing the reputation of the School should be adopted. Experience has shown that the publicity secured as the result of good research work is the most effective way of increasing the reputation of an educational instituion of the higher grade.[18]

Establishment of teaching hospitals gave universities control over powerful community institutions. For all these reasons, university presidents eagerly allied themselves with medical reformers, undertook to raise endowment for a salaried medical faculty, and willingly suffered the pains of accommodating collegiate ways to the utilitarian ideals of medical practitioners.

The actual experience of reform in any particular school depended on when the process of reorganization was begun. For the early innovators, pressures for change grew out of the internal improvements of the 1890s. Higher-quality instruction in the laboratory sciences sharpened the faculty's desire for better-prepared students. Better students required still higher-quality courses and a more professional faculty. For the schools entering later into the process of reform, external competition was a more important stimulus than internal circumstances. The driving force behind reorganization was the pressure of competition, the need to prevent competitors from cornering the regional market for high-quality medical training. The last schools to reform were forced to do so to meet the legal requirements of the medical profession and licensing boards. It was simply a matter of survival.

The experience of reform also depended on the position of a school within the system. Schools attached to well-endowed universities could afford to take a radical step into reform. Harvard jumped from a high school to a B.A. degree requirement in 1899. The Cornell Medical School opened in 1898 on a graduate basis. Like Johns Hopkins, these schools were designed to be small, elite schools serving the minority of students who were willing to spend the time and money for training both in the liberal arts and medicine. Both Harvard and Cornell consciously emulated Johns Hopkins. Some less well endowed schools that took such a radical step just barely survived – Western Reserve, for instance.[19] Reorganization was slower and more improvised at the best large teaching colleges, such as Michigan, Rush, Columbia, or Pennsylvania, whose reputations and financial health depended on large audiences, not endowment. In these schools, reform proceeded gradually from a high school standard to an optional six-year B.A.–M.D. dual degree program to a two-year college requirement. The synergism between reform ideals and financial crisis is most evident in this group of schools. State universities often established separate two-year courses in the bio-medical sciences, sending their students to a nearby city for clinical work. This was the case at California, Illinois, Wisconsin, Indiana, and Chicago. Because they were public institutions, state universities were more subject to the crosswinds of medical politics.

The experience of reorganization was almost endlessly varied, yet everywhere it involved the same basic problems and issues: accommodating utilitarian and academic goals; achieving a balance between the biomedical and clinical sciences; bridging the gap between the old generation of physician–teachers and the new generation of research-minded professionals. Every proprietary school in its own way had to relinquish financial independence and a large, diverse market and accept an uncertain partnership with academics and a limited collegiate market.

The medical market was the crucial factor in the escalating cycle of reform. The pool of college students with the means and desire for graduate medical training was limited and had not yet begun to grow in response to improved professional opportunities. When reformers introduced a collegiate entrance requirement, they committed themselves to competing for a smaller, more select market and usually suffered an abrupt decline in enrollment and consequent financial crisis. Invariably, ambitious schools responded to crisis by redoubling their efforts to compete more effectively for the top of the market, offering still higher-quality courses, and raising their requirements yet again. This cycle of financial crisis and escalating expectations was the engine of change, and in a remarkably short time, the old market system was replaced by the new.

The new symbiosis between colleges and professional schools depended on a growing pool of college graduates who saw medicine as an attractive career. The number of college students enrolled and the percentage of the college-age cohort enrolled increased steadily up to World War I and rapidly after about 1910 (see Table 6.2). The reliance of medical educators on the strategy of escalating quality reflected their confidence that this trend would last. Indeed, they took vigorous steps to ensure that it would by promoting the ideals of professional service and mobilizing resources for preprofessional science programs. More people were going to college in the expectation of going on to medicine and other professions.

The reform coalition was crucial to the success of the strategy of escalating quality. University presidents and deans could intervene in the premedical market as well as in the policies of medical schools. They redesigned college curricula to meet the new demand from medical schools and insisted that medical schools stick to their commitments to academic standards. They managed to control both supply and demand simultaneously; this is why the old market system was replaced so quickly by the new.

Table 6.2. *Attendance in American colleges and universities (1870–1950)*

Year	Enrollment	Percentage of 18 to 21 cohort
1870	52,000	1.7
1880	116,000	2.7
1890	157,000	3.0
1900	238,000	3.9
1910	353,000	4.9
1920	598,000	7.6
1930	1,101,000	11.8
1940	1,494,000	15.2
1950	2,297,000	27.2

Biomedical scientists pursuing their professional interest alone would never have been able to succeed as well. This is the difference between the United States and Britain or Germany. In Europe, individual discipline builders mobilized resources as best they could; in America, they were carried along by a wave of systematic institutional reform.

Although it is not possible to give a full account of the variety of medical reform, selected case studies will reveal how the process worked.

EASTERN LEADERS: COLUMBIA AND PENN

Columbia's College of Physicians and Surgeons (P&S) is a good example of how a large and prestigious medical college was led from improvement to reform. P&S had virtually no endowment and received no aid from Columbia College, but its large enrollments produced sufficient income to pay a salaried preclinical staff and the mortgage interest on new laboratories.[20] The medical faculty and President Seth Low fully expected that further improvements would pay for themselves by attracting more students. As students became more expensive to train, however, this simple economic equation began to fail. A turning point was reached in 1899 when the faculty began to be troubled by the fact that a third to a fifth of each freshman class dropped out, discouraged by the difficulty of the preclinical science courses. As Dean James McLane realized, this was the result of raising the degree requirements without raising the requirements for entrance. Sophisticated laboratory courses in physiology and anatomy were being taught to students who were no better prepared in basic chemistry and biology than those who had taken the textbook and lecture courses of the 1880s.[21] Students and faculty were demoralized; moreover, the loss of a student after one year meant the loss of three years of tuition fees. Dean McLane's committee recommended that the admission requirements be raised to admit only students who could finish the course, arguing that the increased number completing the degree would more than pay for the reduced numbers in the first year. The phenomenon was in fact not new: as the best medical school in New York City, P&S had always tended to lose students to New York University or Bellevue, which were academically less demanding.[22] So long as the first-year lecture courses were taught by unsalaried staff, the cost of this attrition was low. But laboratory teaching by full-time professors involved a much greater investment in each student, and the cost of dropouts became less acceptable.

McLane's plan was not the only possible solution to the problem of attrition and deficits. Some members of the medical faculty suggested that the way to cut costs and keep students was to cut back on the expensive laboratory teaching, especially in physiology and anatomy. A special committee was appointed to consider these proposals, chaired by McLane. John G. Curtis, professor of physiology, lobbied vigorously for smaller, more select classes. Not surprisingly, McLane's committee again recommended that the best strategy was more, not less, scientific training and higher, not lower, academic standards.[23] The faculty accepted McLane's report and agreed to raise the requirement for admission to one college year in 1902.

The minutes of the medical faculty do not reveal why there was so little support for retrenchment, but no doubt one compelling reason was the increasing local competition. In 1898 Cornell University founded a medical branch in New York City, taking advantage of the secession of a group of the most progressive faculty from the NYU–Bellevue Medical College.[24] Cornell emulated Johns Hopkins: three years of college work were required for admission, and from the start, it had a substantial endowment. It was designed to appeal to the academic elite of medical students and also proved to be an attraction for research-minded faculty at Columbia. Dean McLane cited an example in 1899 in which a junior man at P&S was offered twice his current salary to come to Cornell.[25] Whereas some clinicians may have wished their colleages in anatomy, physiology, and physiological chemistry to have less influence, they did not want to lose them to Cornell. The conservatives might have preferred more students, not more scientific ones, but they did not want their best students enticed away to Cornell. They might not subscribe to the highbrow ideals of Cornell, but they had little option but to emulate them. The strategy of escalating standards easily won the day.

The first steps in raising the admission standards were taken cautiously. The Committee on Entrance Standards recommended only that P&S require a high school diploma, as did Columbia College and the School of Mines. They rejected the idea of requiring courses in basic physics, chemistry, and biology, despite urgent pleas by Curtis and Chittenden (the acting head of the Department of Physiological Chemistry). It was finally agreed to require either a certificate from a five-year "gymnasium" course, one year of college, or an examination in mathematics, Latin, and modern languages. The faculty rejected a proposal to give double credit to basic science electives, and chemistry, physics, and basic anatomy continued to be taught as freshman medical courses.[26]

McLane's committee did not expect that these requirements would greatly diminish freshman enrollment. They predicted a 25% loss but did not doubt that this loss would be made up by the greater number who would complete the M.D. degree program. Their expectation was based on previous experience with the four-year degree and improved laboratory courses:

The experience of this school in the past has uniformly shown that a raising of the education standard has increased rather than diminished the numerical strength of the classes as an *immediate* result of such changes, and that the *ultimate* effect has always been a decided advance in the material prosperity of the Institution.[27]

They were mistaken: the effect on enrollment was disastrous. The number of freshmen in the first year was nearly halved in 1902 and nearly halved again by 1904. Total enrollment in 1908 was 322, or 41% of the peak 795 in 1899.

But the enrollment crisis only precipitated still more radical reforms. In 1904 a member of the 1898 committee proposed that physics and inorganic chemistry be required for admission in 1907.

The faculty agreed. In 1905 the optional six-year combined B.A.–M.D. program was increased to seven years.[28] In 1908 two premedical years were required for admission. Despite annual deficits in the preclinical departments, President Nicholas Murray Butler supported every one of these reforms. Whereas the medical faculty accepted academic standards, the university accepted full financial responsibility for enabling P&S to live up to these standards. Thus the nominal affiliation of P&S with Columbia became, in practice, a functional union.

In 1908 the first moves were made to reorganize the clinical branches, with Dean Samuel Lambert playing a leading role. A plan for affiliation with Roosevelt Hospital was scuttled in 1908 and again in 1910 by a group of physicians who objected to the university's having any voice in hospital affairs. In 1911 P&S and Presbyterian Hospital agreed to affiliate, and Edward Harkness gave $1.3 million to endow research and clinical teaching.[29] It took over a decade more to work out the political and financial problems of creating a complete teaching hospital, but we need not be concerned with that story here.

The upward spiral of innovation is unusually clear in the case of P&S. Up to a point, internal improvements in the preclinical sciences were instituted without altering the college's institutional structure or its relation to the market and the university. The decision in 1899 to increase the requirements for admission went beyond internal improvement. External market relationships were altered in ways that could not be managed within the old institutional framework. From that moment, innovation did not cease until the proprietary college had been transformed to a university professional school.

Could the reformers have been as unaware as they seem to have been of the long-term consequences of that first step? The documents do not suggest that they were consciously emulating Johns Hopkins or the German universities. Competition played a role, but it was local competition. The reformers spoke more of continuities than of radical breaks with tradition and justified reform in terms of economic efficiency. Such arguments were aimed, of course, at clinicians, who would not have been won over by being shown all that must follow. Perhaps the reformers did know what they were doing. Yet there was a quality of sleepwalking in this early phase of reform, when the final shape of the new system could not be clearly seen and when reorganization was primarily a local affair. A decade later a very different rhetoric prevailed: open commitment to radical change, large expenditures, the highest ideals, and the most comprehensive programs was the order of that day. But for the pioneers, reform meant improvising solutions to problems created by earlier improvements.

A similar cycle of reform took place in the University of Pennsylvania Medical School. Penn, too, was a large, traditional, and prestigious teaching school, which had set the pace in improving laboratory departments. In 1896 the medical faculty decided that the requirement for a high school diploma should be strictly enforced, with no "equivalents" permitted. Laboratory instruction was expanded, and smaller and more practical classes were initiated in the clinical fields. The result was a sharp drop in enrollment. In the hope of attracting more Penn undergraduates to medical study, the university established an optional seven-year combined B.A. –M.D. program in 1899, but enrollments continued to decline, from 883 in 1897 to 472 in 1902.[30] The university had guaranteed to meet temporary deficits resulting from the higher admission standard, but it was becoming clear that the crisis was not a temporary one. The medical school had no endowment, and the university's modest endowment could not support more deficits. In 1902 Simon Flexner saw no hope for relief through higher quality:

Already a new college entrance requirement has cut the classes below the danger point, so that there is already heard a cry for greater leniency in enforcing the entrance requirement. I do not think there will be any yielding on that point, but there is equally no outlook for a betterment of the class by adding to the entrance conditions, even to the extent of Michigan or Rush.[31]

Flexner was proved wrong, however.

In 1902 a committee was appointed to investigate the cause of the decline in enrollment. It reported that the lack of modern teaching laboratories in physiology, pathology, and pharmacology made it difficult for Penn to compete for the best students. E. T. Reichert, Flexner, and Horatio Wood (pharmacology) were asked to submit plans for improved facilities, and in 1904 a new laboratory building was completed.[32] In 1906 the faculty voted to require basic physics, chemistry, and biology for admission in 1908, a full year of college in 1909, and two years in 1911.[33] The pattern of innovation was the

same as at P&S: internal improvements, disruption of the traditional relationship with the high schools, and closer relations with
the university's premedical programs. The strategy adopted was to
compete for a smaller, more select market by offering higher-quality
services.

Penn was slower than P&S to institute these new practices,
perhaps owing to its symbiotic relation with Philadelphia's Central High School, which had a science course tailored for entrance
into local medical schools. (In 1910 Dean Allen Smith used this fact
to argue against a college requirement for admission.[34]) By 1910
reformers felt that Penn's position as a progressive school had
slipped. The preclinical faculty were aging, and the new Department of Research Medicine, under pathologist Richard Pearce, was
an island of clinical research in a school dominated by conservative
teacher–practitioners. Dean Charles Harrison Frazier, an active
member of the AMA Council on Medical Education, and Provost
Harrison (Frazier's uncle) were increasingly concerned with the
inbreeding and complacency of the clinical faculty and the lack of
organized research in the preclinical disciplines. Aware of the escalating standards of the reform movement, they knew that Penn was
vulnerable to criticism and must act before its weaknesses were
publicly exposed. Abraham Flexner's impending visit of inspection in March 1909 provided the reformers with the occasion they
needed.

Harrison and Frazier took their case secretly to the trustees,
using the threat of Flexner's exposé to generate a sense of crisis.
Harrison discreetly advised Vice-Provost Edgar Fahs Smith not to
interfere on behalf of his brother Allen Smith, the medical dean.
David Edsall, professor of therapeutics and an active reformer, was
drawn in to plan the reorganization of the clinical branches. Physician and one-time physiologist Wier Mitchell lobbied among the
trustees, who agreed to a wholesale reorganization of the faculty.[35]

The reformers' campaign was aimed at the chairs of medicine and
surgery, but the biomedical departments were the first to benefit
from it. In January 1910, Harrison pressured James Tyson to retire
from the chair of medicine, making way for Edsall; John Marshall's
chair of chemistry was abolished to make way for a new chair of
physiological chemistry, and Alonzo Taylor was called from Berkeley. Alan Smith was transferred from the chair of pathology to
comparative pathology, and Howard Ricketts, from Chicago, was

appointed in his place (but died before he could take the chair). Edsall's place in therapeutics was taken by pharmacologist Alfred Newton Richards, from Northwestern. Edsall, Richards, Taylor, Ricketts, and Pearce were all young and militant advocates of medical science and research. The faculty council was reorganized to give university officers more control over medical policy, and clinical professors were allowed to give only half time to private practice. The medical faculty was informed of these new policies in a special meeting of the trustees in March 1910.[36] Edsall wrote Simon Flexner of his astonishment and delight: "You...would not recognize the atmosphere any more....I could not ask [for] a broader and more progressive spirit than they have shown in everything."[37]

Opposition soon erupted, however, led by the professor of surgery, William White, and fueled by anger at Harrison's Machiavellian tactics. Tyson's friends, the old young Turks of the 1890s, backed White. Alfred Stengel, director of the Pepper Laboratory for Clinical Research, refused Edsall access to the facilities. Harrison resigned under pressure, and his successor, Edgar Fahs Smith, immediately began to undo the intended reorganization. Allen Smith was restored to the vacant chair of pathology. Wier Mitchell resigned, tired of the "constant hot water in the faculty." There was a move to restore Marshall to the chair of chemistry. With his support melted away and unable even to lecture, Edsall accepted a well-timed call to Washington University in 1911.[38] (A first call in 1910 and the resulting show of alumni support for Edsall had triggered Harrison's putsch.) Planning his second offer to Edsall, W. H. Howell wrote a friend: "Edsall, Pearce, Taylor, and Richards are all alone against fourteen. Pennsylvania is surely doomed and it seems so strange when a year ago everything seemed more promising there than anywhere else."[39] Reformers in other schools saw the "fiasco" at Penn as a setback for progressive ideals. Cornell physiologist Graham Lusk wrote a discouraged note to biochemist Philip Shaffer: "The fizzle of affairs at the University of Pennsylvania shows how difficult it is to get good results in the East. Such results can only be obtained when the scientific man possesses the real power."[40] Edsall gave Flexner a postmortem:

Penn is doing badly enough. They have legislated Pearce and Taylor out of the Medical Council by making a new Executive Faculty, thus eliminating all the "young Turk" element except Richards who is not aggressive. . . . White seems to be in almost absolute control of the Medical School.[41]

But the tide of change was too strong. The two new biomedical departments thrived under Taylor and Richards. White soon retired, and within a few years, the faculty had accepted most of the reforms that Harrison and Frazier had tried to thrust upon them.[42]

THE MIDWEST: ST. LOUIS AND CHICAGO

The Washington University Medical School enjoyed a position in Saint Louis similar to P&S in New York or Penn in Philadelphia. It was the largest and most progressive of a half dozen local medical colleges. Its rather modest improvements were advanced by local standards: salaried professors of chemistry and anatomy; a diagnostic pathology laboratory to serve city physicians and (it was hoped) to stimulate research; and a volunteer library. Loosely affiliated with the university since 1891, in 1899 it absorbed the Medical Department of the Missouri Institute of Science and became a university faculty. In 1900 its graduates won 19 of 25 staff appointments in city hospitals.[43] As reform spread to the Midwest, however, the reform group at Washington University began to measure their achievements not against local competitors but against Harvard, Penn, and the Rockefeller Institute. The problem was the familiar one, to live in university style on the resources of a proprietary school:

The great bar to our taking the position the Medical Department of W. U. should occupy, is lack of money. How are we to get it? Practically all our income is from tuition fees. The cost of giving the best medical education is nowhere met by the tuition fees, and we could only increase our income materially by so lowering our requirements for entrance to and exit from our school as to attract a poorer, though larger class of students. This cannot be considered. We must therefore have a revenue from outside sources and this means an endowment.

We need many things; the salaries of our paid instructors are inadequate. We should be able to command the best men in each department, and to offer them facilities for original research. We need to improve our equipment, our teaching plant. We need a library for our students and we need a hospital of our own for ward teaching. . . . With the means at their disposal the Medical Faculty have done well to bring the school to its present position, but with Harvard spending $500,000 on a building for Physiological and Pathological Laboratories, the University of Pennsylvania erecting a new and very complete Laboratory Building, and Rockefeller giving $200,000 to establish a Laboratory for Medical Research, we must advance or recede.[44]

Improvements had been done on a shoestring, without help from the university. The two salaried professors, W. H. Warren (chemistry) and Robert Terry (anatomy), were squeezed between better and more expensive teaching and static budgets. They improvised, paying out of their own pockets for microscopes for a new laboratory course in bacteriology.[45] But improvised improvements simply made the long-term problem more intractable. By 1906 a debt of $51,000 stood in the way of organic union with the university, which was struggling to raise endowment for its own reform and was in no position to make any commitment to the Medical Department. The situation was the same in many such schools, rich in ambition but poor in resources; forced by its affiliated status to keep up with university standards but unable to draw on university endowments. As the reform movement gathered momentum, the ante to play in the national medical education game seemed increasingly out of reach. The gap between expectation and achievement became a chasm.

Reorganization at St. Louis followed the same script as in Philadelphia, with less melodramatic stage business. The crucial figure was Robert Brookings, the chairman of the university board of trustees. In 1906 Brookings turned his attention to the financial reorganization of the medical school. He and trustee Adolphus Busch offered to pay off the accumulated debt and to assume responsibility for raising the $200,000 required for organic union if the medical faculty would relinquish administrative control. It was an offer the hard-pressed medical faculty could not refuse. Union was complicated by local medical politics, however. When the medical school was formed by merger of two rival colleges in 1891, it inherited two contentious faculties supported by two bodies of alumni, who blocked every move for organic union. These contending medical factions also made it impossible for Brookings to appeal to the local philanthropists who had given millions to the university.[46] It was clear by 1909 that no insider could bring the factions together and that some outside authority was needed to overrule both factions. Abraham Flexner provided the needed shock.

Brookings was unprepared for Flexner's devastating report of his visit to the medical school: the clinical departments were "wretched"; the preclinical departments were old-fashioned and had no connection with the clinical branches. Indignant, Brookings went to see Flexner and was persuaded by him that only a complete reorganization would do. Washington University was a strategic outpost in Flexner's plan for a rationalized national system of medical schools. His strategy was to build up the strongest school in each region to the level of Johns Hopkins, to serve both as a source of model physicians and as a pacesetter for other schools in the region. He hoped Washington University would become the Johns Hopkins of the Southwest. Robert Terry was undoubtedly correct in his suspicion that Flexner deliberately overstated the failings of the medical school to stimulate Brookings into supporting his very ambitious and expensive plan.[47]

Brookings and Flexner then applied the same tactics to the medical faculty. Flexner made a dramatic appearance and laid before the faculty his vision of the "manifest destiny" of the school in the Southwest. Flexner's application of the carrot and the stick was irresistible. Traditional medical rivalries were forgotten for the moment; the medical faculty resigned en masse so that reconstruction could begin from the ground up.

The ultimate goal of reorganization was a salaried clinical staff and a university hospital. However, the first step was the complete reorganization of the preclinical departments. Of the original preclinical faculty, only Robert Terry was reappointed. The chair of chemistry was abolished and the new Department of Biological Chemistry was organized for Philip Shaffer from the Cornell Medical School. Joseph Erlanger was called to physiology from Wisconsin; Eugene Opie to pathology from the Rockefeller Institute; George Dock to medicine from Tulane; John Howland to pediatrics from Columbia; and David Edsall from Penn. All the new men were outsiders, free of local political loyalties; all had reputations as researchers. As Dock wrote to Opie on the eve of their assembling, "I doubt if any other school can offer so many attractions to any one who wishes to combine teaching and investigation as will the one now planned."[48] Together they planned and carried out the organization of the new hospital and the new clinical faculty, attending to everything from high policy to the details of laboratory design.

Reorganization of the clinical departments proved more difficult than the preclinical disciplines. Delay gave the old clinical faculty time to repent, and Shaffer (then dean) urged Howland and Edsall to hasten their arrival in St. Louis, fearing a repetition of the counterrevolution at Penn.[49] The danger of resurgent factionalism was real: the university still had to rely on local practitioners to teach most of the clinical specialties. Resentment was growing toward the aggressive and sometimes tactless medical carpetbaggers:

There were many men with more experience than the new heads of the departments, and there were many distinguished names among the clinicians in the city. The necessary shifts in titles and appointments were bound to bring resentment. In some cases, the Executive Faculty were unaware of the personal dislocations which resulted from the faculty changes. They were called facetiously by some the "Wise Men from the East."[50]

Opie reported to Howland that the political turmoil was being blown up by local reporters who were all too eager to exploit old medical feuds.[51]

The new men felt at times that Brookings was too anxious not to offend powerful medical interests. Shaffer himself made a discreet but desperate inquiry in 1912 whether the chair he had turned down at Cornell the year before was still vacant.[52] Although these moments of panic passed, some of the faculty were lured back to more peaceful and established institutions. Shaffer wrote to his New York friends:

We have been having trouble here, but I believe it is largely passing and that the undertaking will emerge without any very serious wounds. The trouble has been in large part one of misunderstanding, and that is fast disappearing. As you know we have lost Edsall, and Howland is restless, but that is the greater reason why we should stick tight and see the thing actually accomplished, for it can and will be done.[53]

The Barnes Hospital was completed in 1915 and dedicated, appropriately, by William Welch.

The success of schools like Washington University encouraged others to make equally ambitious plans. In 1910 Richard Beard returned to the University of Minnesota from a meeting at St. Louis, impressed and alarmed at the progress being made by Washington University:

Realizing, as we must, that [Washington University] is simply putting itself into form to accept the invitation of the Carnegie Foundation to become the center of medical education in the Southwest, I cannot escape the conclusion that what Missouri and St. Louis have done, Minnesota and the cities of Minneapolis and St. Paul and Duluth could do; that the very same opportunity awaits the University of Minnesota, to become, in fact, as it is in prospect, the medical center of the Northwest. The argument of this Washington University achievement, which is passing into history, is inescapable in the obligation it puts upon us. We have the occasion and it is a large one. Have we not the men who, refusing to await the slow process of development which is shared at the best with other hungry colleges, will undertake a similar campaign for a complete University Hospital system in the immediate future. Relying upon the state for land and for hospital maintenance, why should we not go out and get, from private sources, the means necessary to build and equip a hospital system as Washington University, Harvard..., Johns Hopkins...and others have already done?[54]

The increasing availability of endowment money from large foundations and private philanthropists, plus the threat of competition from other schools, made it necessary to act quickly. Within a year, President George Vincent had initiated a complete reorganization of the university's affiliated medical college.[55] The wave of reform thus spread from St. Louis north to Minnesota, south to Texas,[56] and throughout the state universities of the Midwest.

Reorganization of the preclinical departments generally proceeded with dispatch because it was to the advantage of every interest group to see these subjects as academic disciplines. When it came to the clinical branches, however, several strong interests felt that these were not sciences and did not belong under university aegis. Physician–teachers were by no means the only opponents of clinical reform. At the University of Chicago, professors of the biological sciences strongly opposed attachment with Rush Medical College. In California, Illinois, and other states where populist sentiment was strong, state legislators vigorously opposed any public investment in clinical schools on the grounds that it was simply subsidizing a privileged and well-paid professional elite. This attitude gradually changed as reform leaders succeeded in persuading people that clinical specialties were true sciences and that clinicians served the public as well as themselves.

In many cases, political and ideological differences between the biomedical and clinical sciences resulted in the creation, as an expedient, of separate faculties. The universities of Chicago and California both took this course, for somewhat different reasons. In these geographically split schools, however, ideological and financial pressures ultimately forced a complete union.

Rush Medical College was one of the largest and most progressive medical schools in the 1890s.[57] In 1896 the eminent German bacteriologist Edwin Klebs was appointed to lecture on recent German research to a few select students. The majority of the Rush faculty were not stars of this magnitude, of course; improvement was uneven. Prior to Jacques Loeb's arrival in 1900, physiology was a lecture course without demonstrations, and there were no laboratory facilities.[58] The chairs of chemistry and pathology were still the only full-time salaried chairs in 1896, and the high school requirement was not enforced. Klebs was a token of what Rush hoped to become.

The key to these hopes was affiliation with the new University of Chicago and access to the Rockefeller millions. After nearly six years of negotiations, affiliation with the university was consummated in 1898. Systematic development of the preclinical departments began at once. Part-time physician–teachers were removed, and preclinical teaching was put in the hands of university faculty.[59] President William Raney Harper hoped to put the clinical faculty on an academic basis as well. In 1901 he promised anatomist Joseph Flint that he would have a salaried chair of surgery by 1903, a promise that one outsider dismissed as a "gold brick."[60] The high school requirement was strictly enforced, and in 1899 Harper proposed that one year of college be required for admission in 1905. E. Fletcher Ingals, professor of laryngology and rhinology and the leader of the reform group at Rush, was cautiously optimistic:

I think that [1905] is as soon as we could well require five years...and I believe that at that time there will be no difficulty in doing so. If we find that Johns Hopkins and Harvard have been able to maintain their classes we need have no hesitation in making this further requirement at that time. If they have failed we can withdraw the proposition soon enough to save us from disaster, though as you suggest it is not at all likely that we should have to make such a move as this.[61]

Like his counterparts at P&S and Penn, Ingals underestimated the effect of even these modest steps toward putting Rush on a university basis.

Rush had 1,100 students in 1898, and providing laboratory instruction in physiology, pathology, anatomy, and chemistry to classes of 250 students was a far cry from letting Klebs cultivate small groups in the latest research. By 1901 expenses of the new laboratory building were $10,000 more than had been expected, and a $20,000 deficit was projected for 1902. At the same time, the stricter entrance standards began to cut into enrollments and tuition fees, Rush's sole source of income. Murmurs of dissatisfaction from the clinical staff grew louder, and Ingals feared an eruption if the expenses of the preclinical departments could not be drastically reduced, and soon.[62]

The articles of affiliation barred Rush from using university endowment, so there was no help there. But Ingals began to eye the new, spacious, and well-equipped Hull Biological Laboratory at the university campus, with its endowment of $2 million. Because Loeb and others were already teaching the preclinical courses at Rush, Ingals and Harper agreed that it would be more efficient if the preclinical courses were simply transferred to the university. Rush would lose the tuition income of the freshman and sophomore classes to the university, but Ingals calculated that the reduction in operating expenses at Rush would more than offset the loss in fees.

Although the Rockefellers had previously declined to endow a full medical school, the university, in effect, assumed financial responsibility for half the Rush course. Ingals and Harper saw this division of labor as a step toward a university medical school:

I do not think we will be a whit behind either Johns Hopkins or Harvard...There is a belief among the most thoughtful members of our faculty that the University...is a better place to teach most of the fundamental Chairs than the ordinary medical college and although this will be distinctly a part of the Rush Medical course, yet it will be done under University influences and according to ideal methods.[63]

A grant of $50,000 from John D. Rockefeller, Jr. enabled the Hull Laboratories to be equipped for large-scale teaching, and the preclinical sciences became departments of the university.[64]

This division of labor did not resolve the fundamental issues of reform, however. Financial pressures and professional conflicts soon led to a more intimate union between Rush and the university. Transfer of the preclinical departments to the university budget eased the immediate pressure on Rush, but not for long. Students entering Rush were held to the same requirements as university freshmen, and the high academic standards of the university scared medical students away. Enrollment dropped from 1,100 in 1898 to 750 in 1903.[65] In 1904 two full years of college work were required for admission to Rush. Enrollments plummeted, and because 90% of Rush's income still came from tuition, deficits quickly became unmanageable.

Ingals managed to reduce a projected deficit of $24,000 in 1905 to $3,600 by imaginative one-time economies and a gift of $10,000 from a friendly alumnus. But when another deficit of $14,000 was projected for 1906, Ingals had no tricks left in his bag:

Our present standard makes it nearly impossible to increase the number of students from other colleges and thus we shall be forced to face a large yearly deficit until the classes at the University become about 75% larger than now or until Providence intervenes in our behalf. [66]

Ingals could no longer apply the traditional remedies of proprietary institutions. Mortgaging the property was out of the question, as any debt would preclude union with the university. Assessing the faculty for donations had been a common way of raising funds when the faculty had received dividends. But the clinical staff had received no compensation at all for three years and had already given $4,000. They could hardly be pressed to pay for the privilege of giving up half their practices for teaching and research. Ingals did request donations of $250, with distaste and misgivings:

I have a little fear that this call for money will cause some members of the Faculty to range themselves with the few who are in favor of lower standards for the purpose of securing larger classes; but I do not think it possible for this faction to obtain a controlling voice. If it unhappily should succeed, nothing would remain for the rest of us but to resign and sacrifice all that has been done. [67]

The more Rush adhered to university ideals, the less appropriate was this kind of charity.

The obvious solution was to raise endowment for the clinical departments from local philanthropists; but the proprietary status of Rush closed this door too. At the time of affiliation, the board of trustees, which then consisted entirely of Rush faculty, was replaced by business and civic leaders to emphasize that Rush had become a public service institution. But the articles of affiliation were carefully drafted to avoid any definite commitment to Rush by the university, at the insistence of the Rockefeller family. The public image of the proprietary medical college was not as easily changed as its legal basis, however. Medical schools that trained men for a lucrative profession were not regarded as fit objects of charity by those who patronized private colleges and universities. A $1 million endowment drive initiated by Frank Billings in 1899 ended in failure in 1903. The Rockefellers perceived medical research as a public service but balked at helping to turn out large numbers of physicians.[68] Harper's plea that medical research and medical training were inseparable fell on sensibilities not yet accustomed to the idea of a university medical school.[69]

Affiliation with the university also resulted in a subtle but profound change in the attitude of Rush alumni. Institutional loyalty depended on local professional rivalries; few Rush alumni felt any loyalty to the university. Individuals who had been most sympathetic to improvement lost interest in reform. In 1904 Ingals reported to Harper that Arthur Bevan, professor of anatomy and a leader in the AAMC, was disaffected. So too was Dr. Nicholas Senn, whose family had built the new pathology laboratory. There were murmurs that Dean Dodson, who had a half-time university salary, was giving too much weight to university interests.[70] Fearing revolt, Ingals announced to the new president, Harry Pratt Judson, that tinkering with existing institutional machinery would no longer do.[71]

Competition finally forced the university to commit itself to a complete medical school. The University of Illinois and Northwestern were both eager to attach Rush. Edmund James had been trying since 1898 to unite the state university with its affiliate, the Chicago College of Physicians and Surgeons, but had been thwarted by opposition from populist legislators and sectarian medical interests.[72] (In 1902 the homeopaths got an injunction against a merger, forcing the college to close temporarily.) Meanwhile, a group of Rush faculty were lobbying vigorously to become part of the state university, in the hope that Rush would thus remain a large teaching school.[73] Discouraged by the prospects at P&S and aware of the rumors of secession at Rush, James discreetly broached the possibility of affiliation with the University of Illinois.[74] Ingals and Judson realized that union with Rush must be consummated if the University of Chicago did not want to be left with only a two-year preclinical course. Within a year, the decision was reached to create a complete medical school and university hospital at the university's campus, with full-time clinical chairs based on the Johns Hopkins model. Rush was to be reorganized as a postgraduate medical division.[75] Segregation of the preclinical and clinical sciences thus came to an end at Chicago.

THE FAR WEST: UNIVERSITY OF CALIFORNIA

A similar story unfolded on the Pacific Coast. Toland and Cooper Medical Colleges in San Francisco were the two leading medical colleges in California and, like Rush, had begun to make improvements in the late 1890s. Cooper acquired a German pathologist, William Ophüls, in 1898; the Toland faculty, eager to keep abreast of their arch rival, took the initiative for organic union with the state university.[76] Their initiative was eagerly picked up by the new president, Benjamin Ihde Wheeler, who was eager to build a complete university at Berkeley. The Toland faculty relinquished control over its finances and became a faculty of the university. The dean, A. A. D'Ancona, acted as business agent and liaison. Wheeler planned to make California a center of medical science, ". . . ranking with the medical departments of the University of Berlin, of Heidelberg, or Paris, . . . and of Johns Hopkins and of Harvard. . . ."[77]

One by one the preclinical departments were organized. Pathology was first in 1899: the reigning clinician–pathologist was dismissed and Alonzo Taylor was called from Penn to organize teaching and research in experimental pathology. Phoebe Hearst was persuaded to give $24,000 to equip a pathology laboratory and pay half of Taylor's salary. In 1901 Wheeler and Taylor together planned the reorganization of the Department of Anatomy and succeeded in enticing Joseph Flint from Johns Hopkins, where he had worked with anatomist Franklin Mall. Mrs. Hearst was again asked for $14,000 for a histology laboratory. Taylor, Wheeler, and Flint then proceeded to create the Department of Physiology. Jacques Loeb was wooed away from Chicago by the promise of more pay and opportunity for research. A local physician, Dr. M. Herzstein, was persuaded to fit out a physiological laboratory. Flint personally visited each one of the regents to lobby for yet another salary in the university budget.[78] By 1902 the preclinical departments were all in the hands of salaried academic scientists, imported from the best Eastern schools.

President Wheeler was clearly the constant guiding hand in the "academization" of the preclinical departments. There were no local entrepreneurs in the biomedical sciences, and the progressives on the clinical faculty would never, by themselves, have been able to overcome the rooted political opposition to a state role in medical education. Wheeler's strategy was to be patient but relentless and vigilant, seizing every opportunity and always "keeping the pressure on" both the clinicians and the politicians.[79] Local competition spurred Wheeler's ambitions. Though not affiliated with Stanford University until 1910, Cooper Medical College was led by progressive physicians who were willing to back their ideals with cash. Cooper had made much improvement in the biomedical sciences by 1901 and forced Wheeler to immediate action:

The Cooper Medical College, which does not rely upon its earnings alone but which receives regular assistance from Dr. Lane, now has a pure pathologist, and is sending an anatomist to Johns Hopkins and abroad to be trained in that department. They will then have their scientific departments well filled, and that fact, with the advantages of the Lane Hospital, will in the minds of the profession place their school upon a better basis than is the Medical School of the University.[80]

Given the political vulnerability of a state university, private support from the medical community seemed to many a more promising basis for reform than the state legislature. Wheeler was aware of the challenge to his political skills.[81]

In 1902 Wheeler unveiled an ambitious plan for reorganizing the clinical branches and building a university hospital – three plans to be exact: one based on the $1 million he hoped to obtain from Mrs. Huntington; one modeled on the Johns Hopkins Hospital, for $3 million; and a third, costing $5 million, that would equal the complex being built at Harvard.[82] Wheeler planned to require two college years for admission as soon as the market could bear it, and proposed an optional six-year B.A.–M.D. program to increase the local supply of qualified students. His strategy was to preempt Cooper in clinical instruction and draw graduates of Stanford's two-year program in the preclinical sciences: "The only students we care for are the well-trained men and in case the hospital plans materialize we should need a good group of students of our own training much sooner than 1905."[83]

Alonzo Taylor was less optimistic about the prospects for clinical reform, recognizing that it depended on changes in institutions that university presidents could not control. The quality of research in the preclinical sciences depended on better scientific teaching in the colleges and greater cooperation of local hospitals in providing clinical materials for teaching and research. Most important, the cultured middle classes had to be made to accept the cultural value of medical science and to provide recruits and the endowments necessary for training medical scientists.[84] Taylor proved the shrewder prophet. The time was not ripe for Wheeler's grand scheme. Harvard got Mrs. Huntington's million, and the hospital remained a paper plan. But the preclinical departments thrived, and the two-year college requirement went into effect as planned in 1904.

Dean D'Ancona and most of the clinical teachers supported the academization of the preclinical sciences. They expected that putting the preclinical staff on the state's payroll would permit the medical school to use its entire tuition income for improvements in the clinical departments. Indeed, that was probably their principal interest in reform. D'Ancona was dissatisfied with the irregularity of bedside teaching by busy practitioners. He hoped that more regular and continuous teaching could be assured by offering small salaries to ambitious young practitioners.[85] In view of the glut of physicians and their generally modest standard of living, this was perhaps not an unreasonable hope; but things did not work out as expected.

Division of the preclinical faculty between Berkeley and San Francisco satisfied no one. Taylor was located in San Francisco but was increasingly anxious to join the academic circle he had helped to create at Berkeley. Loeb taught only at Berkeley, leaving an assistant to teach medical physiology in the city.[86] Flint was also at Berkeley, but the big anatomy course was taught in the city, on the medical school budget. D'Ancona discovered, to his chagrin, how expensive it was to teach anatomy as a scientific discipline. The cost jumped from $1,020 in 1901 to $5,400 in 1902, a sum the medical school could ill afford. Higher entrance requirements had resulted in a sharp decrease in enrollment, reducing the school's income by $4,000.[87] The expected improvements in clinical teaching did not materialize. Having sold the regents on these expensive reforms, Wheeler was embarrassed by the obvious financial inefficiencies of operation. No one was happy with the widening gap between the values of the laboratory men and the clinicians. The clinicians objected to the separation of preclinical teaching from clinical practice, especially in pathology. Taylor complained that his teaching and research suffered in the clinical context: "Our situation constitutes an isolation from physics and chemistry, as well as from physiology, that is in every way bad."[88]

To keep the laboratory men happy and spare the medical budget, Wheeler resolved to move the preclinical departments entirely to

Berkeley. The regents and the medical faculty approved, and transfer was completed in 1906, when the great earthquake and fire conveniently destroyed the school's facilities in San Francisco.[89] The preclinical sciences thus became university departments, separated from the clinical context. Pressures for economy and efficiency reinforced policies based on conflicting academic values. However, consistency of administration only made more obvious the basic flaws in the policy of segregation.

The University of California Medical School was "almost annihilated," in Wheeler's words, in the great enrollment crisis. The lowest ebb came in 1908 when only two physicians were graduated.[90] Wheeler kept the school alive, but only by laying aside his plans for reform. In 1907/8, income from tuition was only $7,943, whereas the state subsidy was $33,397. Hospital receipts of $40,527 did not cover the $48,629 put into improvements. Wheeler tried to raise $1 million for hospital endowment, but by 1909 pledges totaled only $110,000.[91]

The dissatisfaction of the clinical faculty with the divided school erupted in 1908 in an attempted counterrevolution against the biomedical group. It was an opportune moment: Flint had resigned and Taylor was on leave in Upsala. The clinical faculty was nervously watching Cooper Medical College, which had not raised their admissions standards and was flourishing.[92] For physicians accustomed to thinking in terms of local rivalries, this seemed a disastrous trend. This time of trouble was also a chance for the remnants of the preclinical faculty to settle old scores. The most vehement opposition came from Dr. Robert Orton Moody, who had taught surgical anatomy before being replaced by Flint. Relegated to a minor role in osteology, Moody lobbied in faculty meetings to restore anatomy to the clinicians and was supported by a group of them.[93]

Opposition to the academics produced a temporary alliance between the older generation of preclinical teachers and clinicians who preferred their conservative style and interests to the independent style and unfamiliar research interests of Taylor and Loeb. An ad hoc committee was appointed, chaired by Moody, to lower the premedical requirements and to investigate the charges that the preclinical courses were not answering the needs of clinical instruction. Dean D'Ancona was sympathetic with these complaints, and in October 1908, he sent a bill of particulars to Wheeler.[94]

Alonzo Taylor bore the brunt of D'Ancona's criticism. The clinicians felt that Taylor was too little concerned with practical pathological anatomy and clinical pathology, failed to provide diagnostic services for city physicians, and neglected autopsy work in favor of research in pure physiological and pathological chemistry. Taylor defended himself in a long letter to Wheeler, arguing that diagnostic and clinical pathology belonged in clinical medicine and that his duty was to advance experimental pathology.[95] The local defense was left to Jacques Loeb, who responded to attack by firing off a vituperative letter ridiculing the older generation of physiologists and pathologists whom the clinicians so admired:

You will notice that [D'Ancona and his group] praise Dr. [William] Ophüls as an ideal pathologist. Ophüls . . . is a fairly good representative of the Virchow school of pathology which 30 years ago was considered modern. . . . No University school will envy Cooper for having a pathologist like Ophüls, while a pathologist of the accomplishments and the horizon of Taylor would be considered an ornament by the leading University medical schools in Europe and the East. Perhaps one day (when it is too late) it will dawn upon the instigators of D'Ancona's letter that their nearest approach to University standing will come through the fact that for a little while they were forced to endure Taylor as a colleague.

You will also notice that they commend the services of Moody for the medical school. I have met Moody on several occasions recently and can conscientiously say that he is about the most ignorant and stupid Biologist whom it has ever been my good fortune to meet. He is overloading our students with worthless technical instruction. . . . In order to make the reorganization of the medical school complete they ought to propose to you that the janitor of the Anatomical Laboratory be requested to give a course in medical Physiology.[96]

Having thus vented steam, Loeb announced that he would not waste his time "in fighting ignorant and . . . unscrupulous men," and refused to meet further with Moody's committee.[97]

Wheeler assured Taylor and Loeb that there would be no backsliding on academic standards.[98] But he also realized that D'Ancona's demand for closer relations between the clinical and preclinical fields was legitimate. By 1910 medical reformers saw the growing isolation of the biomedical sciences as the chief impediment to reform in the clinical branches. California got bad marks on this point in the Flexner Report. Henry Pritchett, president of the Carnegie Foundation, lectured Wheeler in 1909 that high entrance requirements and excellent biomedical courses did not make a medical school:

In talking with your men I have been interested to see that those in the Berkeley side felt that the clinical men knew little of what they were doing, and those in the clinical side felt that the men engaged in the first two years had scant appreciation of the demands of medical training. It is clear that the university has not quite solved the problem of coordinating the two parts of the medical school.[99]

Wheeler was aware that the separation had been "advantageous in every respect except that the Medical School seems to be cut in twain."[100] The difficulty was knowing how to bring the twain together again.

Taylor and Loeb were violently opposed to being exiled to the hospital in San Francisco; the clinicians were equally set against the idea of a complete university school at Berkeley, knowing full well that few of them would survive such a reorganization. Wheeler strongly favored bringing the entire school to the campus. Pritchett felt that the preclinical men should move, because a teaching hospital had to be located in the city.[101] The issue was never resolved. A new hospital complex was built in San Francisco in the mid-1920s, but the preclinical departments remained in Berkeley.

CONCLUSION

The same problems appear over and over in the records of other medical schools between 1900 and 1910: university presidents eager to have a medical school but unwilling to commit university resources to what seemed a bottomless sink; faculties split between salaried, research-minded preclinical staff and practitioner–teachers in the clinical branches; veiled or open antagonism between generations; frustrated deans unable to tap either medical or university philanthropists; and alumni uncertain of their loyalties and responsibilities. Traditional differences in professional values and goals were exacerbated by the economic consequences of half-way steps toward reorganization. Premedical requirements were tailored to the needs of the preclinical departments, but the clinical departments suffered the consequences of radically reduced enrollment and income. Small elite classes suited the academic goals of the preclinical men but not the needs of the local medical interests. Universities and medical schools could no longer function separately but had not yet discovered how to give up their separate institutional ways.

The economic crises that were precipitated by collegiate entrance requirements forced both sides to commit themselves to complete union. Clinicians realized that improvements in clinical teaching could not be financed internally without giving up control of appointments to university administrators. University leaders realized that only a full commitment of university resources would prevent collapse or secession of clinical faculties. Once this accommodation occurred, the pace and style of reform quickly changed. The Carnegie Foundation and the General Education Board took up the cause of reform. Matching grants from foundations primed the pump of private philanthropy. Reform agencies systematically encouraged competition, set standards, and rationalized the system on a national scale. The change in atmosphere from 1900 to 1910 is striking. In 1900 modest, improvised plans stood the best chance of success. By 1910 philanthropists were moved by grandiose plans for regional Johns Hopkinses. Reform spread to schools that previously could never have aspired to high academic standards but that now had to in order to survive in a market where academic quality was the principal means of competition.

By 1920 American medical students were spending more years in training than students in any European country. They were devoting more time to studying the basic and preclinical sciences. In Germany, the six-year course was the norm: two collegiate-level years in *Gymnasium* (with little laboratory work, however) and four in the university. In Britain, the six-year course was divided a little differently: four in the university in the basic sciences and physiology and then two in hospital schools. (In 1919 collegiate requirements made it difficult for British medical students to transfer to American schools, to the unconcealed gratification of some educators on seeing the tables turned.[102]) In America, a six-year course was the norm by 1915; but even then it was common practice to spend eight years, four in college and four in medical school. In 1920, 40% of new medical graduates had B.A. degrees; 70% did by 1930, although few schools required a B.A. for admission. Competition was the cause. More young people were going to college; after 1920 the supply of qualified applicants grew so fast that schools began to impose ceilings on class size. Students responded by spending four years in college, mainly in scientific or biomedical studies. Thus the eight-year course (nine including the intern year) became the rule.

The style of the preclinical sciences was shaped by two key features of the educational system: (1) Their location in medical schools, rather than colleges, entailed close linkages to clinical medicine; (2) the availability of students well prepared in basic chemistry and biology (with laboratory experience) enabled biomedical professors to teach specialized courses in an academic style. The balance between disciplinary and utilitarian goals in the biomedical sciences reflected these opposing influences. Service roles pulled toward clinical problems; a clientele socialized in academic values pulled toward academic approaches to problems. Walter Fletcher and Wilmot Herringham were struck in 1921 by how American colleges taught the sciences as cultural subjects. The great advantage of the American system, they felt, was that premedical students were exposed early and intensively to laboratory science. They also noted the American tendency to emphasize the clinical aspects of physiology, biochemistry, or pharmacology. They approved but also noted the disadvantage that these disciplines were not developed as broad biological sciences. Fletcher also disapproved of the American tendency to create special departments of biochemistry and pharmacology separate from physiology.[103] These were shrewd observations of the differential effects of institutional context on scientific styles. Specialization of disciplines like biochemistry was made possible by the length of the medical course of study and the location of the preclinical departments in university-controlled medical schools.

In Germany, students entering medical study from *Gymnasium* had only one summer's laboratory experience. Organic and physical chemistry and general physiology vied with the biomedical sciences in a crowded course, leaving little room for new biomedical specialties. In Britain, the biomedical sciences were part of a collegiate course, but separation from the clinical branches left both weaker. German and British institutions did not encourage recruitment to the biomedical disciplines and made it difficult to mobilize resources on a large scale for new specialties. American institutions, with their blend of academic and utilitarian ideals and symbiosis of college and medical school, had greater potential for systematic discipline building. Preprofessional science courses prepared American medical students to accept physiology and biochemistry as basic applied sciences. Professors' chronic complaints of ill-prepared students tell as much about their high expectations as about the actual quality of premedical instruction. Biomedical departments could adopt an academic style because it was generally accepted that the biomedical sciences provided good mental discipline for clinical practice, training the faculties of observation and inductive reasoning. [104] This belief mirrored the market relationship between premedical and medical institutions and the heady ideologizing of the reform movement.

At the same time, improvement in the biomedical sciences was justified by their relevance to clinical teaching and research. In America, the biomedical sciences ("preclinical" may be the more apt term after 1915) were basic applied sciences, infused with academic ideals but firmly rooted in the medical market. They lacked the high academic style of European sciences but had considerably more potential for growth and specialization.

7

From medical chemistry to biochemistry: the emergence of a discipline

The reorganization of medical institutions created opportunities for growth and innovation in all the preclinical disciplines. Because the reform movement emphasized intellectual quality and uniform standards, competition for regional or national leadership became a powerful argument for higher budgets. Discipline builders were liberated from local medical politics. Workers in all disciplines were encouraged to acquire specialized academic credentials and to engage in fashionable lines of research. Each discipline adapted these new resources to its particular needs, but the basic strategies are similar in all.

As universities gained control of the preclinical sciences, they established academic criteria for appointments and promotion. The AMA Council on Education in 1909 was unanimous and vehement in their opinion that physiology and biochemistry should be taught by full-time specialists: "The old but still prevalent idea that almost any young practitioner with time on his hands could do as professor of physiology cannot be too forcibly condemned."[1]

More sophisticated medical students made it possible for anatomists, physiologists, and biochemists to teach more specialized courses and to teach them as basic experimental sciences. The new professionals had much higher expectations than the pioneers. For example, Henry Pickering Bowditch had had to bootleg laboratory instruction into his lectures on medical physiology; his disciple, William T. Porter, saw lectures and medical application as incidental to pure experimental physiology.[2] Here is the difference between the generations: what had been academic frosting for the pioneers was cake for the new professionals. Research achievement became as important as teaching skills in building the reputation of a school. Contribution to medical knowledge was perceived as a better way of improving medical practice than churning out large numbers of general practitioners. Young Ph.D. biochemists began to expect time and reward for research, even in large teaching schools. Pathologist John Aub looked askance at the offer of a chair at Northwestern:

The man in charge would have but little time to devote to research, and it is research alone which will bring a young man to the position. What should it profit a man to obtain a professorship if he lose his research soul?[3]

New academic roles encouraged new priorities and styles of biomedical research. Problems of process and function had greater prestige than problems of morphology; experimental methods were favored over description, and a comparative approach infused problems of human biology. In anatomy there was a tension between descriptive gross anatomy and experimental cytology and embryology. General or cellular physiology became an important subfield of physiology. The traditional stock-in-trade of physiological chemists, the analysis and description of chemical substances, was overshadowed by a concern with the enzymatic processes in living tissues. Chemical theories of growth, metabolism, infection, and resistance were widely discussed.[4] Experimental pharmacology, drawing upon both physiology and biochemistry, replaced traditional descriptive *materia medica*. Pathological anatomy was regarded as less fundamental than the physiological and biochemical processes that gave rise to symptoms and lesions. Bacteriologists became more concerned with the chemistry and physiology of infection and resistance, less with morphology and classifications. In all the sciences, the issues were the same: description versus experiment, static versus dynamic, structure versus process, and discipline versus clinic. The increasing reference to chemistry and biology in the biomedical disciplines reflected the new symbiosis between medical schools and universities.

In medical chemistry and *materia medica*, the differences between the old and new generations were so great that the new men saw themselves as the pioneers of entirely new disciplines, pharmacology and biological chemistry. A young biochemist–pharmacologist, Carl Alsberg, saw clearly the advantages to him of the generation gap:

Chairs in [pharmacology] in our medical schools are held by elderly practitioners who lecture upon materia medica and therapeutics. Many of the chairs will soon be vacant and will be filled by professional pharmacologists. Adequately trained pharmacologists are, however, exceedingly rare in America at present.[5]

Alsberg felt that the opportunities in physiological chemistry were less good. In fact, medical chemists were also being rapidly replaced by biochemists. In training, expectations, career patterns, and scientific outlook, medical chemists and biological chemists, like teachers of *materia medica* and pharmacologists, were distinctly different species. In these two cases, the medical reform movement established virtually new biomedical disciplines.

MEDICAL CHEMISTS AND BIOCHEMISTS

Like many groups cast aside in the name of progress, the medical chemists have been treated unsympathetically by historians. Depicted as ill-trained amateurs interested only in routine clinical testing and boiling up urine, the medical chemist was a familiar figure in the rhetoric of reform.[6] He was the mythic antagonist of the new professional, defending old habits against scientific progress. Like most stereotypes, this one does have elements of truth. Most medical chemists were trained not as physiological chemists but as chemists or physicians. Most took no interest in physiological chemistry for its own sake. Physician–chemists regarded medical chemistry as a place to bide their time while waiting for a more prestigious chair of medicine. Others were busy practitioners specializing in toxicology and forensic medicine, a lively and lucrative trade. Among medical school chemists were many who did not aspire to or failed to make careers in the newer, more prestigious specialties of organic and physical chemistry. Most courses in medical chemistry consisted almost entirely of elementary inorganic chemistry, with a bit of organic and physiological chemistry thrown in toward the end, along with urinalysis and toxicology.

Like most stereotypes, however, the image of the medical chemist has been exaggerated for ideological effect. Some were as competent and up-to-date as professional biochemists. Some were teaching physiological chemistry prior to reform. Medical chemists rendered valuable services in public health boards and city coroners' offices, and were active promoters of medical reform. Our stereotypical view of the medical chemist is that of the generation of biochemists who competed with them for chairs and laboratory rights. It was the biochemists who survived to tell about the victorious campaigns for medical science, and it was very much in their interest to dramatize the failings of their predecessors' training and academic style. They tarred the best medical chemists with the same brush as the worst. In this competition between two generations, with different professional experiences and ideals, revolution, not evolution, was the strategy of choice for the challengers, and they had all the political advantages on their side. The medical chemists were indeed out of place in the new academic medical schools; but their role was nicely adapted to the realities of the old-time medical college.

Medical chemists came in two varieties: physicians turned chemists and chemists who applied their skills to medicine. For physician–chemists, teaching physiological chemistry was often a small part of their varied roles. S. M. Morris, M. D., known as "Old Test Tube" to his students, taught chemistry at the Texas Medical School, maintained a large medical practice, and ran a commercial analyst's business on the side. (His clients included the owners of the first wells from the Texas oil fields.)[7] A less colorful but more typical physician–chemist was Arthur E. Austin, a Harvard graduate (M.D.) who was professor of chemistry and toxicology and subsequently professor of clinical medicine at Tufts Medical School. Austin was a capable practitioner–teacher, interested in new laboratory methods of diagnosis and therapeutics. There were many like him. Rudolph A. Witthaus, M.D., professor of chemistry and toxicology at the Cornell Medical School, was a famous New York medical jurist, author of the standard work on forensic medicine, and an active medical reformer. He was one of the group that seceded from NYU to found the Cornell Medical School and he guided the school through its most difficult years.[8]

Until quite late, most medical chemists were trained primarily as physicians. In 1900 there were 246 teachers of medical chemistry in 149 medical colleges: 170 regular faculty and 76 instructors and assistants. Of these 246, 144 (59%) had the M.D. degree only (54 also had B.A. or M.A. degrees). Another 30 (12%) had both M.D. and Ph.D. degrees. (Though highly sought after, these hybrids remained a small minority.) Of the 72 individuals with nonmedical degrees, only 25 had Ph.D. degrees and 47 had bachelors' or masters' degrees. Thus a total of only 55 of all medical chemists in 1900 had Ph.D. degrees and nearly half of those also had medical credentials.[9]

Within a decade, most medical schools insisted on the Ph.D. degree as the standard requirement for appointment in biological chemistry.

The varied roles of the medical chemists continued to be viable in smaller schools trying to reform on shoestring budgets. In 1898, for example, a young graduate of Johns Hopkins was lured away from a country practice in Nebraska to teach pharmacology at Creighton Medical College. To supplement his small salary, he taught chemistry (and Latin!) and was offered a job in the coroner's office:

There is not a man in the city of Omaha who could or would undertake a complete toxicological examination of a dead body. The doctors all tell me I could make money in the courts if I could do such work and that the chemist must be a physician. You know how much [chemistry] I have had. Do you think that by . . . going to some good school in the summer I could work up enough to do such work in a few years?[10]

It was logical as well as economical to combine toxicology, forensic medicine and clinical analysis with teaching general chemistry.

Medical colleges also attracted professional chemists, who saw medical chemistry as an applied science analogous to agricultural or pharmaceutical chemistry. Before the academic chemical specialties were established in universities in the 1890s, chemistry was primarily an applied science, flourishing in schools of agriculture, pharmacy, medicine, and mining or engineering. These schools continued to offer professional opportunities for Ph.D. chemists; perhaps not academically prestigious jobs, but respectable and sometimes quite lucrative ones. It was common practice for academic chemists to also serve as professors of medical chemistry. Among these medical chemists were some of the best American chemists of the day.

Charles F. Chandler, professor of chemistry at Columbia, exemplifies this type of medical chemist. Trained in analytical and applied chemistry at Göttingen, Chandler taught chemistry in the Schools of Mines, Pharmacy, Dentistry, and Medicine and in Teachers College; he did professional work for the New York Board of Health, was a popular forensic and toxicological expert, and ran a large and profitable industrial consulting practice.[11] The course and textbook developed between 1887 and 1894 by Chandler and his understudy, Charles E. Pellew, was basic chemistry, slanted to the interests of medical students.[12] It was a natural style for versatile technical chemists. Edmond O'Neill, head of the College of Chemistry at the University of California, likewise was interested in industrial and agricultural chemistry as well as medical chemistry. He was city chemist and was active in the coroner's office.[13] John H. Long, professor of chemistry at Northwestern Medical School from 1882 to 1918, was trained in chemistry at Tübingen, served as chemist for the Illinois Board of Health, and was active on the AMA Council on Education.[14] Victor Vaughan was a medical chemist with a special bent toward sanitary chemistry and health reform. Charles A. Doremus played similar roles in the New York University–Bellevue Hospital Medical School.

Unlike the new chemical specialties, which cut across many fields of application with a limited range of methods, older specialties like medical, pharmaceutical, and agricultural chemistry were defined by their special areas of application and their special audiences. This way of organizing a discipline was appropriate for a system in which academic and professional colleges were separated, each with its own roster of basic science teachers. These applied styles of chemistry were a vertically integrated package of basic chemistry, appropriate parts of organic, physical, or biochemistry, and strictly technical applications to the analysis of fertilizers, feeds, soils, drugs, urine, and other clinical materials. The role of the medical chemist was perfectly adapted to the scientific institutions of late-nineteenth-century America.

As colleges of medicine, agriculture, and pharmacy became university schools, this mode of specialization ceased to fit institutional realities. Academic reformers insisted that medical and other professional students should have the same basic chemistry as college students, plus advanced work in organic, physical, or physiological chemistry, where it was relevant to medical or professional problems. The consolidation of central university departments of chemistry serving diverse professional schools encouraged a different organization of disciplines. Specialties were defined by particular theories and methods, not special areas of application. The older and more diverse specialties seemed unprofessional. In fact, the applied science style lasted a decade or so longer in medical schools than it did in universities before being superseded by the new specialties. It was only in this decade that there was a marked difference either in style or status between academic and medical chemists.

There was some small niche for physiological chemistry in the traditional medical curriculum. It was often slipped into the final weeks of the basic chemistry course, although at a rudimentary level. Contemporary textbooks give a rough estimate of its weight and quality. Elias Bartley's popular *Textbook of Medical and Pharmaceutical Chemistry* (sixth edition, 1906) devoted 150 of 670 pages to physiological chemistry, and even that was mainly a list of organic compounds; the bulk was elementary physics and chemistry. Most schools offered advanced electives in toxicology and urinalysis but only rarely in physiological chemistry as such. So long as medical colleges had to provide students with general chemistry, opportunities for biochemists to develop specialized roles were sharply limited. Teaching remedial general chemistry was not an appealing career for ambitious biochemists. Medical chemists had little incentive to specialize in biochemistry. Clinical or forensic medicine offered more stable and attractive careers to physician–chemists. Academic specialties or industrial work were more promising careers for Ph.D. chemists. Medical students had no vocational incentive to become biochemists.

In these circumstances, specialization was more likely to hinder than help a young man's career. For example, the dean of the University of Texas Medical School asked J. J. Abel in 1908 whether a candidate for a post in medical chemistry was overspecialized:

As you know, the smaller medical schools cannot require a college course, or training in the scientific subjects for admission to the course in medicine....Most of our students have never studied chemistry before coming here and we have to give a course in general inorganic chemistry during the first year in order that they may understand the work in medical chemistry during the second year....Has Dr. Whitney had a broad training in chemistry or has his work been exclusively in physiolgical and pathological chemistry?[15]

There was a market for general chemists or clinical chemists but not for biochemists. This was the case generally until about 1905.

The situation was dramatically changed when medical schools introduced collegiate entrance requirements. Because incoming students were required to have already taken general chemistry, this subject quickly disappeared from the medical curriculum. It was superseded by more specialized courses in biological chemistry, and medical chemists were replaced by professional biochemists. General chemists and physicians did not possess the appropriate credentials to teach specialized courses in biological chemistry, and specialists were suddenly in short supply and, consequently, in great demand. As the reform movement gained momentum, specialization became a good strategy for advancing a career. What had been a marginal role for medical chemists became the basis for a new biomedical discipline.

Another letter from Abel's files reveals how new institutional structures favored specialization. When Arthur Austin left Tufts in 1905 for a chair of medicine and toxicology at Texas, the faculty proposed that his understudy, Frederick Hollis, take charge of general chemistry and that a medically trained biochemist be hired to teach the second-year course in physiological and pathological chemistry. Hollis had a Ph.D. degree in physiological chemistry from Yale and was eager to take over the advanced clinical work. He also realized that it would be professional suicide to stay on as a general chemist: "I shall try to see if there is an opening elsewhere, as I feel that it would be foolish to look forward to considering my main work in general chemistry, which, it seems to me, is not likely to remain long a part of a medical school course."[16] Hollis was right: only specialized biochemists had any prospects in the new medical market. Schools like Tufts that continued to hire only biochemists with M.D. degrees found it increasingly difficult to compete.[17]

As general chemistry disappeared from course rosters, second-year courses in physiological and pathological chemistry were shifted into the first year and expanded into systematic, theoretically oriented treatments of the subject. Applied clinical biochemistry was offered as an elective in the clinical years. In the old medical college, physiological chemistry had been squeezed into the narrow space between elementary and applied chemistry; the new symbiosis with universities allowed biochemistry to expand into a full-fledged preclinical discipline, coequal with anatomy, physiology, and pathology.

Some medical chemists saw the changes taking place in their institutions as an opportunity to improve their own academic status. Some had already been picking up advanced training in physiological chemistry and had played active roles in the movement for higher admission requirements. John A. Mandel, Doremus's assistant chemist at NYU–Bellevue, had spent summers in Berlin studying physiological chemistry and translated Olof Hammarsten's famous textbook.[18] John Marshall, Dr. Theodor G. Wormsley's understudy at Pennsylvania, had a Ph.D. degree in chemistry from Tübingen in addition to an M.D. degree and postgraduate experience in physiological chemistry in Germany. He had thoroughly modern views of the role of biomedical science and, as dean, had tried hard to put these ideals to work.[19] Long's counterpart at Washington University Medical School was William H. Warren, Harvard Ph.D. chemist and industrial consultant, who had been called in to organize the new chair of chemistry and the new laboratory course in 1898. He too had acted as dean, promoting premedical science requirements and a greater role for the laboratory sciences in clinical medicine.[20] Elbert Rockwood, professor of chemistry at the Iowa Medical School, began as a chemist, studied medicine, and received a Ph.D. degree in physiological chemistry from Yale at the age of 44.[21] Many medical chemists looked forward to a gradual evolutionary change from medical to biological chemistry. They embraced progressive ideals and improved themselves, in the hope that specialization in physiological chemistry would be the avenue to academic status.

These hopes were not ill-founded. The medical chemist's role was gradually becoming more specialized, even before reform. Physiological chemistry was occupying a larger part of general chemistry courses; for example, at Harvard it was about half and half by 1900. Edward S. Wood's second-term course in "medical chemistry" was mainly devoted to urinalysis, but the list of collateral reading included textbooks by Halliburton, Hoppe-Seyler, Hammarsten, and Sheridan Lea. In 1896 it was retitled "physiological chemistry."[22] Charles Pellew's 1894 textbook was described as "true physiological chemistry," and only 61 of 284 pages were devoted to inorganic chemistry. It was quite reasonable for medical chemists to expect a gradual evolutionary improvement of their roles.

In fact, the change was not evolutionary but revolutionary. Most medical chemists did not inherit the new departments of biological chemistry. There were some exceptions, of course: Mandel retained the chair at Bellevue, as Long did at Northwestern. Abraham L. Metz was professor of chemistry and medical jurisprudence at Tulane until 1919. In most schools, however, medical chemists were displaced by a new generation of professional biochemists. Those with medical training switched to other clinical specialties. At Texas, Morris saw the handwriting on the wall: realizing that he had neither the training nor the taste for biochemistry, he vacated his chair in 1907 and retrained himself as an otorhinolaryngologist.[23] Arthur Austin returned to Tufts in 1908 as a professor of clinical medicine. Those with Ph.D. degrees in chemistry turned to industrial consulting or technical work. At California, O'Neill became a professor of technical chemistry. Charles Pellew became a consulting chemist. William Warren left Washington University to teach college chemistry and subsequently became an industrial chemist. Some medical chemists set themselves up as professional public analysts. Wood's associate professor at Harvard, William B. Hills, set up a commercial business doing urinalyses for life insurance examiners.[24]

Other medical chemists accepted lesser service roles in the new departments. At Iowa, Elbert Rockwood taught a variety of courses in toxicology, sanitary chemistry, and clinical chemistry. John Marshall was demoted and reassigned to teach general chemistry in the schools of Veterinary and Dental Medicine, where general chemistry was still part of the professional curriculum. This was a common way of dealing with tenured medical chemists whose roles had become outmoded.

Some medical chemists found a haven in academically less prestigious medical schools, where clinicians continued to favor the older style of medical chemistry. At Tufts, for example, Austin and Hollis were succeeded by a string of physician–chemists. As late as 1950 the Department of Chemistry was staffed almost exclusively with doctors of medicine, none of whom were members of the American Society of Biological Chemists. Other schools had a similar policy, apparently: the American Society of Biological Chemists took note in 1920 that in some medical schools, including grade A schools, biological chemistry was taught by individuals who were not eligible for membership in the society because they did not have a degree in biochemistry or did not publish research.[25]

Within the brief span of a decade, departments of medical chemistry in leading medical schools had been reorganized as departments of biological chemistry, staffed by a new generation of professional biochemists. Philip Shaffer looked back with amazement at the sudden enthusiasm for biochemistry after decades of neglect.[26] Chittenden marveled in 1908: "The time was, and only a few years ago, when it was a rarity to find a laboratory of physiological chemistry attached to a university. Now, such laboratories are to be seen on all sides."[27] The marvel is how thoroughly a whole generation of medical chemists was succeeded by a new generation of biological chemists and how little competition was offered by other departments with a potential stake in biochemistry, especially chemistry and physiology. It was in this brief period of rapid change that the American pattern diverged from the European pattern of dependence on organic chemistry or physiology.

There are two questions here: Why did reformers cast biological chemistry as a preclinical science rather than a collegiate premedical science? Why did they make it an independent discipline rather than a part of physiology?

BIOCHEMICAL OPTIONS

It seems to have been taken for granted that biological chemistry belonged in medical schools not colleges. The latter option was simply not seriously discussed. It was occasionally suggested that physiological chemistry was part of organic chemistry and could be made a premedical requirement: Gustav Mann, British-trained professor of physiology at Tulane, did so in 1909.[28] But no medical school gave up biological chemistry, and colleges generally made no move to capture it.

The rationale behind this division of labor is illuminated by arguments presented to the Association of American Medical Colleges in 1906 for and against giving credit for preclinical courses taken in college. There was a desperate need at the time to get more college-trained students into shrinking medical classes. Yet medical educators were clearly averse to any measure that shifted preclinical subjects from medical schools to colleges. The idea that physiology or physiological chemistry could be taught just as well in colleges was seen as a fatal precedent: why not then teach anatomy, or therapeutics, or even pathology in colleges as well, leaving medical schools only the clinical branches? This seemed to AAMC delegates to subvert everything for which they had been striving, perhaps heralding a return to the two- or three-year medical course. Reformers had fought hard for the four-year course and for expansion of the biomedical sciences in the medical curriculum. They did not want to lose these prestigious disciplines to colleges, which had done nothing to promote physiology or biochemistry. Some argued that reliance on colleges would enable the less progressive medical schools to avoid investing in facilities and professional staff in the preclinical disciplines.[29] (In fact, much of the pressure for transfer credits was coming from the poorer medical schools.)

The fundamental issue at stake was where exactly the line should be drawn between collegiate and professional training. The AAMC delegates agreed that there was a difference between "pure" chemistry or biology and the "applied" medical sciences. The first gave mental discipline, breadth, and a scientific outlook; the others imparted specific practical knowledge. Consequently, they thought that there should be a fairly strict division of labor. Basic sciences were inappropriate to the practical ends of medical schools; liberal arts colleges could not be expected to instill a single-minded purpose into their students. Frederick S. Lee, professor of physiology at Columbia, argued that the medical sciences, for purposes of medical instruction, should be treated as applied sciences:

By this I do not mean to advocate narrowness. It is true that medical anatomy, medical physiology and medical chemistry are terms which too often signify limited conceptions. But there is nothing in the phrase, "applied science," which prevents its subject matter from being treated in a broad-minded and liberal spirit....[I]n such a spirit our students of medicine should be taught the relation of the knowledge which they acquire daily to the practical needs of the practitioner. Theoretically this can be done in the college; practically it is not done there. It is reserved for the instructor in the medical school, who is constantly in the clinical atmosphere and with whom the clinical application of the scientific fact is not merely a remote obligation.[30]

There was a clear consensus in the AAMC as to which disciplines belonged in medical school and which did not. In Lee's view, human anatomy was a medical study (excepting embryology and histology); general chemistry was a pure science; physiology and physiological chemistry were borderline cases, but belonged in the medical school:

Physiological chemistry...touches at all points on pathology. It is the daily task of the physician to cope with derangements of metabolism, to deal with problems in pathological chemistry....Moreover, normal physiologic products are daily becoming more important as therapeutic agents. No course in physiological chemistry would...be complete if it did not deal with the pathological bearings of the subject. Such a presentation of the science is rare, if not altogether wanting, in other than medical schools.[31]

Bacteriology, pathology, and pharmacology, Lee felt, were unambiguously applied sciences. C. Judson Herrick, professor of zoology at Dennison College, presented a taxonomy of the sciences that agreed closely with Lee's.[32] Frederick Waite, a biologist and professor of anatomy at Western Reserve, held similar views. In short, it was the general opinion circa 1906, that physiological chemistry was an applied science and properly belonged in the medical school, not the liberal arts college.

Lee, Waite, Herrick, and others based their argument less on abstract ideals than on the current practices in colleges and medical schools. In principle, colleges could teach all the biomedical sciences but in practice, they did not. Waite took an explicitly pragmatic view: only subjects that colleges were *in fact* teaching better than the medical schools should be college subjects.[33] Because Waite had visited some 75 colleges and 40 medical schools since 1903, recruiting for Western Reserve, his statements are reliable evidence of current practice. Inorganic chemistry was universally well taught in colleges, Waite found; organic chemistry less well, but better than in most medical colleges. (He estimated that two-thirds of colleges gave a course equivalent to the AAMC standard.) Physiological chemistry, in contrast, was not a regular collegiate subject: only one in five colleges and universities without a medical school taught physiological chemistry in a way that would satisfy medical school requirements: "It is properly a technical subject and belongs in the second year of the medical school. While it can be taught in some institutions, it is inadvisable for many of the liberal arts colleges to attempt to do it."[34] Physiology, anatomy, and general bacteriology Waite thought could be divided between colleges and medical schools. In practice, however, they were already medical school subjects and they remained so.

Why then did physiological chemistry become a preclinical discipline in the medical curriculum? For three reasons: because it had traditionally been part of the medical curriculum and was taught in a way that linked it closely to pathology and therapeutics; because at a time when there was a sudden demand for physiological chemists, there were few to be found outside medical schools; and because medical reformers did not want to abandon a strategically important discipline. There was no intellectual reason why the scope of biological chemistry could not have been defined differently, as belonging to biology, or organic chemistry, or general physiology.

No principle prevented it from being split between "general" bio-chemistry in college and clinical biochemistry in medical schools, as it was in Britain. Ideals reflected current American practice. Had medical educators decided that physiological chemistry belonged in college, it would have been equivalent to deciding not to have it at all. Colleges were discouraged from teaching biological chemistry because it had always been clinically oriented. Both sides felt ambivalent about the emerging partnership between colleges and medical schools, and there was lingering mistrust. Biological chemis-try had political and symbolic significance for medical reformers at the crucial moment when its location was being decided. Posses-sion was nine-tenths of policy. The scope and style of biological chemistry were shaped by what medical chemistry had been.

The architects of the modern medical school had every reason to support biochemists' claims to equal status with physiology or pathology in class time, staff, and budgets. Physiologists and pa-thologists routinely testified to the vital importance of biochemis-try to their own disciplines. Clinicians' insistence that biological chemistry be taught by chemists with M.D. degrees testifies to their belief in its importance to clinical medicine. Deans and univer-sity presidents, glancing anxiously at what their competitors were doing, took it for granted that a full-fledged department of biologi-cal chemistry was an indispensable part of a quality medical school.

The real issue for most medical schools was where physiological chemistry belonged among the medical sciences: in independent departments, in departments of physiology, or in departments of chemistry? University leaders were not immune to the belief that German ways were best, even if they did not fit American practices. The official position of the AMA Council was that biological chemistry was a part of physiology.[35] Some physiologists did man-age to keep control of biochemistry, at least temporarily, and some biochemists saw attachment to physiology as a step up the academic pecking order from medical chemistry. Most physiologists accepted the independence of biochemistry, however, and combination with physiology remained a minor pattern in American medical schools. Chemists made no serious claim. Independent departments were the rule.

The most important reason for this distinctive pattern was again the strong tradition of medical chemistry: ideals followed practice. Medical chemistry had always been an independent department, and physiological and pathological chemistry had always been a part of medical chemistry. The departmental infrastructure, budget lines, and laboratory facilities were all in place for biological chemists to simply take over from their predecessors. Where medical chemistry was for some reason relatively weak and physiology was strong, the European pattern often prevailed. Often, this was where Europeans happened to have local influence, for example, in the case of Jacques Loeb. But in most places, medical chemistry set the pattern for the new generation.

Ironically, it was the backwardness of American medical colleges in the biomedical sciences that made possible the sudden success of biological chemistry in the 1900s. When medical chemists disappeared, biochemists took their places. The independent department was the result of the reform impulse acting upon an established, independent institution. Biochemistry did not evolve gradually out of physiology, as in Britain; it was not split between organic chemistry and physiology, as in Germany. In the United States, biological chemistry emerged like a butterfly from the cocoon of medical chemistry.

Some recurrent features of this metamorphosis are exemplified by Columbia and Harvard, two of the first to reorganize their departments of chemistry, in 1898 and 1904. The structural connection between the new college entrance requirements and the establishment of biochemistry is especially clear at P&S, where biological chemistry was established before there was an audience for it. The role of a death or resignation in providing the occasion for reorganization is a recurrent theme. So too is the vital role played by physiologists in seizing these occasions, formulating strategy, and generally acting as midwives to the new discipline. University chemists were, in contrast, not actively involved. In no case was there any serious opposition to plans for an independent department of biological chemistry. In most cases, however, there was considerable uncertainty as to exactly what the emphasis of biological chemistry should be in the medical context: pure chemistry and biology, or pathology and clinical medicine?

COLUMBIA P&S

Reorganization at P&S was precipitated by Charles Chandler's unexpected resignation in 1897 from the medical faculty.[36] John G. Curtis and T. Mitchell Prudden saw the vacancy in the chair of chemistry as a "precious opportunity" to reorganize it as a department of physiological chemistry, independent of chemistry, and with closer connections to physiology and pathology.[37] Chandler had no real interest in physiology or pathology and had apparently not been cooperative. Curtis was determined that the position not simply be filled by Pellew or some other medical chemist. He immediately invited Chittenden to make a tour of inspection and arranged for a formal committee to reconsider the role of chemistry in the medical curriculum.[38] An independent, specialized department of physiological chemistry was, for Curtis and Prudden, the strategy of choice to ensure the development of chemical physiology and pathology. Curtis hoped to entice Chittenden himself to New York:

Chittenden is the only man whose researches have given him a commanding position in this country as a master in his corner of science, and it is only such a man who should be called to a professorship at Columbia of the Chemistry of Living Matter; for these last words indicate the important fact that the work of such a Professorship is vital as furthering the work not only of Physiology and Pathology in relation to medicine, but of these sciences on their purely biological side, and of zoology and botany no less. Neither Prudden nor I could think it wise to plunge into the endless uncertainties involved in inviting over an Englishman or a German.[39]

Curtis was aware that Abel had tried and failed to get Chittenden to Johns Hopkins, and Henry Bowditch had recently complained to him of the need for better physiological chemistry at Harvard.

Lack of qualified men was not the only impediment to Curtis's plan: there was also the lack of a qualified audience. Because P&S did not yet require college work for admission, students still had to be instructed in general chemistry. It was hardly a tempting prospect for a physiological chemist, as Chittenden made plain to Curtis, and Curtis in turn to Low: "We cannot get the man we want largely because... inorganic, organic and physiological chemistry are entangled together. Would it be possible to disentangle them?"[40] Disentangling physiological from medical chemistry required that the medical college be reorganized on a graduate basis:

We are accepting students in numbers who are unfit to study medicine, and who are dropped by examination at the end of the first year, but who pay $200 each which, obviously, we can ill afford to do without. This situation retards our headway as a first class institution, like a sail towing behind a yacht.[41]

Because it was not yet possible for the university to insist on a college entrance requirement, Curtis proposed that the instruction in inorganic and organic chemistry be transferred temporarily to the university's Department of Chemistry, leaving physiological chemistry to be taught in a new department at P&S.[42] Curtis looked forward to the day, however, when inorganic chemistry would be made a prerequisite for admission.

President Low favored Curtis's plan and won the cooperation of the Department of Chemistry.[43] But the basic structural problem remained: the presence of general chemistry in the medical curriculum forced physiological chemistry into the position of an advanced specialty. Reluctantly, Curtis and Prudden accepted the fact that physiological chemistry, included by Chandler in his freshman course, would have to be shifted back to the sophomore year, replacing the required course in toxicology. The gains were clear: the vacant chair would not revert to medical chemistry for lack of a specialist to claim it; physiological chemistry could be developed separately rather than as an addendum to general chemistry; general chemistry would be taught as a pure science rather than as applied medical chemistry; a precedent would be set to make it a premedical requirement as soon as possible; and, finally, responsibility for the medical applications of chemistry was placed where Curtis felt it belonged, in the medical faculty.[44] The disadvantage was that physiological chemistry did not yet have the status of a discipline equal to physiology or pathology, as Curtis had hoped. It was structurally a substitute for toxicology, not general chemistry.

Curtis's aim was not simply to promote physiological chemistry; he saw the reorganization of chemistry as the entering wedge for further reform. His committee strongly endorsed collegiate entrance requirements: "applicants would then enter the Medical School properly to begin at once the study of Physiological Chemistry."[45] In most medical schools, the establishment of physiological chemistry followed structural reorganization; at P&S, it was a vehicle for reorganization. It was for this reason that President Low gave such strong support to Curtis's plan. Discipline building and reform politics went hand in hand.

It remained for Curtis to find an instructor in physiological chemistry, and he again turned to Chittenden. William J. Gies, who had just received his Ph.D. degree, was a capable teacher but not an experienced entrepreneur. Curtis persuaded Chittenden to commute to Columbia as part-time director to organize the department and to supervise Gies until he was ready to take charge.[46] Gies was an ambitious and energetic man and, by 1900, was attracting growing numbers of students, turning out research, and building a network of local contacts. With the occasional protection of Dean McLane in the rough and tumble of university politics, the department thrived.[47] In 1901, with Chittenden's assent, President Butler appointed Gies adjunct professor and department head.[48]

Although college chemistry was not required for admission to P&S until 1904, Chittenden began early to reinstate physiological chemistry as a first-year course. He had insisted on the right to permit students prepared in chemistry to take physiological chemistry as freshmen, and the number of freshmen qualifying for exemption increased rapidly from 1 out of 146 in 1898 to 17 out of 160 in 1899 and 20 out of 112 in the first term of 1900.[49] It was harder to make the privilege of a few into a general requirement. In 1902 the curriculum committee rejected a proposal to require chemistry for admission, and when one year of college work was required in 1903, the faculty declined to make chemistry a specific requirement. In practice, however, most entering freshmen had already taken chemistry. In January 1904, Gies reported that 50 to 60 freshmen were enrolled in physiological chemistry out of a class of 98.[50]

The ever-present pressures for economy and efficiency worked to Gies's advantage. In 1904 President Butler warned the medical faculty that freshmen with exemptions in physics and chemistry were largely wasting their first year, an inefficiency the university could ill afford, as each student now cost the university money. Gies seized the opportunity, proposing that his department take over the teaching of general chemistry, along with the requisite laboratory space and equipment. The chemists did not object, and Butler, desperate as always to balance the budget, was only too eager to go along.[51] In December 1904, the medical faculty agreed to make physics and chemistry an explicit requirement for admission as of 1907. Almost simultaneously, Gies petitioned the faculty to make physiological chemistry a freshman course, and in 1905 it finally occupied the place in the medical curriculum that general and medical chemistry had nearly a decade before. The status of Gies's department was recognized in 1907 with a new name, "Biological Chemistry."[52]

Reform ideals, professional interests, service roles and audiences, and economics were all important forces in the transition from medical to biological chemistry. At first the ideals of Curtis, McLane, and Low outstripped the curricular need for physiological chemistry and the willingness of the medical faculty to accept reform. By the early 1900s, the faculty's conception of what was possible began to lag behind the reality of the student marketplace. Audience demand and pressures for efficiency became more important than ideology. Finally, structural reorganization of the entire school gave biological chemistry full status as a biomedical department, with an assured service role in the medical curriculum.

HARVARD MEDICAL SCHOOL

At Harvard the process of innovation was less complicated by structural problems because the B.A. degree was required for admission. The prospect of an endowed chair made finance less a problem than it was at P&S, which had virtually no endowment. Politically, however, the establishment of biological chemistry at Harvard was more complicated. Physiological chemistry had been developed by the departments of chemistry and physiology for nearly a decade before reorganization. Henry Bowditch and Walter B. Cannon played midwives' roles, as Curtis had, but were decidedly interested parties. The medical chemists had the advantage of possession and felt threatened by the physiologists. The Cambridge chemists had their own ideas of what should be done. There was no Chittenden to dominate the scene, only contending rival interests.

Physiological chemistry began to evolve in the European pattern when Bowditch introduced laboratory instruction in chemical physiology in 1892. But when W. T. Porter introduced his more ambitious laboratory course in physical physiology in 1896, chemical physiology was transferred to E. S. Wood's Department of Chemistry.[53] Physiological chemistry was an attractive area for expansion for Wood, and specialized roles soon evolved. The entire second term of Wood's course was devoted to physiological and pathological chemistry. Between 1898 and 1902, a senior elective was given by pharmacologist Franz Pfaff, who was designated "instructor in pharmacology and physiological chemistry." At its height in 1903, the Department of Chemistry had no fewer than three specialized positions. Besides Wood and his associate professor, William Hills, there was an instructor in physiological chemistry, Robert L. Emerson. His assistant, Carl Lucas Alsberg, came in 1902 from two years of study in physiological chemistry and pharmacology at Strasbourg. An instructor in clincial chemistry, Henry F. Hewes, had two assistants in chemistry. All seven had M.D. degrees.[54]

The physiologists soon repented of having let physiological chemistry slip into the chemists' camp and tried unsuccessfully to reestablish a claim. In 1900 Albert P. Mathews was appointed to a new instructorship, undoubtedly intended for chemical physiology because Mathews had studied with Kossel before taking his doctorate in physiology at Columbia. In January 1901, Porter asked the faculty to move physiological chemistry to physiology but was turned down. In April 1901, Bowditch won approval for a course in "chemical physiology" to be taught by pharmacologist Waldemar Koch, but only in the graduate school.[55] Thus thwarted, Koch and Mathews left to join Loeb at Chicago. Not surprisingly, Wood and Hills resisted these incursions into their territory, and in 1902 Bowditch appealed directly to President Eliot's long-standing concern for medical reform:

> To my mind the only chemistry which a medical school ought to teach is physiological chemistry, together with a short course on toxicology. This physiological chemistry should be organized in the same department as physiology, for the reason that...about half of physiology really consists in the study of chemical phenomena. The present incumbents of the chemical department seem to feel a certain sort of jealousy of the physiologists and apparently fear that their importance in the School is likely to be diminished by effecting a closer union with the physiologists.[56]

Reorganization of the medical school had brought physiology an endowed chair, a new building, and research endowment.[57] Bowditch had both means and motive to develop chemical physiology.

Bowditch's anxiety was heightened by impending plans for the development of biological chemistry in the new medical school. A large endowment had been promised for a chair and the B.A. degree requirement made it inevitable that biological chemistry must become a full department, growing out of chemistry or replacing it. The new buildings on Longwood Avenue were nearly finished, and it was clear to everyone that the disposition of roles and laboratory space would determine how much territory each department occupied for many years. Wood obviously hoped to inherit the new chair and department, and Bowditch just as obviously hoped to prevent it. Bowditch's increasingly vocal dissatisfaction with the medical chemists reflected his fear that Wood had time on his side. The new chair had to be claimed now.

The immediate need was to remove general chemistry from the curriculum. In October 1904, a committee chaired by Eliot decided to split chemistry into two parts: physiological chemistry in the first year and clinical chemistry in the second, thus eliminating general chemistry. This plan offered an opportunity to detach Wood from physiological chemistry. Walter B. Cannon, Bowditch's young protégé, proposed to Eliot that Wood be restricted, as professor of clinical chemistry and toxicology, to teaching the second-year course and that a professor of biological chemistry be appointed at once to develop the new freshman course, with Alsberg assisting. Cannon aimed to preempt Wood's claim and establish his own department's claim to chemical physiology, and he appealed to Eliot's commitment to leadership in medical reform:

Unless there be a change, the Medical School will come prominently before the country with chemical physiology not represented, with no one to compare with Chittenden and Mendel at Yale, Gies of Columbia, Abel and Jones of Johns Hopkins, or Vaughan of Ann Arbor.... Furthermore, making a change now will probably cause less feeling than certainly will be caused if there is any attempt two or three years hence to disturb established places in the new buildings.... Unless, therefore, a man at present in the Department of Chemistry is to take in a few years the most important scientific position in the School, the reasons seem to me cogent for attempting to secure immediately the best man available for that position.[58]

If Wood were to keep his hold on the new basic course in physiological chemistry, he would have a strong claim to the new chair of biological chemistry. The physiologists' strategy was to argue, on the basis of quality and standards, that the chair be occupied at once by the "best man," that is, by a professional physiological chemist.

Bowditch backed Cannon's argument with specific suggestions as to how the salary for the new professor might be procured through imaginative use of existing endowments. As John Curtis had discovered, however, the problem was not the lack of funds but the lack of a "best man." Bowditch therefore proposed as an expedient that a physiological chemist be appointed in physiology:

As [Cannon's] plan may arouse some opposition it would perhaps be thought best to appoint a really expert physiological chemist in the department of physiology with the title of Instructor or Asst. Professor of Chemical Physiology. Such a man can be had (for less than the salary formerly paid to Dr. Hills) in the person of Dr. Folin now employed at the McLean Asylum in Waverly. This plan would have the advantage of securing at once the services of a really competent leader in research work and of giving us more time to look about for a full professor of "Biological Chemistry."[59]

Bowditch could not have been trying to attach the new department to physiology. His aim was to ensure that it would not be dominated by Wood's chemists but by specialists sympathetic to physiologists' interests. However, Eliot was apparently not willing to kick Wood upstairs.

The situation changed in the spring of 1905 when it was discovered that Wood was dying of cancer. Wood's understudy, Hills, had already left in 1904, and Carl Alsberg had an offer from Gies of an assistantship at Columbia. Dean Richardson informed Alsberg that chemistry would be completely reorganized and asked him to stay.[60] Eliot's first thought was to put the department in the hands of a pure chemist, and apparently he asked T. W. Richards to take charge. However, Charles Loring Jackson persuaded Eliot that Richards's own work was more important – and healthy – than the political turmoil of the medical school.[61] The chair of biological chemistry remained vacant, even as chemistry disintegrated. Makeshift arrangements were made. Alsberg administered the department, though still an instructor. He was assisted by Lawrence J. Henderson, who was transferred part time from the Department of Chemistry at Cambridge, where he continued to teach a course in biological chemistry.[62] A graduate of the Harvard Medical School, Henderson had just returned from two years with Hofmeister at Strasbourg.[63] In 1907 Eliot appointed Otto Folin as research associate professor of physiological chemistry, but Folin continued to work part time at the McLean Hospital.[64] The shape of the new department reflected the complicated politics and improvisations that brought it into existence. It was the work of many hands, and its exact character remained unclear.

Alsberg, Henderson, and Folin had quite different talents and styles. Henderson had done important work on the thermochemistry of organic compounds with Richards, and as a pure chemist, he found physiological chemistry lacking in organizing theories and methods. On being appointed to the medical school, he took up physicochemical studies of electrolyte balance in blood, which he thought more appropriate to a medical context. But his enthusiasm for kinetics earned him the nickname of "little k."[65] Folin, in contrast, had studied analytical and organic chemistry (with Stieglitz) and specialized in urinalysis and metabolism. Eliot's brief for him in 1907 rested on his achievements in "the practical subjects taught in the Medical School," namely nutrition, metabolism, urinalysis, clincial analytical methods, and metabolism of fever.[66] Of the three men, Folin was closest to the style of the old medical chemists. Carl Alsberg was trained in both chemistry and biology at Columbia and, according to Henderson, spoke enthusiastically for the "biological point of view." (Henderson was uncertain as to what exactly he meant.) He was eclectic in his research interests and seems to have depended on his collaborators for problems. He worked with Phoebus Levene on protein chemistry, with Henderson on acidosis, and with Folin on protein metabolism.[67]

There were also marked differences in personality and style among the three Harvard biochemists. Alsberg was New York–German–Jewish intelligentsia;[68] Henderson was Boston–Yankee intelligentsia. Both were culturally sophisticated intellectuals, with broad interests and a taste for philosophy. Henderson was always more at home in Harvard Yard than at the Medical School.[69] Folin, in contrast, had emigrated from Norway as a boy to escape a drunkard father and a life of poverty. He worked his way through the University of Chicago, was reserved, self-reliant, and had little of Henderson's or Alsberg's cultural polish. Jacques Loeb recalled:

While he was studying he had to teach chemistry in a veterinary school in Chicago in order to earn his living. . . . He had more outside work to do to earn his bread and butter than most of our students put into their own specialty. Of course the hard struggle shows somewhat in the personality of the man. He does not possess that amiable and graceful relaxation which characterizes the man of the world.[70]

Folin was unassuming, an enemy of snobbery, and completely devoted to his students and his profession. Not surprisingly, relations with his colleagues were uneasy.

Although he was officially the senior man, Folin had no official duties within the department. He recognized Alsberg's and Henderson's abilities and got them raises in salary and promotions.[71] According to Walter Bloor, who was close to Folin at the time, Alsberg and Henderson hoped to get Henderson's friend Edwin Faust appointed to the new chair and "shelve" Folin as research professor.[72] Folin had Eliot's trust, however, and was becoming more involved in medical teaching. Alsberg, meanwhile, edged himself out. He had apparently been led to believe that he was in line for a chair of pharmacology. In the fall of 1908, with an offer from the U.S. Department of Agriculture in hand, Alsberg pressed Eliot, complaining that he had had inadequate facilities and too little time for research.[73] Unperturbed, Folin told Eliot that Alsberg was a good teacher and administrator, though "extraordinarily ambitious for power" and "unusually impatient of limitations."[74] Eliot would not be bluffed, and Alsberg resigned. A week later, Folin left McLean and became full-time chief of the department.[75]

Left shorthanded by Alsberg's departure, Folin began to press Henderson to give his full efforts to the medical school, gently at first, but with increasing insistence. Henderson was unwilling to give up his attachment to Harvard College and found himself more frequently in conflict with Folin's ideas of developing biological chemistry.[76] In October 1908, Folin refused to back Henderson's promotion to instructor if he did not give up teaching biochemistry at Harvard College. This provoked an outcry from the Harvard chemists, who protested that Henderson was attracting the more thoughtful young chemists to medical careers. Henderson was a member of their inner circle. Charles Loring Jackson was one of the first to recognize the importance of Henderson's work on blood and wrote glowingly of him to Eliot as a "second Richards."[77] Jackson and Richards saw Henderson as the herald of progressive biological chemistry in the medical school and almost certainly considered Folin's work on urinalysis and metabolism as simply more of the old medical chemistry.[78] They had pointedly ignored him ever since his arrival in Boston in 1902.[79] Folin agreed to withdraw his objection for that fall but made it clear to Eliot that he expected Henderson's "complete withdrawal from Cambridge after this year."[80] Eliot did not interfere.

In 1909 Folin was appointed Hamilton Kuhn Professor of Biological Chemistry. Henderson was deeply disappointed; he did not resign but stayed away, in part to let Folin organize the department in his own way and in part because Folin's way was just not his: "All my Medical School teaching became irksome and...the long hours of teaching elementary, routine biological chemistry in the laboratory came to seem an intolerable waste of time."[81] Henderson spent more and more of his time at Harvard College, where he taught biological chemistry and the history of science and ultimately became involved in general physiology, industrial physiology, and social theory. By 1915 Folin had made the Department of Biological Chemistry into a flourishing and influential school, with a strong emphasis on analytical methods and clinical applications.

Why did Folin's conception of biochemistry prevail over the alternatives? Chance events and personalities should not obscure the underlying structural reasons. Folin's conception of biochemistry was most in keeping with the actual needs of the medical school. Walter Bloor pointed to Folin's unexpected success as a medical teacher: this was probably crucial. Folin was a productive researcher and his interests were highly relevant to physiology and clinical medicine. Eliot clearly saw him as the best fitted to lead a medical department, and the Cambridge chemists had no real leverage in medical affairs. Wood was thus succeeded by the man who most resembled the old medical chemists.

VARIATIONS ON A THEME

Elsewhere, the transition from medical to biological chemistry was not complicated by the presence of so many talented and ambitious men. But the sequence of events was the same in most schools: gradual evolution of specialized roles within medical chemistry; structural reorganization and disappearance of general chemistry; rapid replacement of medical chemists by biological chemists. The pattern is clearest at Pennsylvania and Washington University.

John Marshall's Department of Chemistry at Penn cultivated physiological chemistry well before the 1910 putsch brought in Alonzo Taylor. A specialized role for a demonstrator of physiological chemistry was created in 1903, when Marshall appointed Philip B. Hawk, a student of Chittenden's and the first graduate of Gies's school (Ph.D., 1903). Like Gies, Hawk was an ambitious and energetic promoter of his profession. While at Penn, he wrote his *Laboratory Manual of Physiological Chemistry*, based on Chittenden's course at Yale. (Chittenden and Mendel's custom was to give verbal directions; but Hawk discovered that the shorter laboratory time allotted to physiological chemistry at Penn made brief written directions a necessity.[82]) Hawk's was probably the most popular of the various manuals then available, as its 13 editions attest. It gave teachers access to a packaged, high-quality, modern course. Hawk was succeeded in 1907 by William Welker, also a Gies disciple.

Even before general chemistry was officially required for admission to the medical school in 1908, Marshall was devoting more money (and presumably more time) to physiological chemistry than to general chemistry. His budget for inorganic chemistry between 1905 and 1908 was $550 per annum, whereas the budget for physiological chemistry was $950 from 1905 to 1907 and $1350 from 1907 to 1908.[83] Marshall had the title of the department changed to the Department of Physiological Chemistry and Toxicology in anticipation of the new entrance requirement and his new specialized role.

To the reformers, however, Marshall represented the old medical chemistry, and in 1910 he was abruptly informed by Provost Harrison that because chemistry had become a premedical course his services were no longer needed for teaching medical students. Marshall was demoted to associate professor and transferred to the Schools of Veterinary and Dental Medicine, where freshmen still needed to be taught elementary chemistry.[84] An anonymous benefactor endowed a new chair of physiological chemistry in the medical school, and a new department was created to give the new Rush Professor, Alonzo Taylor, a free hand to organize his own staff and research program. Marshall's displacement by Taylor was in part a symbolic act: he was demoted not because of what he did but because of what he was. Reform and progress required a new generation of specialists with the correct credentials and a demonstrated commitment to modern lines of research.

A similar story unfolded at Washington University. There too physiological chemistry was developed as a subspecialty by chemist William Warren. In 1907 physiological chemistry was included in the department title. When the six-year B.A.–M.D. program was introduced in 1909, a full-year course in physiological chemistry was introduced for the freshman year.[85] Warren had been active in the reform movement and had served as dean in the critical years from 1908 to 1911 when the medical faculty was reconstituted. He did not enjoy the fruits of his labors, however. When the decision was made in 1910 to organize a department of biological chemistry and to bring in a trained biochemist, Warren's role was restricted to teaching organic chemistry; it was made clear that he was not a candidate for the chair.[86] In 1911, after a trying year, he secured a job teaching chemistry at Clark University. Warren's trials can be readily imagined, given his awkward situation as a rejected, lame-duck professor. As he wrote his successor, Philip Shaffer:

You will understand, I think, what my state of mind is when I say that I wish to forget that the year 1910–1911 was ever a point of time so far as I was concerned. . . . I am thankful for your efforts in my behalf, though I am more than glad that they proved unavailing. . . . In brief, back to pure chemistry is the sum of it all. I cannot tell you how glad I am that it is so.[87]

Warren's credentials as a chemist (a Ph.D. degree from Harvard) and his background in industrial work had been ideal for the role of medical chemist in 1898 but not for a biological chemist in 1910. He was not a specialist and had no medical training, a lack he himself admitted to be a handicap for a teacher in a medical school.[88] His successor had both.

The selection of a biological chemist was left to the new faculty: John Howland (pediatrics), Eugene Opie (pathology), George Dock (medicine), and Joseph Erlanger (physiology). There was a range of options: organic chemists, physiological or clinical chemists, even pharmacologists. The list of candidates included Carl Alsberg and Walter Jones; Folin and his protégé, Philip Shaffer; Henry Dakin, British-trained organic chemist and assistant to Christian Herter; Joseph Kastle, professor of organic chemistry at Virginia; and Arthur S. Loevenhart, formerly Abel's assistant and professor of pharmacology at Wisconsin.[89]

The choice was between a bioorganic chemist and an analytical chemist with interests in clinical applications. The original plan to combine physiological chemistry and pharmacology favored Kastle or Loevenhart, but when it was decided to have two separate departments, the balance swung toward Folin. Physiologist Joseph Erlanger continued to favor Kastle or Loevenhart, but Opie and Howland favored a clinical biochemist, and with Dock's aid, their counsel prevailed. When Folin declined the chair, Brookings offered

Shaffer a post as pathological chemist in the hospital (perhaps because of his lack of teaching experience). Shaffer declined, and Brookings then offered him the chair.[90] The faculty's main concern was that the new man should cooperate closely with pathologists and clinicians.[91] Walter Jones, a more experienced teacher than Shaffer, was rejected because his narrow interests would "...not bring him into close relation with the other departments."[92] Kastle was rejected for similar reasons. As at Harvard, the choice fell on a man who resembled most closely the medical chemist he displaced. This was true of many schools that reorganized after 1910.

The succession of generations was not always so abrupt. Where the medical chemist was too weighty a presence to be thrust aside, there was a more continuous development from medical to biological chemistry. The Cornell Medical School is a good example of this evolutionary pattern. Soon after the founding of the school, Rudolph Witthaus began to expand physiological chemistry in the curriculum, adapting to the new collegiate entrance requirement. The freshman course in inorganic chemistry continued to be given for students who had not had general chemistry, but extra lectures were added in urinalysis and toxicology. By 1901 physiological chemistry and toxicology occupied 11 weeks of the second-year course in medical chemistry.[93] Specialized roles for physiological chemistry did not evolve, however. Witthaus taught physiological chemistry himself, and the emphasis of the department remained on basic chemistry. When general chemistry became a required premedical course in 1909, Witthaus did not shift physiological chemistry into the freshman year but taught organic chemistry instead. The curriculum in 1909 consisted of 131 hours of organic and only 99 hours of physiological chemistry.[94]

A variety of biological chemistry more relevant to physiology and pathology was meanwhile being developed in the Loomis Laboratory. There an active group consisting of Philip Shaffer, pathologist James Ewing, pharmacologist Robert A. Hatcher, physiologists Graham Lusk and John Murlin, and Silas Beebe (therapeutics) collaborated on problems of chemical pathology and metabolism. But it remained an informal research group. Witthaus held a tight grip on the teaching of physiological chemistry, and in his hands, it was strongly oriented to his own interest in toxicology and forensic medicine. The administration was unwilling (or unable) to force Witthaus into early retirement. Biding their time, the

Loomis group and Dean Schurman laid the ground for Shaffer to succeed Witthaus when the chemist retired in 1911. Witthaus's understudy, C. G. L. Wolf, was informed by the dean that he had no chance of being considered as Witthaus's successor, and he obligingly resigned.[95]

Plans for reorganizing the Department of Chemistry were dashed by Shaffer's acceptance of the post at Saint Louis in 1910.[96] Shaffer's place was taken by Stanley Benedict, a Mendel protégé (1909), and Gies's chief assistant at P&S. Hatcher and Lusk tried to tempt Shaffer back when Witthaus retired in 1911. Lusk wrote him that there was no longer any impediment to completely changing the courses in chemistry.[97] When Shaffer decided he could not desert Washington University, Benedict was given temporary charge of the Department of Chemistry and in 1912, having proved himself, was appointed to the chair. The shape of the department did not immediately change. Benedict himself was primarily an analytical chemist, and not until 1919 was physiological chemistry made a "major subject" equal to organic chemistry in the medical curriculum.[98]

In nearly every case so far, physiologists and pathologists were the leading antagonists of medical chemistry. The decision to reorganize biological chemistry usually came from higher up, from university presidents who wanted modern research men and saw the connection between specialization and medical reform. But it was the preclinical men who decided what biological chemistry would be in practice. In most cases, they selected biological chemists whose work was relevant to physiology or pathology. Their role was not disinterested but neither was it self-serving. They did not want to expand their own territory; rather, they wanted to establish a friendly neighboring discipline with which they could carry on a mutually profitable exchange of ideas and competences. In most cases, their interest was better served by a strong and independent department of biological chemistry within the medical school than by reliance on university chemists.

A DEVIANT MODE: PHYSIOLOGY

In some cases, however, biological chemistry was more intimately attached to physiology or pathology in the European manner. This was a deviant pattern, in the sense that it grew out of special local circumstances rather than the systemic characteristics of American medical schools. There was often a European physiologist directly involved, Jacques Loeb most notably, but others too. Economy was often the main motive for a combined department in smaller schools. This pattern was also prevalent in the two-year preclinical courses of state universities, where there was no tradition of medical chemistry and where the clinical departments were not a strong presence.

The departments at Chicago and the University of California, both founded by Jacques Loeb, typify this Euro–American mode. At Berkeley, Edmond O'Neill had been teaching organic and physiological chemistry to medical freshmen since the mid-1890s.[99] In 1902, however, O'Neill was restricted to organic chemistry, to give Loeb room for expansion in physiological chemistry. Loeb had his eye on Phoebus Levene, Kastle, and Loevenhart: men trained in bioorganic chemistry.[100] Loeb's conception of physiological chemistry was distinctly European.

Loeb's plans failed to materialize. Loeb had been brought to Berkeley on the understanding that he would not have to teach medical students, and his purist ideals cost him a crucial resource for expanding his discipline. Physiology remained part of the separate preclinical program at Berkeley. President Wheeler backed Loeb but was hard pressed just to keep the new biomedical departments afloat and seized every opportunity to cut nonessentials. Without a service role in medical instruction, physiological chemistry was easily regarded as such a luxury. Loeb did not push aggressively to get a physiological chemist. His tendency was to want the best, and when the best did not come forward, to want no one. Alonzo Taylor was more active in trying to recruit a chemist. In 1903 he took the initiative in pressing Wheeler to appoint Arthur Lachmann, professor of organic chemistry at the University of Oregon: "He has a fine training in organic chemistry and it is from that line that the best new physiological chemists have come."[101] Loeb agreed. Wheeler was sympathetic but was not inclined to press his luck with the regents.[102] European ideals did not make up for the lack of vital service roles.

From 1902 to 1906, physiological chemistry as such was not part of the medical curriculum. The medical students in San Francisco were instructed in general and medical chemistry by Franklin T. Green, city chemist and professor of chemistry at the School of Pharmacy. At Berkeley, Loeb taught an advanced course in "chemical biology," advising his students that it was general physiology not biological chemistry. Taylor gave a course in chemical pathology that included a good deal of physiological chemistry. The chemists made no effort to develop biological chemistry. O'Neill was neither an aggressive nor, it seems, a very effective entrepreneur: under his direction, the College of Chemistry was failing to keep up even in the more central chemical specialties.[103] Biological chemistry was done everywhere and nowhere – precisely as it was in Germany.

The situation changed dramatically in 1905 when the first class prepared in general chemistry entered the medical school. Loeb at once proposed to Wheeler that Green be replaced by a physiological chemist:

The change in the prerequisites for the medical students renders the work of Mr. Greene [sic] unnecessary. On the other hand, our medical students have thus far not received the slightest instruction in physiological chemistry and Taylor complains bitterly that this condition of affairs makes his course in pathological chemistry unintelligible to the students. I think we can no longer avoid the issue of appointing a man...in physiological chemistry.[104]

Taylor considered Green unqualified to teach such a course, and Loeb noted his lack of publications. The problem was that Green's salary was only $600, and a specialist in biochemistry would cost $2,400. A simple substitution was out of the question. Loeb and Taylor therefore proposed a less simple swap. There were plenty of young doctors of medicine available who would be glad to teach morphological pathology and dissection for $600. Hire one to relieve Taylor of that responsibility and allow Taylor to teach a new course in physiological chemistry in addition to pathological chemistry.[105] This scheme suited Taylor very well. His main interest had always been chemical pathology, and recently he had become interested in the enzymatic synthesis of proteins and the role of enzymes generally in cell metabolism.[106] Taylor taught pathological anatomy with diminishing enthusiasm and almost totally neglected autopsy work. He was becoming a biochemist and was eager to make his formal duties more congruent with his research interests. He made the right appeal: no university president could resist higher quality at no extra cost. Wheeler approved the scheme, and from 1906 to 1910, physiological chemistry was part of the Department of Pathology.

Politically, the arrangement was unstable. Taylor was still officially responsible for all of pathology, and his medical colleagues finally rebelled at Taylor's neglect of morphological pathology and autopsy. Dean D'Ancona brought their complaints to Wheeler. Taylor was then at Upsala, working with Svante Arrhenius, and was in no mood to abandon his work on enzymatic synthesis of proteins. He replied to Dean D'Ancona's attack with a spirited defense of chemical pathology,[107] but Wheeler agreed with D'Ancona that Taylor must choose one role or the other. In 1909 he releasd Taylor's part-time proxy in pathological anatomy and appointed a bright young instructor of medicine, with strong training and interests in chemical pathology.[108] Taylor acquiesced unhappily in what he guessed was Wheeler's intent: namely, that he drop his course in chemical physiology and resume teaching morphological pathology.[109] Wheeler assured Taylor that he did not intend to force him either way but left no doubt that he must choose to be either a pathologist or a biochemist, not both.[110]

It is not clear exactly what Wheeler's intention was. Taylor assumed he was being invited to organize a department of physiological and pathological chemistry on the Strasbourg model.[111] Wheeler might well have agreed to a new chair and department if Taylor and Loeb had pressed him hard. But he never mentioned this possibility and was no doubt hoping that he would not be pressed and that chemical physiology would continue to be taught by a part-time physician. The division between the clinicians and the Berkeley biomedical group made Taylor's improvised claim to physiological chemistry politically (though not intellectually) untenable. The institutional imperatives of medical schools favored distinct disciplines based on essential service roles in medical instruction. Without an indispensable service role, the Berkeley group had no rationale to develop biochemistry, however essential it was to their research programs. It was financially and politically advantageous for university administrators to use low-paid medical instructors to teach medical biochemistry. As an overhead on physiology or pathology, biochemistry almost inevitably had a weak claim to limited resources, just as in Europe. Perhaps Taylor perceived this, for a few months later he accepted David Edsall's offer of the chair at his alma mater.[112] Loeb too was growing restless, chafing at the medical yoke. He flirted with offers from Columbia and several European universities and, finally in 1910, accepted Simon Flexner's invitation to the Rockefeller Institute. Physiological chemistry remained a minor subdivision of physiology until 1915. European vision and European arrangements resulted in the same problems for discipline builders in Berkeley or Berlin.

Loeb's disciples played a role in establishing chemical physiology at the universities of Cincinnati and Minneapolis, and the pattern of events was much the same. The transition from medical to biological chemistry began at Cincinnati in the familiar way, when the professor of medical chemistry, William H. Crane, M.D., retired in 1909. In anticipation of a collegiate entrance requirement, the university's Department of Chemistry took over general chemistry, and Crane's understudy, Edward B. Reemelin (M.D., 1904) was made assistant professor of chemistry and physiological chemistry. This pattern was interrupted in 1910 when Martin Fischer, Loeb's second in command at California, was appointed to the chair of physiology. Physiological chemistry was then absorbed into physiology and remained there until it emerged as a separate department around 1918 under Albert P. Mathews, Loeb's former colleague at Chicago.[113]

At the University of Minnesota, Richard Beard included physiological chemistry in his course in physiology but did not institute a separate role for a physiological chemist.[114] This European pattern survived the reorganization of the medical school and the introduction of a college entrance requirement. For three years Beard himself continued to teach physiological chemistry. In 1913, however, Beard was ousted from the chair to make way for Elias P. Lyon, formerly Loeb's chief assistant at Rush.[115] Two instructors (both students of Folin's) were appointed to teach the medical school course in physiological chemistry; Lyon himself taught chemical biology. He made an unsuccessful attempt in 1919 to locate a professor of general biochemistry but failed to pursue this lead, probably owing to his increasing responsibilities as dean.[116] Neglected by Lyon, lacking a professor, and without an independent institutional basis, physiological chemistry at Minnesota steadily eroded until finally it was a scandal both in the university and in the profession.[117] In Europe, this syndrome was too familiar to raise many eyebrows; in America, it was exceptional.

In some cases, Europeans were directly involved in combining physiology and physiological chemistry. At Cornell (Ithaca), physiological chemistry had been taught by the Department of Chemistry since the late 1890s, and in 1903 William Orndorff was appointed to a chair of organic and physiological chemistry.[118] It was anticipated that many students would take their preclinical years at Ithaca and then transfer to New York. However, most students preferred to take all four years in New York, and the medical program at Ithaca was gradually absorbed by chemistry and biology. In 1908 Orndorff's chair was split: he was restricted to organic chemistry, and physiological chemistry was transferred to the reorganized Department of Physiology. The British physiologist, Andrew Hunter, was imported to take charge. A. E. Schäffer, who was visiting professor of physiology at Cornell in 1907/08, was behind this change of policy. Both Hunter and Sutherland Simpson, who was appointed professor of physiology in 1908, were Schäffer's students, and Orndorff told Abel that they had both been appointed at Schäffer's instigation.[119] Hunter was succeeded in 1914 by biochemist James B. Sumner, a student of Folin's, but Sumner was never able to advance beyond second fiddle in an ensemble dominated by chemists and physiologists.[120]

Western Reserve's Medical School also came under British influence. When Professor of Medical Chemistry Perry L. Hobbs retired in 1903, it was decided to combine physiological chemistry with the chair of physiology, which had also become vacant. The retiring physiologist, George N. Stewart, was a Canadian trained at Edinburgh (M.D., 1890), and he selected as his successor John J. McLeod, a chemical physiologist at the London Hospital. The British combination of physiology and physiological chemistry did not outlast McLeod's presence at Western Reserve. When he left the United States in 1918, physiological chemistry was taken over by Folin's star pupil, Cyrus Fiske.[121]

Variations on this pattern occurred in several other medical schools: at Virginia, chemists and physiologists had a seesaw rivalry over physiological chemistry from 1906 to 1924.[122] At Wisconsin, where a two-year preclinical program was dwarfed by the large and flourishing school of biochemistry in the Agricultural College, physiological chemistry was combined with physiology until 1921.[123] But even in cases such as these, American biochemists experienced far less difficulty than Europeans did in separating from physiology. In Germany and Britain, the battle for independence dominated the history of biochemistry between 1910 and 1940. In the United States, it was a local aberration. Independent departments were the rule, and dual departments were regarded as compromises with the highest standards of medical instruction.

CONCLUSION

The establishment of independent departments of biochemistry was as swift and thorough as the reform movement that made it possible. In 1909 no fewer than 60 out of 97 medical schools surveyed by the AMA offered courses in physiological chemistry. Only four were reported as being part of a course in physiology. Of the 37 schools that did not offer a course in biochemistry, most were small proprietary colleges that soon foundered in the waves created by the Flexner Report. The rest (Fordham, Louisville, Tulane, Buffalo, Jefferson, and Marquette) established programs and departments within a few years.[124] Some of the courses reported to the AMA as "physiological chemistry" were no doubt courses in medical chemistry, but evidence suggests that good intentions soon became reality. The University of Pennsylvania surveyed 58 leading medical schools in 1911 and concluded that 23 gave biochemistry courses that were comparable to the course given by Alonzo Taylor – a very high standard.[125] Systematically organized pressures for a college entrance requirement and standardized curriculum, the scrutiny of the *JAMA* muckrakers, and the escalating demands of state licensing boards made an independent department of biological chemistry virtually a necessity for every medical school.

The distinctive shape and quality of biological chemistry in America was the result of European ideals and reform zeal acting upon the structure and traditions of the proprietary medical college. The independence of medical colleges from universities and the absence of academic prerequisites gave medical chemists an indispensable role and an independent claim on resources. The same circumstances offered relatively few opportunities for professional physiologists. When reform came, physiologists were in no position to co-opt biochemistry. Reformers' zeal for high academic standards was translated into improved, specialized, and independent departments of biological chemistry. Those same reform ideals, acting in the context of British medical institutions, resulted in specialized subdepartments of physiological chemistry within physiology. In America, biological chemists stepped easily into the roles of the old medical chemists, and these roles shaped their discipline.

The claim of biological chemists to academic status and resources rested primarily on their service role in teaching first-year medical students. American biochemists' research interests were more strongly oriented toward clinical analysis than Europeans' and less toward general physiology. There was no equivalent in America to Hopkins's school. The revolutions of the reform period should not blind us to important continuities: the character of American biochemistry reflected more of the old medical chemistry than the young Turks might have cared to admit.

All this is not to say that there were no real options for discipline builders. There were options, and variant department styles are the rare survivors of what might have been, if not a wholly different system, at least a more varied one. If the academic reform impulse had operated within a more advanced academic system, where the biomedical disciplines were stronger and medical chemistry less entrenched, the European pattern could well have prevailed, and physiologists could have been less midwives and more possessive guardians. Johns Hopkins, Harvard, Berkeley, and Cornell (Ithaca) remind one of European patterns. Had universities been more aggressive in laying claim to biochemistry, could it not have resembled general physiology more than clinical chemistry? Chittenden's school at Yale is just such a case. If the reform impulse had had more of the practical ideals of the old medical college and less of the dazzled idealism of European scientific medicine, what was there to prevent more medical chemists from inheriting new departments, as they did at Tulane and NYU? Could not biochemistry have evolved out of medical chemistry as a combination of organic chemistry and applied chemical pathology? The varieties of biochemistry that emerged at some large teaching schools, like Tufts, Northwestern, or Jefferson Medical College, adumbrate what might have been a system like the London Hospital Schools. Some of these alternative styles will be discussed in later chapters. The point here is that in the American system they were minor variants of a discipline that was shaped by the distinctive structure of the American medical college and the special qualities of the medical reform movement in America.

8

Unity in diversity: the American Society of Biological Chemists

By 1920 departments of biological chemistry were established in most American medical schools. They were equal in status with the older biomedical disciplines and had an equal claim on student time and university resources. Europe had the superstars, but in the United States, even the average medical schools had good facilities and resources for research. Philip Shaffer's ideal in 1915 was a permanent staff of four and a budget of $14,000, including $4,000 for teaching and research.[1] In 1920 Alonzo Taylor had two assistant professors and a budget of $19,650,[2] and a similar plan was proposed by Columbia to the General Education Board.[3] Folin's staff included an associate and an assistant professor, an instructor, and three teaching assistants; his budget was about $16,000, including $4,400 for expenses.[4] Folin eschewed the older pattern of one professor with a retinue of student assistants and technicians. Each professor developed his own line of research and shared equally in training graduate students.[5] In size and general policy, these were typical of the leading departments circa 1920.

The best standard department was a complex institution. In addition to teaching 70 to 120 medical students, Folin's staff managed five to seven doctoral candidates per year, one or two foreign researchers, and two or three advanced medical students. About ten physicians spent a month or so each year on research projects, and Folin kept close contacts with local hospitals. Philip Shaffer gave Abraham Flexner a picture of the typical functions of a department of biological chemistry:

(a) teaching physiological chemistry to medical students, the main course being given (usually) in the first year, and which should be followed by a shorter course in the third or fourth year; (b) the conduct of laboratories in the hospitals for the more extended or difficult chemical examinations and for research (in cooperation with clinical departments) upon the clinical aspects of disease (blood chemistry, metabolism ward, respiratory exchange); (c) giving instruction (preferably individual in character rather than formal courses) to graduate students who are candidates for higher degrees, and contact with University departments outside the medical school. Perhaps there should be added also, provision for instruction in chemical hygiene, now almost universally neglected.[6]

Departments differed in their emphasis on these varied functions: some were almost exclusively devoted to teaching medical students, such as Tufts or Northwestern.[7] A. P. Mathews and Thornburn Robertson emphasized research and graduate training. W. J. Gies cultivated relations with chemists and biologists, whereas Folin and Shaffer developed a symbiotic relation to hospital clinics. But these were variations within a single institutional form.

By 1920 there was little controversy over the substance of the standard course in biological chemistry. Reformers worried about such minor issues as variability in the number of hours (from 128 at Columbia to 297 at Johns Hopkins) and uniformity of scheduling.[8] The typical course of 75 to 80 lecture hours consisted of 15 hours of basic quantitative and physical chemistry, 18 hours on the chemistry of the fats, proteins, and carbohydrates, 30 hours on metabolism and the chemistry of urine, and 12 hours on special problems in chemical physiology and pathology (inorganic metabolism, acid–base balance, secretions, and colloidal chemistry). Emphasis was on fundamental principles rather than clinical applications; laboratory sessions focused on basic analytical procedures and normal metabolism and urinalysis, rather than on examination of pathological materials. The relevance of basic principles to clinical work was constantly invoked, however. In 1920 an American Society of Biological Chemists (ASBC) committee suggested alternating lectures on basic chemistry and on applications to pathology in order to hold students' attention.[9]

Textbooks too achieved a more or less standard form by 1920. The old textbooks of medical chemistry rapidly lost their markets to more specialized texts after about 1910. Laboratory manuals like Philip Hawk's, which gave extensive coverage to the physiology of digestive enzymes, urinalysis, and metabolism, proliferated; European handbooks of physiological chemistry seem to have enjoyed an expanding market. The first American textbook was Albert Mathews's, published in 1915. Like virtually every such text, it was written for medical students; but Mathews also aimed "... to arouse interest in the subject, to stimulate curiosity and inquiry." His personal asides, historical diversions, and occasionally lively style irritated some of Mathews's colleagues, but they apparently appealed to students, and the book went through six editions.[10] Other textbooks by American authors did not appear until the 1930s.

CONSOLIDATING A DISCIPLINE

Increasing standardization was symptomatic of the "professionalization" of biochemistry. Standardization was the banner of the medical reform movement, as it was of other social movements in the Progressive era. A heterogeneous system of medical certification was reduced to uniform national standards. Biomedical disciplines likewise became more homogeneous as standard licensing examinations defined least common denominators of expertise. New journals and professional societies and insistence on specialized credentials sharpened disciplinary boundaries and made poaching more difficult.

Prior to the foundation of specialized departments, journals, and societies, biochemistry was practiced by individuals whose first loyalty was to chemistry, physiology, pathology, or clinical medicine. Because medical chemistry was so narrowly conceived, much of the best biochemistry was done under the aegis of other disciplines. This particular kind of disciplinary diversity presented a tactical problem for avant-garde biochemists: how to unite these varied interests and not lose control to better-established disciplines. Biochemists were also becoming occupationally more diverse. Most nineteenth-century biochemists were academics; between 1905 and 1915, however, nonacademic institutions began to create roles for professional biochemists. Hospitals, medical research institutes, industrial research and development laboratories, government regulatory agencies, and expert commissions all offered opportunities for research careers. This range of occupational roles provided opportunities for discipline builders to broaden their political base. Consolidation of occupationally diverse groups was the strategy of choice for coping with disciplinary competition. Specialized departments, journals, and societies eroded disciplinary diversity by making it more difficult for pure physiologists and chemists to practice biochemistry. Recognition of specialized credentials by employers ensured a protected market for biochemists. Physiologists, chemists, and clinicians, who had been insiders, became external allies; different disciplinary approaches were internalized as biochemical specialties.

Consolidation of diverse biochemical interests countered the threat of co-optation and division inherent in nineteenth-century biochemical institutions. Founders of journals and societies sought alliances with every conceivable constituency. They took care to include representatives of every discipline and of all the applied branches of nutritional, agricultural, and clinical biochemistry. They sought the broadest possible range of research papers for the new journals. The idea was to unite biochemists in a variety of institutional contexts, to win the support of physiologists, clinicians, chemists, and others who were practicing biochemistry without a license, and to maintain the controlling hand.

The sudden popularity of the name "biochemistry" ("biological chemistry" was the preferred American variant) between 1900 and 1910 was part of the strategy of consolidation. No discipline had so many aliases as biochemistry did prior to 1900: animal or zoo-chemistry, phyto- and cytochemistry, physiological, pathological, medical and immunochemistry. William Gies complained that its ambiguous names impeded public recognition of biochemistry as a distinct profession.[11] Perhaps so: certainly the profusion of names was symptomatic of the diverse and disconnected disciplinary contexts in which biochemistry was practiced. Adoption of the terms "biochemistry" or "biological chemistry" was no mere fad but a strategy for discipline building. It signified a break from the traditional dependence of "physiological chemistry" on a single constituency, physiology. "Biochemical" journals and societies staked out a claim to a larger piece of intellectual turf, covering many disciplines. "Biochemical" departments proclaimed their relevance to basic chemistry and biology and a host of agricultural and biomedical fields.

Many of the half-dozen new biochemical journals that appeared between 1900 and 1910 flew the banner of multidisciplinarity at their mastheads.[12] Benjamin Moore organized the *Biochemical Journal* in 1906 as a vehicle for his eclectic biological researches, after John Langley balked at taking them for the *Journal of Physiology*. Christian Herter's policy as editor of the *Journal of Biological Chemistry* (founded 1905) was to publish papers in all the biomedical sciences.[13] The idea was not merely to increase subscriptions: broad-based journals were also a means for uniting a highly diverse discipline. Christian Herter made this point explicitly when he argued that the *JBC* should publish the transactions of the newly established society. Whereas some members feared that Herter was trying to influence society policy, Herter saw it as ". . . simply one further step in the direction of consolidating the biochemical interests here."[14]

Changes in the name of departments were likewise intended to convey the idea of a broadly ecumenical discipline that was not just a handmaiden to medicine. This was Howard B. Lewis's rationale for changing the name of the Michigan department in 1935 from physiological to biological chemistry: "Since we are a university department and are training students from all over the campus, many of them being graduate students in botany and zoology, the use of the term, Physiological Chemistry, emphasized too much the aspect of nutrition and medicine."[15] (A few of Lewis's colleagues balked, but university administrators solidly supported the change in name.) For many biochemists, the term "physiological chemistry" was a disagreeable reminder of their former subservience to physiology and medicine.[16] Adoption of the name "biochemistry" symbolized the strategy of consolidation.

Organizing professional societies was the most overt political means of consolidating biochemical interests. The Biochemical Society was organized by a group of London biochemists in 1911 to strengthen the occupational position of biochemists in botany, agriculture, the brewing industry, medicine, pathology, and public health. A closer union of plant and animal biochemists was of particular concern to the founders, and meetings of the peripatetic society were held at breweries, hospitals, and agricultural stations, as well as universities.[17] The same strategy was used by Abel and Geis in organizing the American Society of Biological Chemists in 1906–7.

The founders of the ASBC appear to have sensed that biochemistry was already being recognized by employers as an occupational specialty and that the time was ripe for insiders to organize institutions to protect and expand their interests. Carl Alsberg wrote, somewhat cynically perhaps:

Whatever the preamble of the Constitution of the Society of Biological Chemists, the real motive for the formation of the Society was trade-unionism pure and simple. The object was and is, to gain recognition for bio-chemistry in Medical Faculties and to drive from chairs on these Faculties men unqualified to fill them. To a considerable degree both objects have been attained; and bio-chemistry has in consequence been greatly elevated. The other types of bio-chemists [other than "mammal physiological chemists"] ought to profit as much by organization and they certainly furnish as good a field for similar missionary work.[18]

At the time (1910), Alsberg was lobbying for a division of biological chemistry in the American Chemical Society, to organize biochemists working in chemistry, microbiology, and agriculture. This was precisely the kind of competition that the ASBC leaders sought to preempt.

FOUNDING A SOCIETY

The principal organizers of the *JBC* and the ASBC were not themselves biochemists, and their aims were not simply those of "trade-unionism." Christian Herter, the founder, editor, and financial backer of the *Journal*, was a physician and pathologist, who devoted his independent fortune to the pursuit of medical research. His private laboratory at 819 Madison Avenue in New York produced nearly one-fifth of the articles in the first few volumes of the *JBC*. Closely associated with the Rockefeller Institute circle, Herter shared the ideals of a cultivated, civic-minded, upper-middle-class elite for whom consolidation of interests was a familiar strategy of social reform.[19]

John J. Abel, who took the lead in organizing the ASBC, was likewise active in a variety of reform projects. He was drawn into the Saltpeter Commission, a body of academic experts appointed by the new Food and Drug Bureau to investigate chemical preservatives in meat products. Abel was well aware of the public visibility and status that organization and public service brought to academic biochemistry.[20] He hoped that the temporary commission, centered at the University of Illinois, might evolve into a permanent research institute for "animal chemistry, bio-chemistry or whatever you choose to call it" endowed by the great meat-packing families:

Rockefeller was induced to see the need of long continued, patient research in the field of infectious diseases. . . . I believe that the great captains of the meat industry could be made likewise to see the enormous role that chemistry, physics, and physical-chemistry are bound to play in the details of their industry . . . and hence in the welfare of our population. You will see that I am an enthusiast on this subject.[21]

Abel hoped that a central institute would stimulate and guide a discipline that had been allowed to develop in a haphazard way. Nothing came of Abel's scheme, but it exemplifies the spirit of an age that had great faith in large-scale organizations and expertise.

As an outsider, Abel was not overly concerned with keeping biochemists in control of a society composed of diverse specialists. William Gies, who shared Abel's enthusiasm for consolidating interests, was much more alert to the problem. In 1899 he had organized the Society of Physiological Chemists of New York City and had already begun to think of consolidation on a national scale.[22] In 1905 he organized a biochemical section of the American Chemical Society, as a preliminary step toward a separate national society.[23] In December 1905, he and Abel planned a meeting, in conjunction with the annual meeting of the Physiological Society, to organize a separate society. Gies feared that physiologists and chemists would want to squash a separate biochemical society. Whereas Abel was inclined to accommodate, Gies urged him to take a strong stand for a separate organization:

I prefer an independent society and will be satisfied with nothing less. I am no more in favor of asking the American Physiological Society to give us a section than I am of asking the same of the American Chemical Society. It would perhaps be more reasonable to ask it of the latter society, for it has already taken steps to organize a permanent biochemical section. But I don't see the point in the sectional business, with something more satisfactory ahead of us. To discuss the matter in the Physiological Society would be the limit of foolishness. What we want is a vigorous, aggressive, *independent* society of biochemical workers banded together for the advancement of biological chemistry in all its relationships, not merely in connection with physiology.[24]

Abel was aware that some physiologists had resented the *JBC*, and he hoped to gain their support for the new society by inviting their advice and consent.[25] Gies convinced Abel that this tactic would be more likely to arouse than to calm opposition. Abel notified Chittenden that the biochemists would not seek the physiologists' consent to the new society but assured him that they did not intend to compete with the physiologists' journal or society.[26] He wrote to L. B. Mendel that "the vital connection" with physiology would not be severed, but he made it clear that the "friendly irreconcilables" would proceed to form a separate society.[27]

To secure the support of chemists, Gies and Abel enlisted such influential medical chemists as John Marshall, Harry Grindley, and John Long, who had strong ties to the American Chemical Society. Gies feared some might object:

Long is a "pretty warm baby" in the ACS and might be very strenuously in favor of a section in...the Chemical Society instead of an independent organiztion. We would lose nothing in that fact, however, for we could put him and Mendel in the elevator and send them to the roof to settle the matter, while we go ahead with the business at hand.[28]

Abel's fear of dissension was not allayed by Gies's flippant and dismissive remarks about Chittenden and Mendel.[29] Gies was an optimist, a salesman, and a biochemical jingoist, and his vehement enthusiasm was not always tempered by tact and balanced judgment. His letters to Abel could fill an anthology of scientific boosterism:

If you will also keep in mind another very common human trait – the desire to have a front seat on the band wagon – you can readily picture to yourself the merry scramble when you sing out "git-ap." Nail your flag for a biochemical society to the top of the pole. Let those who will, join you around it, but let those who won't be given the "glad hand" and best wishes for a happy new year.[30]

Herter was no doubt correct in surmising that opposition to the new society had been, for the most part, a figment of Gies's dramatic imagination.[31] In the end, neither the chemists nor the physiologists opposed the new society. Gies at once wrote to Mendel (who was absent from the organizing meeting), proposing a joint meeting with the Physiological Society.[32]

From the start, efforts were made to recruit members to the society from all branches of biochemical science. Gies made a particular point of including the botanists, zoologists, and clinicians, whom he was courting for his Columbia network.[33] Abel envisioned the ASBC as a society of "chemically trained workers in Biology as a whole and of Medicine (with a sprinkling of organic and physical chemists who have leanings our way)."[34] The society was indeed very diverse: physiological and medical chemists comprised only one-third of the 81 founding members of the society. There were 17 physiological chemists, 14 pharmacologists, 9 chemists, 9 medical chemists, 7 physiologists, 7 pathologists, 6 clinicians, 6 biologists, 2 bacteriologists, and 2 agricultural or animal chemists.[35] The varied affiliation of ASBC members reflects the absence of a specialized infrastructure and the importance of allies in the early phase of discipline building. For at least 10 or 15 years, representatives were systematically elected from nonacademic institutions and allied disciplines, as well as from biochemical specialties such as nutrition, home economics, public health, and agricultural chemistry.

There were two criteria for election to the society; one was disciplinary: "the publication of one paper and good work since."[36] The other criterion was for those who took an interest in promoting the profession, either as ally or employer. In practice, individuals may have been elected because they had influential patrons to speak up for them. Stanley Benedict complained of such practices in 1915. He felt that election should require publication of two papers on different aspects of biochemistry and on topics not suggested by a mentor.[37] This disciplinary standard seems to have been generally met. Physiologists and pathologists, directors of important bureaus and industrial laboratories, and sympathetic clinicians continued to be elected but in diminishing numbers. The society was increasingly dominated by the productive elite of the discipline.

As a professional infrastructure was created, outsiders became less important, and the makeup of the society reflects this trend. Consolidation of biochemical interests by means of separate departments, journals, and societies drew sharper boundaries between biochemistry and other biomedical disciplines. At the same time, however, society members represented an increasingly varied array of internal specialties and nonacademic professional roles.

These changes in the structure of the discipline are reflected in the changing institutional sources of papers published in the *Journal of Biological Chemistry* (see Table 8.1). The proportion of papers from physiology and pathology declined sharply after 1907, as did papers from chemistry after 1930. Contributions from clinical departments rose, however, as more biochemists were employed in clinical research teams.

INSTITUTIONS AND CAREERS

Analysis of the careers of society members also shows the trend toward occupational pluralism and a more exclusive definition of disciplinary identity. After the first few years, fewer and fewer new

Table 8.1. *American university disciplinary sources of articles published in the "Journal of Biological Chemistry"*

Year	Total Number	% of total articles from univ. sources	Percentage of articles from academic departments					
			Bio-chemistry	Medical sciences	Physiology	Pathology	Chemistry	Others
1907–8	65	61	35	—	23	11.0	17.0	7.7
1915	113	55	37	6.2	19	7.1	8.9	18.0
1926	148	63	47	14.0	7	4.0	18.0	10.0
1937	233	69	41	22.0	5	0.4	13.0	14.0
1948	394	71	59	6.9	8	1.8	11.0	10.0
1959	440	73	61	14.0	4	0.5	5.9	12.0

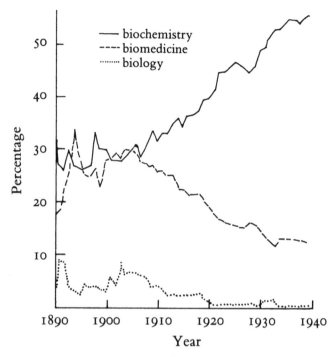

Figure 8.1. Proportion of professionally employed ASBC members affiliated with biomedical disciplines.

members were elected from disciplines other than biochemistry; fewer were employed in other biomedical disciplines (see Figure 8.1). Between 1895 and 1905, more than a quarter of future ASBC members were physiologists or other biomedical scientists. By 1940 the proportion had fallen to one-tenth. Individuals employed as biologists comprised 5% of the membership in 1906 but less than 1% in 1920. These figures do not mean that individuals shifted from physiology to biochemistry: few in fact did so. Rather, fewer physiologists, pharmacologists, and pathologists were doing the kind of research that qualified them for election. New members were much more likely to be biochemists than were older members. Three-fourths of all members admitted (to 1942) from clinical and biomedical sciences had been elected by 1920, compared with one-fourth of biochemists. No fewer than one-third of all biomedical members were founders.

The proportion of society members employed as chemists also dropped sharply, from one-third in 1900 to 15% by 1925 (see

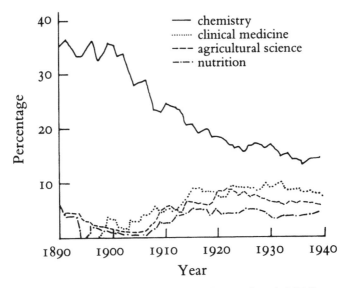

Figure 8.2. Proportion of professionally employed ASBC members affiliated with chemistry and other disciplines.

Figure 8.2). This figure does not mean that fewer chemists were elected but rather that job specifications were becoming more specialized, especially in nonacademic institutions. In the 1890s, government bureaus, hospitals, and chemical manufacturers hardly differentiated between chemists and biochemists. By 1920 specialized roles existed for professional biochemists, in part because of the existence of specialized journals, departments, and societies. These institutions helped promote a more exclusive division of labor. The proportion of ASBC members employed as biochemists increased from less than one-third in 1905 to well over one-half in 1940. If we include biochemists in applied specialties, such as clinical chemistry, agriculture, nutrition, and home economics, then the trend toward disciplinary consolidation is even more pronounced.

Further evidence for the weakening of links with other biomedical disciplines comes from analysis of co-membership in other professional societies. Figure 8.3 shows the percentage of co-membership from successive Ph.D. or M.D. degree cohorts. Over one-half of ASBC members-to-be who earned degrees between 1895 and 1899 joined the American Physiological Society; fewer than one-tenth of those who got their degrees after 1920 did so. Co-membership in the American Society of Pharmacologists and the Society of American Bacteriologists was generally low and slightly declining. The rapid decline of co-membership in the American Medical Association and the downward drift in co-membership in the Society for Clinical Investigation likewise reflect the new division of labor between professional biochemists and clinicians. Fewer clinicians actually carried on biochemical research; fewer biochemists acquired a medical degree. However, the increasing co-membership in the Nutrition Society and the Society of Clinical Chemists reflects the vitality of these applied branches. The old role of physician–biochemist was replaced by professional subspecialties.

In contrast to the decline of co-membership in biological and biomedical societies, more and more younger members joined the American Chemical Society; almost 90% of the 1930–1934 cohort did so. This fact reflects the strong market relation between the two disciplines. Many, perhaps most, biochemists took their undergraduate degrees in chemistry, and a good many had Ph.D. degrees in chemistry. Chemists regarded biochemistry as an applied branch, and recruits to biochemistry brought this outlook with them.

The trend toward occupational diversity is strikingly revealed by the increasing proportion of ASBC members employed in nonacademic institutions. Government bureaus, agricultural experiment stations, industrial laboratories, medical research institutes, and hospitals all began to employ biochemists in greater numbers between 1900 and 1920. Research departments expanded in a period that looked to scientific experts for social progress. Routine occupational roles in fertilizer testing, urinalysis, water analysis, and so on became professional roles integrating research and application. Whereas some of these institutions were attached to universities, their mission was not to instruct but to produce goods and services. Investment in research was justified by practical results: scientific regulation of foods and drugs, new diagnostic tests or therapies, new food products, improved animal feeds. Biochemical research was an overhead on production and service, as it was an overhead on teaching in medical schools. These institutions created a professional market for biochemists and fostered a conception of biochemistry as an applied science.

The pattern of role innovation was similar in each case: a few innovating institutions created roles for professional researchers.

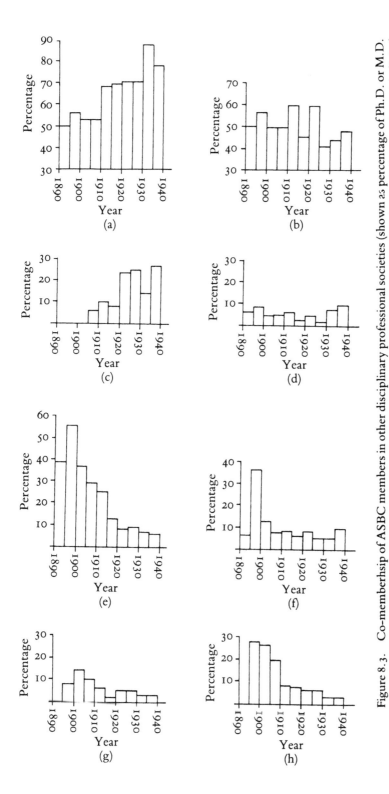

Figure 8.3. Co-membership of ASBC members in other disciplinary professional societies (shown as percentage of Ph.D. or M.D. degree cohorts): (a) chemistry; (b) experimental biology; (c) nutrition; (d) bacteriology; (e) physiology; (f) pharmacology; (g) clinical research; (h) American Medical Association.

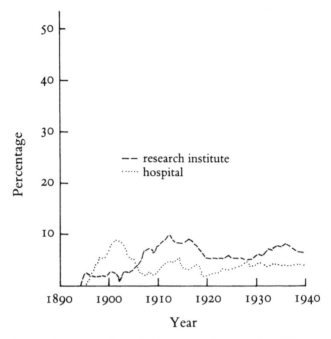

Figure 8.4 Proportion of ASBC members employed in hospitals and medical research institutes (shown as percentage of total professionally employed).

The new market expanded rapidly as existing institutions reorganized to compete for the best research biochemists. After a decade or so of rapid growth, employment opportunities more or less kept pace with growth of the system as a whole.

Hospitals were the first new market for biochemists, beginning about 1895. The numerous hospitals constructed between 1895 and 1915 catered to an urban, middle-class clientele, who accepted the view that the best medicine was scientific medicine. Most new hospitals included laboratories for routine diagnostic testing, but these were also regarded as appropriate contexts for research by professional biochemists. In 1902 hospitals employed almost 10% of ASBC members-to-be. This figure dropped to about 5% by 1908 as other markets opened up (see Figure 8.4).

The federal government had employed a few chemists in various bureaus from the 1860s, but the numbers were limited by political opposition to a strong government role in industrial and agricultural development and public health. Expansion of regulatory func-

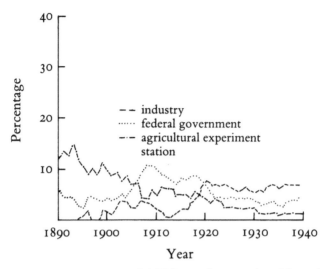

Figure 8.5. Proportion of ASBC members employed in various non-medical institutions (shown as percentages of total professionally employed).

tions created opportunities for more specialized research roles. Around 1904, bureaus began to compete with universities for research biochemists, and the proportion of ASBC members-to-be employed in Washington rose rapidly to over 10% in 1909 and then declined relative to more rapidly expanding sectors (see Figure 8.5). The Department of Agriculture was by far the largest federal employer of biochemists. A 1906 survey of 716 government chemists listed 23 biochemists, 21 of these in agricultural bureaus.[38] A few top biochemists were employed in the Hygienic Laboratory, Joseph Kastle and William Mansfield Clark, for example, but the Public Health Service was much less expansive than the Department of Agriculture in its use of science for regulation. The conservative medical bacteriologists who ran the service resisted expanding into new areas of biomedical research until after 1945.[39]

Conditions for research in government bureaus improved markedly in the early 1900s as civil service codes were extended to scientific jobs and professional criteria replaced patronage and nepotism. As scientists took over administrative posts, bureaus gradually became more supportive of professionals' desire to publish basic research. Carl Alsberg had mixed feelings about accepting a government post in 1908. He feared bureaucratic red tape but expected to have better facilities and technical assistance than he had had in academia. He did not plan to remain long in the Department of Agriculture but felt that a few years there would increase his output of research and improve his professional standing. Alsberg was pleasantly surprised: he was in no way hindered in selecting and publishing his own research, and in 1912 he succeeded Harvey Wiley as chief of the Bureau of Chemistry.[40] William Mansfield Clark, who spent 17 years in the Department of Agriculture and the Hygienic Laboratory, had high praise for government service when he left for an academic post in 1926.[41] In the early 1900s, government bureaus provided many young biochemists with postgraduate research training and a boost into academic careers.

Medical research institutes were the third market to open up to biochemists. The proportion of ASBC members employed in research institutes rose to almost 10% during the period from 1912 to 1914 and then declined somewhat in the 1920s (see Figure 8.4). The Rockefeller Institute for Medical Research employed a large majority of biochemists in this sector, but ASBC biochemists turn up in some dozen smaller institutes.[42] Many of these institutes were attached to teaching hospitals and served as postgraduate research training schools, just as government laboratories had before World War I. This role was facilitated by the provision of graduate research fellowships by the Rockefeller Foundation and other private philanthropies after World War I.[43]

Opportunities for biochemists in industry prior to World War I were severely limited by the virtual German monopoly in the production of pharmaceutical and medical chemicals. When wartime restrictions created a rich and protected domestic market for medicinals and pharmaceuticals, however, American chemical companies rushed to expand research and development. Biochemists were in sudden demand. Between 1916 and 1920, the proportion of ASBC biochemists employed in industry soared from near zero to almost 10% (see Figure 8.5). A sample count of individuals listed as biochemists in *American Men of Science* suggests that two-thirds to three-quarters were employed in industry. Supplying biochemists to industry was crucial to expanding graduate programs in the 1920s. By 1930 university departments were vying for industrial or government biochemists to organize large-scale research programs. Expanding professional markets provided a rich market and a secure economic base for departments with graduate programs. This symbiosis was crucial to the development of the discipline between 1920 and 1940.

The sudden obsolescence of the medical chemists plus the demand from other institutions created a bonanza for young biochemists. In 1905 Gies noted that "...the demand for competent physiological chemists now greatly exceeds the supply."[44] In 1913 he noted ruefully: "There is increasing demand for biological chemists all over the country, and I am repeatedly asked to make nominations to positions that pay larger salaries than I myself receive."[45] Ten years earlier, a half-dozen biochemists had applied eagerly for the assistantship at Johns Hopkins, including Mathews and Folin.[46] With a doctorate in chemistry with Julius Stieglitz and research experience with Kossel, Salkowski, and Hammarsten, the best Folin could do in 1899 was a job teaching analytical chemistry at West Virginia. In 1907 Folin declined a position at the Rockefeller Institute to take the Harvard offer.[47] Two years later, having just declined the chair at Washington University, Folin marveled at the readiness of Harvard to meet any offer: "The encouraging feature is the general desire in so many places to get the best men and willingness to pay for them. It seems especially so to me as I never had an offer till about three years ago."[48]

Owing to the scarcity of senior biochemists, beginners like Gies, Alsberg, Hawk, Jones, Shaffer, and Benedict were given responsibilities and rewards very early in their careers. As Abraham Flexner observed, it was the young who profited from the boom in the preclinical sciences: "The rewards of early promise or of early performance have been alike great and prompt. It is unlikely that the pace will permanently keep up."[49] Pharmacologists likewise enjoyed a seller's market, as Abel noted in 1908.[50] New institutional structures made disciplines thrive that had been the neglected stepchildren of the old system.

The sudden demand for biochemists put a considerable strain on a supply system that was adapted to scarcity and survival, not abundance and growth. Medical school departments emphasized undergraduate teaching and had small, informal graduate programs. Professors depended on graduate students or newly fledged graduates for teaching and research, rather than a staff of experienced junior colleagues. This arrangement was appropriate to a slow-growth market and enabled Mendel, Gies, and Mathews to turn out research and a modest number of experienced teachers with a bare minimum of investment. As demand increased, however, the turnover of assistants became uncomfortably brisk. At Columbia, Gie' found it difficult to keep his best instructors for more than a few years before they received offers of higher pay and more independence. Between 1906 and 1910, he lost no fewer than nine assistants, among them A. N. Richards and Stanley Benedict.[51] Competition for Yale graduates was equally keen. From 1908 to 1916, Chittenden and Mendel exported 16 assistants to 14 different institutions. Half a dozen soon occupied chairs, among them Stanley Benedict, Israel Kleiner (NYU), Victor Myers (Western Reserve), Byron Hendrix (Texas), William C. Rose (Illinois), and Howard B. Lewis (Michigan).[52] Mendel was torn between spreading the Yale influence and keeping experienced individuals for teaching and research.[53] The University of Chicago, which had relied on its singularity as a research university to acquire good faculty cheap, was hard pressed to match offers of higher salaries and better facilities in new departments.[54]

As medical school departments were expected to mount large research programs, they were no longer able to rely on poorly paid student assistants. Pressures built up to invest in full-time junior staff, and this change took some of the pioneers by surprise. In 1911 some Columbia faculty complained to Dean Lambert about Gies's inability to keep his best young staff, the scattered and superficial quality of his research, done mainly by inexperienced students, and his failure to appoint an assistant professor.[55] Gies was stunned. He protested that these qualities were not the result of mismanagement but of his role as feeder of the system and his policy of keeping the expenses of training and research to a minimum; he expected to lose his best students.[56] In fact, Gies had made a vice of efficiency: he was autocratic and disliked delegating power; although complaining of shortage of funds, he had regularly turned money back to the dean each year. These habits were well suited to the slow-growth market of the 1890s but not the boom market of 1910 to 1930. Growth and investment in quality were the new order of the day. Victor Vaughan and Walter Jones were likewise trapped in patterns of behavior learned in the pioneering years, and their departments rapidly fell behind.

The shift from a loose coalition of disciplinary interests to a discipline run by and for professional biochemists caused some of the midwives to lose interest: Herter and Abel, for example. Soon after the ASBC was delivered safe and sound, Abel withdrew from society affairs to organize a pharmacological journal and society –

projects he had long had in mind.[57] In 1909 he also withdrew from the Saltpeter Commission, to the dismay of his biochemist colleagues.[58] Although Herter continued to edit the *Journal of Biological Chemistry* until his death in 1911, he too felt that he had outlived the midwife's role. As early as 1907, Herter's interest turned to organizing clinical research. He became involved in planning the new Rockefeller Institute Hospital and dreamed of domestic competitors for the German journals of clinical research.[59] In one of his periodic attacks of depression, Herter lamented his anomalous role as an amateur in an increasingly professionalized world:

I am coming to have a realization that my work is of a very second rate or third rate order and that it would not be missed if I should quit it. If I should continue to do something in the experimental way it will be simply to please myself, as I have gotten into a sort of experimental habit, of which it is difficult to break oneself. I have always worked largely from a sense of duty but now I feel this much less and think it will be wiser to spend what time may remain to me in the pursuit of my real aims, which are much more humanitarian and literary than scientific.[60]

In his better moments, Herter felt reconciled to his role. In 1910 he wrote to Abel about his biochemical assistant, Henry Dakin:

I have not succeeded in doing much work personally this winter in the lab, but Dakin is carrying it along very successfully. He does everything in a chemical way so much better than I do that I am growing quite prepared to be satisfied with looking on. After all, there is much satisfaction to be had in that way and we ought to feel pleased instead of discouraged if we can facilitate the work of better trained and more modern young workers.[61]

The midwives had no place in the nurseries of the new discipline.

CONCLUSION

Although fewer chemists, physiologists, and clinicians actually practiced biochemistry, as consumers and partners they continued to shape the practice of biochemistry. Chemistry was the main source of recruits to biochemistry; clinical medicine provided jobs and service roles; general physiology offered important biological problems, though few opportunities for institution building. The disciplinary styles and programs current in the 1920s and 1930s were shaped by the institutional relations with chemistry, biology, and clinical medicine. The clinical style, which dominated most medical school departments, reflected biochemists' service roles in medical teaching and clinical diagnosis and research. The styles that were later known as bioorganic and biophysical chemistry were nurtured by the continuing recruitment of organic and physical chemists into biochemistry. Most chemists felt that biochemistry was an important market for pure chemists; almost none felt any responsibility to put it on their departments' budgets. A biological style, focusing on basic problems of intermediary metabolism and bioenergetics, thrived in a few departments or research institutes that did not depend on medical service roles. But the lack of such roles undercut attempts to foster "general biochemistry" in departments of general physiology. It was not until after 1940 that general biochemistry infiltrated medical school departments, as basic research and graduate programs were expanded to capture government grants and a booming university market.

In the following chapters, I shall show how institutional contexts shaped the ways in which biochemists envisioned and practiced their discipline. The central theme will be that intellectual programs are also political programs for building and maintaining institutions. Institutional missions, service roles, and supporting constituencies all influence intellectual priorities. The dominance of the clinical style in American biochemistry from 1920 to 1940 reflected the political economy of American medical schools. Biochemists' deference to chemical ideals reflected their dependence on chemist recruits; their indifference to biological problems reflected the absence of a constituency in biology. Ideas and research programs are professional strategies, and one cannot separate their intellectual and political aspects.

9

The clinical connection:
biochemistry as applied science

The most significant pattern in the history of American biochemistry prior to 1940 is its close connection to clinical medicine. The first generation of American biochemists to acquire international reputations were known for their achievements in clinical biochemistry; for example, Otto Folin, Stanley Benedict, and D. D. Van Slyke. Most departments of biochemistry were in medical schools and their prosperity depended on their service roles in medical instruction and clinical research in hospital laboratories and research wards. Biochemists regarded clinical medicine as a crucial source of important and fundable research problems, employment for their students, and political support for their profession.

This view may appear to contradict the idea, developed in Chapter 7, that biological chemists liberated themselves from clinical medicine in the period of reform. The drama of succession should not distract us from the underlying continuity. Biochemists freed themselves from a particular kind of relationship only to reestablish the relationship on a new basis. What had been either a hybrid or dependent role became a more or less equal partnership. In the process, clinicians as well as biochemists were obliged to adapt their disciplinary ideals.

As long as there was little opportunity for medical chemists to build a specialized discipline, there was no great problem of reconciling divergent disciplinary goals. Many of the old medical chemists were clinicians, so no role conflict existed there. The rest were applied chemists, who practiced their profession in a context dominated by clinicians and seldom doubted the propriety of clinicians calling the tune.

This one-sided relation disintegrated as collegiate entrance requirements in chemistry made room for a new generation of biochemists whose primary loyalty was to their discipline, not to clinical medicine. Encouraged by university reformers and the rhetoric of "scientific medicine," biochemists asserted their independence from clinicians and looked to closer relations with basic chemistry and biology. Professional self-awareness and creation of professional institutions were facilitated by a militant revolt from the dominance of clinicians. The period from 1900 to about 1910 was a low-water mark in the relations between biochemists and clinicians. The old dependent relationship was broken before a new and more equal partnership was formed.[1]

Historians differ in their interpretation of this split between the biomedical sciences and clinical medicine. Gerald Geison sees physicians' continuing skepticism of the utility of physiology as the manifestation of a deep and permanent fault line.[2] Russell Maulitz admits the tensions but believes that they are the superficial perturbations of a stable partnership.[3] In fact, the tension is integral to the partnership: their place in the system obliges biomedical scientists to accommodate basic science with clinical application. Each generation of clinicians must strive to balance the demands of science and craft, laboratory and ward, but never once and for all. The terms of the partnership are always open to renegotiation as circumstances change. The historian's task is to chart and explain this continually evolving symbiosis.

A new relationship between biochemistry and clinical medicine was already beginning to emerge by 1910, as the last clinician–chemists were replaced by consultant biochemists. This partnership depended in part on internal developments in the disciplines but more crucially on changes in professional roles and institutions. Although fewer biochemists had medical degrees, they were generally more able to exploit opportunities for cooperation with clinicians. Application of chemistry to clinical medicine, once limited to urinalysis and toxicology, expanded to a broader range of problems in internal medicine: the physiology and pathology of digestion, respiration and transport, metabolism, electrolyte balance, and hormonal control of metabolism. Biochemists were better trained, more specialized and free of the routine teaching of basic chemistry that had preoccupied the medical chemists. They had access to research facilities and had professional incentives to delve into research on physiological and pathological processes. Likewise, the academic clinical investigators who began to appear after 1900 were more receptive than their predecessors to the uses of biomedical science. A transitional generation of practitioners – William Osler's generation – brought systematic observation and scientific method to the bedside. Clinical faculties were reorganized and chairs of medicine, surgery, pediatrics, and neurology were occupied by a new generation of clinicians trained in physiology and biochemistry and imbued with the ideal of clinical research. These clinician–scholars looked to biomedical scientists as indispensable partners in clinical research, complementing their knowledge of diseases.

Each partner accommodated his professional role and ideology to the needs and expectations of the other. Professional biochemists trained clinical investigators and developed ever more sophisticated diagnostic procedures. Hospital physicians provided biochemists with abundant experimental materials and attractive research problems. Clinicians enjoyed the prestige of academic connections and an aura of "objective" and "disinterested" science. Biochemists, physiologists, and others enjoyed larger resources and the prestige of participating in the progress of medicine. Clinicians learned to live with independent specialists; biochemists learned to adapt clinical imperatives to their disciplinary goals.

BIOCHEMISTS AND CLINICIANS AT ODDS

Advocates of scientific medicine were acutely aware that academic reform of the preclinical sciences threatened to cut off clinical medicine from its scientific roots. Hybrid roles in medicine and physiology, pathology, or chemistry ensured that at least some clinicians would develop some scientific capacity. Professionalization of the preclinical sciences made it more difficult for clinicians to pursue scientific interests by producing a sharp division of specialized roles. Pathologist Samuel J. Meltzer, a leading reformer, felt that younger clinicians were less capable than their elders. "Brainy young men" were leaving clinical medicine for the biomedical sciences, which offered better opportunities for research careers. Clinicians were allowing borderline specialties like pathology and microscopy to be taken over by scientific specialists, depriving themselves of opportunities for research.[4] The problem was most acute in such leading schools as Harvard, Chicago, and Johns Hopkins, where the gap between preclinical and clinical reform was widest. Progressive clinicians sympathized with the reform of the preclinical sciences but worried that physiologists and pathologists were training a generation of clinicians who were less able to utilize the preclinical sciences in the practice of medicine.

Some biomedical scientists regarded the growing gap between the laboratory and clinic as an inevitable consequence of progress. For example, Alonzo Taylor argued that the modern physiologist should not be expected to know what was current practice in the clinic:

> The more active the departments of physiology and pathology, the farther will they be from the view-point in these subjects held by the clinical teachers, trained in the earlier generation of physiology and pathology; this has been so the world over, it will always be true. . . . In Johns Hopkins, Halstead used to complain bitterly of the anatomy that Mall taught; Osler said he could not teach heart disease on the basis of the current teaching in physiology; in Harvard last year, Cabot was very bitter on the unclinical nature of Councilman's pathology, etc. [5]

Taylor and Jacques Loeb argued that separation of the preclinical and clinical sciences was inevitable and desirable. [6] They assumed, of course, that scientific reform of the clinical branches would not succeed in the near future. They were good strategists but bad prophets.

Cooperation between laboratory and clinical factions was impeded by institutional spheres of influence. Clinicians were jealous of their rights and privileges in hospitals and were suspicious of overtures by biomedical scientists. William Gies tried repeatedly to initiate cooperative research with hospital clinicians at P&S. Despite strong support from the college and medical school deans, his initiatives failed. A project on cancer research had to be abandoned when Gies was not granted access to clinical material. A study of the role of enzymes in oedema was stymied by the lack of cooperation from clinicians at Roosevelt Hospital. [7] Biochemist Philip Shaffer encountered similar resistance at Washington University in 1913. As the official chemist to the new Barnes Hospital, Shaffer proposed that a resident pathologist–chemist be appointed to the Metabolism Ward to perform routine clinical analyses for the hospital staff and to do biochemical research under Shaffer's direction. [8] The request was refused, in part perhaps for financial reasons, but more likely for political ones. The right of the medical faculty to appoint hospital staff was being hotly debated at the time, and an initiative by the academic staff, however well intentioned, was bound to seem politically threatening. It was the same at Columbia. [9]

Many clinicians felt that biochemists without medical degrees were not qualified to handle clinical material. At Tufts Medical School, Frederick Hollis was frozen out of clinical work at the hospital because he did not have a medical degree.[10] Tufts was a conservative place, of course; but even progressive clinicians resisted incursions of biochemists into their domain. Harvard's Dean Henry Christian, a leader in the clinical reform movement, felt that the medical side of Otto Folin's department was "decidedly weaker than it should be" and doubted that a chemist without medical training could fill the need.[11] Christian hoped that Folin's program would train a generation of clinicians who could teach clinical biochemistry. Many agreed with him. In 1917 the AMA Council on Medical Education pronounced that biochemists with M.D. degrees should be preferred over those with Ph.D. degrees for medical school positions.[12] These hopes were not fulfilled. Only rarely did a physician elect a career as a professor of biochemistry; there were too many opportunities in clinical research or practice. Medical schools had to rely on the ability of biochemists to acquire a taste and capacity for clinical work. Confidence in a cooperative division of labor came slowly, through actual experience of cooperation in classrooms and hospital wards.

Among biomedical scientists, opinions differed as to the costs and benefits of a clinical connection. At the University of Chicago, for example, opinion was sharply divided whether or not to accept the offer of the Rush medical faculty to be reorganized as a university faculty.[13] One group strongly opposed a merger, fearing that the clinicians would frustrate graduate programs in the medical sciences. This group included botanist John M. Coulter, zoologist Judson Herrick, anatomists Robert Bensley and Preston Keyes, bacteriologist Edwin O. Jordan, and biochemist Albert P. Mathews. Physiologist Anton J. Carlson and pathologist Harry Gideon Wells favored the union, arguing that physiology and pathology could not survive without a clinical connection. Carlson pointed out that since 1907 over half of those with doctorates in anatomy, physiology, and pathology had entered the university as medical students.[14] Wells foresaw an immediate exodus of medical and premedical students and a complete collapse of teaching, recruitment, and research in the biomedical disciplines.

Wells also observed that it was already easier to get money from philanthropists for medical research than for research in pure science:

Philanthropy is just coming to realize its opportunities in medicine, and it is scarcely open to question that. . .large gifts will be made in the immediate future, as they have been in the immediate past. If the University were to discontinue its medical departments it would fall far from the current of present-day progress.[15]

Rush already had two well-endowed institutes for medical research, the Sprague and McCormick institutes. Wells, who had both M.D. and Ph.D. degrees, saw more clearly than his biological colleagues the advantages of a clinical connection, and he proved the better prophet. Accommodation came much sooner than the pessimists had predicted.

ACCOMMODATION

Many biochemists undoubtedly shared A. P. Mathews's fears that clinicians would dominate any partnership that might develop between them.[16] Many others, however, were convinced that the opportunities of a clinical connection outweighed the dangers. Philip Shaffer saw the benefits of a clinical connection:

Participation in the hospital by Biochemical staff keeps them in touch with clinical problems, gives them opportunity to test out with human subjects their "theoretical" ideas, and allows them to *grow* as members of a *medical* staff; it also maintains a much needed check upon the chemical thinking and technique of the members of the clinical staffs – both sides profit from the constant contact and exchange of ideas. Another great advantage is that the students continue in more or less close relations with Biochemistry throughout the hospital years and see its interest and its usefulness to medicine, as is rarely the case without a professional biochemist in the hospital laboratory.[17]

Shaffer left Cornell and an almost guaranteed chair in 1910 for the promise of closer connections with clinicians in the new hospital at Washington University.[18]

By 1910 ambitious young biochemists regarded a clinical laboratory as a necessity. Biochemists who had ready access to patients had a real advantage in terms of research materials and facilities, especially in the growing area of metabolic research. In 1907 Otto Folin welcomed Eliot's suggestion to work two days a week at the Massachusetts General Hospital, as a chance to increase his research productivity.[19] As a consulting pathological chemist, W. J. Gies helped organize the new biochemistry laboratory at Belleview.[20]

Frederick Hollis resigned from the Indiana Medical School in 1911 because he was discouraged from doing clinical work; he declined another position for the same reason.[21] R. A. Hatcher tried to lure Shaffer back to Cornell in 1911 with assurances that there would be improved hospital facilities and more opportunity for cooperation with the new research men in the clinical branches.[22] Rufus Cole tried this bait to lure Frank Underhill to the Rockefeller Institute Hospital in 1910.[23]

On the clinician's side, accommodation with the biomedical scientist was facilitated by a new conception of clinical science and a new role of clinical investigator. The new generation of academic clinicians was trained in the laboratory sciences but did not migrate out of clinical medicine. These clinicians adopted some of the values of the biomedical scientists but not their professional goals. Research was important; not just passive observation, but active experimentation in laboratory and ward. Practical healing was combined with a search for the fundamental processes of diseases. The new clinical scientists saw their unique objective as "the natural history of diseases, their physiology and pharmacology." They regarded disease states as complex objects, requiring distinctive methods of description and explanation, different from those of the biomedical sciences.[24]

Clinical science was frequently likened to the engineering sciences.[25] As engineers developed basic theories of materials and design out of the methods and ideas of physics, so clinicians constructed theories of disease states from basic physiology and pathology. It was not simply a matter of applying basic science but of creating new basic applied-science disciplines. Clinical scientists' ultimate purpose was to cure the sick, just as the aim of engineering was to build dams or machines. The ideal clinical investigator was thoroughly trained in the basic and preclinical sciences and had performed research in physiology or biochemistry; but he was concerned with the problems of the ward, not those of the laboratory.

This conception of clinical science made possible a symbiosis with the preclinical sciences. There was less need to cling to old hybrid roles and less fear that scientific-minded clinicians would abandon the ward for the laboratory. The biomedical sciences thus became less threatening. As direct competition diminished, mutual expectations became more realistic. As long as only physiologists and biochemists had the skills to do clinical research, it was easy to lay the blame for the sad state of clinical science on their impracticality, as Samuel J. Meltzer did in 1904.[26] But as institutions for training and employing clinical researchers developed, it became less essential that physiologists and biochemists themselves be clinicians. Quite the contrary: in 1909 Meltzer emphasized that clinical science was not applied physiology or biochemistry; rather, it drew upon physiology and biochemistry, as these sciences drew upon biology and chemistry, without being reducible to applied chemistry or biology. Meltzer was glad to see physiologists becoming more interested in clinical problems; but ultimately clinical science needed clinical scientists:

It is time . . . that the men who tackle these problems must have a thorough training in the sciences allied to medicine, but the centre of their activities must be within clinical medicine itself. They must have a bringing up within medicine, their minds must have been filled up with thinking, worrying, brooding over practical and theoretical problems of clinical medicine.[27]

Biomedical scientists might help train clinicians and consult in clinical research, but as partners not competitors.

Accommodation between the preclinical and clinical sciences was more or less worked out by World War I. Lewellys Barker, professor of medicine at Johns Hopkins, wrote in 1913 that biomedical scientists and clinical investigators were increasingly aware of what could and could not be expected of each other. The work of biochemists complemented the work of clinicians, without overlapping or competing.[28] Meltzer observed that clinicians were learning to use physiology and pathology without feeling that they were becoming physiologists or pathologists. Medical chemist W. H. Warren welcomed the mutual dependence of laboratory and clinical men and urged that medical schools restructure their curriculum to encourage this interdependence: "The best laboratory man will be the one who has an adequate conception of clinical purposes because he has clinical experience; . . . the best clinical man will be the one who is most familiar with laboratory procedures."[29]

Reintegration of the preclinical and clinical sciences, referred to in the early 1900s as the "problem of correlation," generated vigorous discussion and much tinkering with the medical curriculum. Some clinicians felt that the responsibility lay with laboratory scientists, whereas some preclinical scientists felt that clinical applications were the responsibility of clinicians.[30] Although the majority of both sides favored cooperation, it was not easy to discover institutional means for accommodating their different goals.

David Edsall was one of the most persistent advocates of "correlation." In 1907 he persuaded the Pennsylvania medical faculty to try a scheme of cooperative teaching in the preclinical sciences. The idea was that young clinicians would intercede at intervals in the basic courses in biochemistry, physiology, and pathology and lecture on the clinical relevance of the basic theories being discussed. Edsall hoped to kill several birds with one stone: clinicians would be encouraged to keep up in basic biomedical science; students would take their basic courses more seriously, learning diagnostics and therapeutics from first principles, not by rote; and a new generation of clinical teachers and investigators would be created.[31]

Edsall's idea did not work as planned. Correlation courses simply became short courses in diagnosis, apart from the preclinical sciences. Physiological chemistry was omitted from the scheme because it was felt that freshmen were not ready for clinical subjects. No one was pleased, and in 1910 Edsall agreed that the correlation courses should be abolished.[32] Other correlation schemes had even more serious flaws. Having clinicians teach the preclinical sciences was unacceptable to Edsall and others because it seemed to revive the rejected role of the clinician–physiologist or clinician–chemist. Offering refresher courses in the basic sciences to third- and fourth-year medical students aggravated the problems of a curriculum already bloated with specialized courses. Most schools simply organized intermediate electives in applied clinical pathology or physiology, either in these departments or in departments of medicine.

For purists like Alonzo Taylor, the latter scheme had the advantage of placing the responsibility for clinical instruction with clinicians, thus freeing physiologists and pathologists to pursue pure science: "As a member of the faculty I am interested in having these important courses taught; as Professor of Pathology I am not concerned with them."[33] Other biomedical scientists were eager to be responsible for clinical applications. Yale physiologist Yandell Henderson saw courses in clinical physiology as a great opportunity for discipline building.[34] Bacteriologist Alexander Abbott felt that however easy and agreeable it was to teach the preclinical sciences as pure sciences, it was the clinical applications that mattered: "I do not wish to be misunderstood, but in teaching the . . . preclinical sciences, the department should be limited entirely to the applied sciences."[35]

"Correlation" became less an issue as an informal symbiosis developed, clinicians becoming more scientific, as laboratory men became more practical. In 1914 a committee at the Cornell Medical School resolved that instructors in medicine, surgery, obstetrics –gynecology, and pediatrics must have research experience in one of the preclinical sciences and be willing to devote one-half time to clinical research in the laboratories of pharmacology or biochemistry. The committee also specified that the preclinical scientists would organize correlation courses on clinical applications, open their laboratories to clinicians, and participate in clinical research. The biochemists were expected to "perfect themselves in clinical diagnosis and therapy." The committee noted that the preclinical departments had already put these ideals into practice.[36] Stanley Benedict's staff in chemistry instructed clinical interns in the chemistry and physiology of hormones, metabolism, and kidney function, worked on improving laboratory procedures for testing renal efficiency and diabetes, and cooperated with clinicans in therapeutic treatment in the wards. Abel saw the same spirit of cooperation at Johns Hopkins:

Obstetricians, gynecologists, surgeons and internists of the hospital are in almost daily consultation with my bio-chemical friends Jones and Koelker. . . . I should wish to see bio-chemical institutes as a training place for the physicians of the future. Note the chemical researchers at present emanating from all departments of medicine.[37]

Training was the key to the symbiosis between biochemists and the new generation of scientific clinicians. By helping to train them, biochemists ensured that young clinicians would be more sympathetic to their discipline than their predecessors had been. Biochemistry departments depended on the good will of clinicians. Department chiefs like Philip Shaffer saw clinical laboratories as indispensable for recruiting and employing biochemists. Cooperation with clinicians was crucial to expanding the market for professional biochemists in hospitals and departments of medicine. Shaffer hoped to corner and protect the market for clinical training, thus stimulating supply and demand at the same time:

The next generation of leaders in all clinical as well as laboratory subjects must have long apprenticeships in one or more of the pre-clinical subjects;

the dearth of men of such training is now a sharply limiting factor. . . . The only way to supply such men is to provide abundant fellowships, assistantships and instructorships in all pre-clinical departments. . . . The remedy in my judgment calls for two steps: (1) reasonable adherence by universities to the policy of appointing to clinical as well as preclinical positions only those with sound scientific training in preclinical subjects, especially in physiology and bio-chemistry. . . and (2) that greatly increased provision be made in fellowships and other staff positions.[38]

Some young clinicians sought training in biochemistry laboratories; many more, in physiology and pathology. Otto Folin, Walter Jones, and Philip Shaffer were glad to have clinical workers in their laboratories, confident that they would one day return the favor.[39]

Clinical departments began to appoint biochemists quite early in the reform period, perhaps in imitation of German practice.[40] In 1908 so much biochemical work was being done in the Department of Medicine at Harvard that Henry Christian petitioned for special laboratories and fellowships to train physicians in biochemistry. Medicine at Washington University in 1913 included medical associates in immunology and biochemistry. Dock and Shaffer hoped to tempt Cyrus Fiske, doctor of medicine and Folin's star pupil, with an offer of a joint position in medicine and biological chemistry.[41] In 1917 John Howland turned to Shaffer for someone to head a new chemical laboratory in pediatrics at Johns Hopkins.[42] Shaffer sent Howland his star student, William McKim Marriott, who instructed Howland in biochemistry as he received instruction in pediatrics. In the early 1920s, demand in departments of medicine for biochemists with M.D. degrees far outstripped the supply. By the 1930s, it was common practice for clinical departments to have biochemists with Ph.D. degrees on their staff.

Positions in medical departments were plum jobs for biochemists, requiring no routine teaching and providing ample funds and facilities for research. A. Baird Hastings's appointment to a post in the Department of Medicine at Chicago in 1928 drew envious approval from a physiologist friend:

I want to congratulate you on your moving up in the scale of things academic by going into a clinical department. . . . I can see a very great advantage, from the point of view of the sort of support one can get for research projects, to be gained by being in a department of medicine. One might do exactly the same sort of experimental work in another capacity and it would not have the same public approval that research work in the

Department of Medicine will have. Popular sympathy gives a department of medicine a lot more support than it would a department of biochemistry, I should imagine. It looks to me as though the departments both of Medicine and Surgery at Chicago are more or less duplications of a physiological staff, but I think it is a fine idea and envy you your opportunity and I wish I could land in a Physiology post on such a staff.[43]

The partnership between biochemists and clinicians was not all sweetness and light, however: when resources became scarce, old rivalries surfaced. The early 1920s were such a time. Postwar inflation had seriously eroded academic salaries, and physicians' salaries had increased fourfold.[44] Medical graduates were going into practice rather than academic medicine, and university departments were still struggling to make do with staffs depleted by the wartime draft. Gies's department at Columbia was stripped of its junior staff; at Saint Louis, Shaffer was reduced to one assistant and student helpers, and lamented that "If . . . provisions [for higher salaries and graduate fellowships] are not made fairly soon, we shall have no young bio-chemists."[45] Folin too saw the postwar manpower shortage as a serious threat to the next generation of biochemists.[46] The "crisis in the preclinical sciences" was the subject of heated debates. Many preclinical scientists felt that the preclinical sciences were being overshadowed by their clinical fields and that they were becoming second-class academic citizens. Some blamed the reformers who had pressured schools into investing heavily in full-time clinical chairs, arguing that the full-time plan had not fulfilled its promise and that the preclinical departments had suffered as a result.[47] The "commercialization of medicine" was lamented as young physicians chose practice over academic careers. In 1920 the National Research Council made an official investigation, deploring the decline in status and support of the preclinical sciences.[48]

Riding the tide of prosperity and power, clinicians complained about the excessive standardization of the Flexnerian reform movement and the "inflexibility" of the medical curriculum. Their point was that the preclinical sciences, for historical reasons, had been over-emphasized at the expense of contact with patients: the purpose of medical schools was to train doctors, not scientists. Moderates in the AAMC agreed that the reform of the preclinical sciences probably had resulted in students less able to diagnose and treat patients. Many medical schools reduced the time given to courses in biochemistry and other preclinical sciences.[49] A conservative clinical pathologist, smarting from the greater prestige of academic pathologists, seized the opportunity to denounce the interlopers as "lay professors," laboratory diagnosis as "pseudo-science...a menace," and laboratory men as "faddists."[50]

Pioneers of clinical science shifted their emphasis from science to practice, from the laboratory to the ward. One of the founders of the clinical laboratories at Johns Hopkins, Charles Emerson, fulminated against preclinical scientists who felt that clinical medicine was merely the application of the preclinical sciences at the bedside and who considered ward work to be inferior to work in the laboratory: "Why are the laboratories not the training ground for the ward rather than supercilious rivals?"[51]

Yet despite the complaints from both sides, no one suggested a divorce. The loudness of the squabble is an indicator of the value of the relationship for clinicians and preclinical scientists alike. Biochemists did not take issue with the assertion of the AMA that biochemists with M.D. degrees be preferred over those with Ph.D. degrees, all else being equal. They asserted that if medical schools wanted more clinically alert biochemists, then they must provide the means to train them. This was the message that a blue-ribbon committee of biochemists gave to the AAMC.[52] The clinicians never questioned the biochemists' role in training clinicians. Biochemists willingly accepted a greater responsibility in exchange for influence and respect in the medical world and ever-increasing material support.

BIOCHEMICAL DIAGNOSIS

Training clinical investigators was one indispensable role for biochemists in clinical medicine; another was providing biochemical methods of diagnosis. Urinalysis was a time-honored part of medical practice. However, the number of really useful procedures was surprisingly small: glucose and acetone were sure signs of diabetes, uric acid of gout; it was thought that the amino acids leucine and tyrosine were indicators of pathological liver or kidney functions; albumin, pentose, phenyl-keto-propionic acid and a number of other compounds were symptomatic of rare metabolic diseases, such as phenylketonuria, made famous by A. E. Garrod. Many other substances were found in urine, but they were curiosities and could seldom be associated with definite diseases.[53]

By 1900 clinical chemistry was one of a family of applied clinical sciences, which included clinical pathology (autopsy) and the newer fields of bacteriology, immunology, serology, and radiology. The remarkable innovations in bacteriological staining and immunological tests for tuberculosis, syphilis, diphtheria, and other diseases overshadowed the old craft of urinalysis, which had changed little since the 1860s. Physicians' new enthusiasm for laboratory methods in the 1890s was probably stimulated by these rapidly developing fields. Around 1900 the pace of innovation in clinical chemistry also began to pick up, carried along by the rapid progress of the newer sciences.

Owing to their lower status as "applied sciences," clinical pathology and chemistry and other activities of the diagnostic laboratory have been largely ignored by medical historians.[54] We know that many more physicians were relying on laboratory methods around 1900. We know that improved and new analytical methods began to appear, and a casual inspection of hospital reports reveals that the number of analyses done each year began to soar after 1900. At the same time, modern clinical laboratories became a regular feature of hospital design. But the details of when and by whom new methods were actually introduced into practice are a story still to be told. This much is clear: the renaissance of clinical analysis coincided with the institutional reform of biochemistry. The prosperity and prestige of biochemists depended to a large degree on their role in developing useful diagnostic methods. Philip Shaffer witnessed the biochemistry boom:

When in 1910 I went to the department of biochemistry in Washington University...research in the subject was limited to that department, almost one might say tolerated in that department. Now there is not one department in the whole medical center that does not rely heavily upon biochemistry. [The new diagnostic methods]...brought biochemistry into a form usable by practicing physicians – office equipment, so to speak – to aid diagnosis.[55]

The earliest innovations in clinical procedures were mostly improvements in existing methods, making them faster, simpler, and more accurate with much smaller samples. Otto Folin's introduction of colorimetric methods (which he adapted from practices he had observed in German breweries) and his improved procedures for creatinine and urea in urine were soon in use everywhere. These simplified procedures made it possible for physicians who were not trained chemists to use them routinely – office equipment in aid of diagnosis. Physicians looking back to the 1890s recalled that a routine urinalysis and hemoglobin assay were almost the only tests that clinicians carried out; most others were regarded as difficult and unusual.[56]

Later innovations in analytical methods went hand in hand with advances in the physiology of metabolism. The discovery of how the acidic products of incomplete glucose metabolism caused acidosis and diabetic coma increased clinicians' and chemists' interest in acid–base and salt balance. Many traditional urine tests proved not to be specific for pathological states, and by 1910 it was recognized that the chemistry of the blood was better diagnostic evidence than urine.[57] Reliable micromethods for blood analysis were devised after 1910, again largely by Folin and his school. Improved tests of liver and kidney function, utilizing special diet regimens, became essential for presurgical diagnosis. The period from 1900 to the mid-1920s was one of rapid innovation in clinical biochemistry.

The advent of routine laboratory diagnosis was a controversial issue in this period. In 1902 Charles A. Emerson, resident physician in charge of clinical laboratories at Johns Hopkins Hospital, took a rather mixed view of this new medical fashion:

Clinical laboratories are growing in favor and influence: publishers have produced a super-abundance of text-books which purport to "make clinical chemistry easy," medical journals accept at sight articles on almost any chemical subject. . . .

At a recent large medical congress so much time was spent on the chemical side of internal medicine that one not interested in that subject must have had to exert unusual efforts to look interested and knowing. Does the "practical man" care to know how a hen synthesizes uric acid?

But chemical education does not emanate alone from medical schools, medical journals, and medical congresses; every practitioner gets a free course through the mails. He is bombarded with pamphlets giving a detailed account of some recent "*Arbeit*" in chemistry, and advertising a new food or new preparation. The whole practical medical world, in fact, is studying chemistry.

But it is not alone medical men who are turning chemists, for the pathologists are also studying chemistry. Their hemolysins, bacterio-hemaglutins, anti-hemaglutins, toxophores, heptophores, complementophilic groups, and intermediary bodies are now or soon will be playthings of "pathologic chemists.". . .

The growth of the physiological chemistry laboratory is of the utmost importance to clinical medicine, for now the clinical laboratory will be provided with methods which are of practical use to the clinical man, and with men well enough trained to use them.[58]

John Long noted in 1904 how many clinicians were using sophisticated chemical terms and concepts. Although they were bewildered by chemical jargon or skeptical of the details of, say, Ehrlich's theory of immune reactions or Martin Fischer's theory of nephritis, clinicians had no doubt that biochemistry was indispensable to diagnosis and therapeutics.[59]

In 1908 Lewellys Barker, professor of medicine at Johns Hopkins and a pioneer in the use of laboratory methods, warned that traditional bedside diagnostic skills were in danger of being lost in the enthusiasm for "scientific" laboratory procedures:

[It] would be a grave error to deprive ourselves of what is good in the old because of the helpfulness of the new. That such a fear should be expressed...shows how tremendous a hold laboratory methods are taking of the minds of developing clinicians.[60]

Between 1900 and about 1915, physicians spilled a volume of ink on the relative merits of laboratory tests and bedside diagnosis. Unsympathetic physicians condemned laboratory science as "pseudoscience" and blamed it for the plague of commercial nostrums. The somewhat overblown controversy was symptomatic of the larger conflict between two generations of clinicians, eyeing each other suspiciously from opposite sides of the clinical reform movement. It ceased to be a controversial issue as the reform movement succeeded.

As early as 1910, reformers like Abraham Flexner held both sides up to ridicule:

Occasionally champions of the laboratory prejudge the issue by calling pathology a real or pure or more or less accurate science, as against the presumably unreal or impure or inaccurate data secured from the patient himself. It becomes a serious question of professional etiquette who should speak first or loudest – the pathologist, armed with his microscope, or the clinician, brandishing his stethoscope. To parallel the dispute, one must go back to the two knights who, meeting at a cross-road, disputed at the hazard of their lives the color of a shield which, as neither had stopped to reflect, had two sides. It is as profitable to discuss which was the right side of the shield as to raise the question of precedence between the laboratory and the bedside.[61]

George Dock wrote in 1917 that "the old question as to the relative value [of laboratory and clinical methods] in general is as dead as the doctrine of the four elements."[62] Clinical biochemistry was no longer the fashion for the clinical avant-garde but the office equipment of every clinician.

CONTEXTS FOR RESEARCH: OPTIONS

The context in which clinical biochemistry developed was the hospital laboratory. The modern hospital itself was a new institution in the 1900s. It was unclear at first exactly what its role should be in supporting medical research and exactly what a clinical laboratory should be. There were various experiments in laboratory organization. In the late-nineteenth century, clinical chemistry was generally part of the pathology laboratory – the autopsy room. Later occupants of the enamel and stainless steel temples of medical science recalled the old pathology laboratory as a dark, cramped, evil-smelling basement room filled with the aroma of boiling urine. The image had an almost primeval quality: "born in obscurity . . . emerged from the sunless gloom of the hospital basement," and so on.[63] Between 1900 and 1915, however, the pathology laboratory evolved into an important and complex institution.

By 1920 a clinical laboratory in a large hospital was a distinct administrative unit or service directed by a chief resident physician. It usually consisted of four or five divisions: clinical pathology, bacteriology, serology and immunology, biochemistry, and radiology. Each division was staffed by trained, often salaried, professionals. The main function of these laboratories was to provide routine laboratory tests for diagnosis or therapy, but the professional staffs were also expected to cooperate with the clinical staffs, to instruct interns and medical students in advanced analytical procedures and to do research.[64] In teaching hospitals, professors of pathology or biochemistry often served as consultants to the clinical laboratories, as the growing expense of large laboratories and the increasing prestige of research forced hospital boards to accept a university connection and academic standards of achievement.[65]

The centralized clinical laboratory was only one of a variety of hospital laboratories. Many hospitals had small, often makeshift laboratories attached to individual wards, where attending physicians could perform routine tests on their patients, check a diagnosis, or monitor drug therapy. The ward laboratory embodied the belief of the Oslerian generation of clinicians that laboratory methods were a vital part of the physician's role and should not be relinquished to a laboratory staffed by specialists. William Osler established ward laboratories at the new Johns Hopkins Hospital in 1899. Routine tests were carried out by attending physicians, and more complex procedures and research problems were referred to William Welch's pathology laboratory.[66] Whereas central clinical laboratories were increasingly staffed by professional scientists, ward laboratories were designed to keep medical science in the domain of the physician.[67]

A third variety of clinical research laboratory was associated with chairs of experimental or research medicine established at a few leading medical schools after 1900. These laboratories reflected the idea of a division of labor between the practical clinician and the specialized clinical investigator, at a time when the academization of clinical faculties seemed a far distant prospect. The William Pepper Laboratory was established at the Pennsylvania General Hospital in 1895. Laboratories of research medicine were modeled on those of the academic preclinical sciences. For example, the Ayer clinical laboratory at Penn (1903) was designed by Simon Flexner for work with patients, complementing his facilities for experimental work in the pathology laboratory.[68] A laboratory of experimental medicine was established at Western Reserve in 1908 to enable physiologists to work on clinical problems.[69] However, the movement never really caught on. As academic clinicians took over chairs of medicine and surgery, special, exclusive research departments were no longer necessary and stood in the way of clinicians' ambitions for research roles.

The most important institutions for clinical research after about 1920 were laboratories organized within the medical and surgical services of large hospitals. These laboratories reflected the belief of the clinical reformers that research was part of every clinician's duty, not just professors of experimental medicine. The laboratories were directed by professors of medicine and surgery in their dual role as chiefs of medical services and were staffed by resident physicians and salaried professional scientists. They provided a context in which laboratory scientists and clinicians could cooperate.

Unlike the central clinical laboratory, those in the medical services were organized around specific problems rather than scientific disciplines and were organized solely for research. In the central laboratories, research was incidental to the service function of routine diagnostic testing. With no control over patients and deluged by routine work, these laboratories gradually became merely service organizations. The low status of clinical pathology and clinical chemistry as medical specialties made it difficult to attract able medical researchers. The shortage of interns in World War I showed hospital administrators that routine testing could be done as well by technicians as by professional biochemists and more cheaply.[70] Even the William Pepper Laboratory eventually degenerated into a testing laboratory.[71]

THE DIAGNOSTIC LABORATORY

Between about 1905 and 1915, however, some biochemists saw the diagnostic laboratory as an ideal institutional context for large-scale research. Facilities for research in academic departments of biochemistry were modest, and budgets were tied to medical teaching. Many felt that research could only be done by professionals who did not try to combine research with teaching but who linked research to income-producing services. Independent research institutions such as the Carnegie and Rockefeller institutes set the fashion in the prewar decade. The transformation of industrial testing laboratories into laboratories for basic and applied research was beginning to occur at places like General Electric and AT&T. The agricultural experiment stations had succeeded in establishing a large-scale research capability on the basis of routine testing of fertilizers, milk, and animal feeds, and many biochemists were familiar with this model. The modern hospital was yet another of these large institutions in which knowledge was turned into goods or public services. The Progressive ideology of utility and service fed biochemists' high hopes for hospital laboratories in which research was conjoined with routine diagnostic testing.

The similarities among these applied science institutions were occasionally noted by the creators of hospital laboratories. Lewellys Barker may have had industrial precedents in mind when he created special clinical laboratories of pathology, biology, physiology, and biochemistry at the Johns Hopkins Hospital in 1904:

It is just as necessary for physicians and surgeons to have their own special laboratories attached to their wards . . . as it is for aniline dye manufacturers to have chemistry laboratories attached to their plants for solving their special problems, or for breweries to have bacteriology laboratories and skilled bacteriologists continually at work to maintain and improve the standard of their products.[72]

Hospitals and corporations were responding in similar ways to the opportunities of applied research. In his roles as analyst, researcher, and trouble-shooter, the clinical biochemist very much resembled his confreres in experiment stations and industrial laboratories.

Otto Folin's experience made him one of the most vocal advocates of hospitals as contexts for biochemical research. The McLean Hospital for the Insane, where Folin was employed from 1900 to 1907, was one of the very first to subsidize research. As early as the mid-1880s, superintendent Edward Cowles envisioned the private hospital as a locus for research. A laboratory of physiological chemistry was established in 1889, and research in pathological chemistry was initiated in 1891, in part owing to encouragement by Harvard physiologist Henry Bowditch. This work consisted largely of urinalysis, carried on by resident physicians with occasional consultation from the Harvard medical chemists. A larger laboratory was built in 1895, and Cowles began to think of a special research department run by a professional biochemist. Reassured by Russell Chittenden "as to there being a proper field for research here for an expert in physiological chemistry," Cowles appointed Folin in 1900, thus realizing his "long-cherished purpose."[73]

Cowles believed that insanity was caused by chemical toxins resulting from deranged metabolism or bad diet and that the clues to these disorders were to be found in the urine (a rather common belief at the time). Folin quickly dispelled any hope of finding specific toxins in patients' urine. In the course of his work, however, he did discover how inadequate the standard methods of urinalysis were and how vague a conception physicians had of "normal" metabolism. At Henry Bowditch's suggestion, Folin devoted himself to improving analytical methods and to a systematic study of the "normal" products of nitrogen metabolism, using patients fed on a standard diet.[74] Besides his valuable new colorimetric methods, Folin conceived a new theory of nitrogen metabolism, which distinguished between a constant "endogenous" metabolism and a variable "exogenous" metabolism.[75] Folin believed that the "endogenous" metabolism was a measure of the body's true metabolic state, which had escaped previous researchers because the much larger "exogenous" metabolism fluctuated with diet.

This theory was the key to Folin's conception of the special role of hospitals for the new discipline of biochemistry. Hospitals provided groups of people whose diet could be controlled and whose urine could easily be collected throughout the day, which was an essential part of Folin's method. Hospitals also provided cases of abnormal metabolism and opportunities for systematic collection of data on a large scale:

For the next few years the conception of a dual protein catabolism . . . will be threshed out on the basis of work on fever patients and on normal persons, with the help of occasional investigation of such suggestive conditions as pregnancy, convalescence, progressive paralysis, gigantism, and dwarfism. This will clear the ground and . . . sharpen our wits and our tools for work on the more difficult chronic diseases, such as rheumatism and gout, and the chemically more complicated diseases, such as nephritis, atrophy of the liver, and diabetes. . . . I regard the whole subject of diabetes, and especially the acid-intoxication theory, as a most fruitful field for purely chemical work.[76]

In hospitals, as in industrial laboratories and agricultural experiment stations, research could serve both theoretical and practical ends – an ideal whose time had arrived in 1907.

A number of progressive hospitals had already begun to appoint biochemists, especially in New York and Massachusetts, states active in the public health movement. Phoebus A. Levene and Samuel Bookman, both students of Emil Fischer's, were appointed as chemists at the Pathology Institute of New York State Hospital in 1896, with the idea that the institute would train clinical scientists for other state hospitals. Lyman B. Stookey, trained by Russell Chittenden, was appointed in 1902. In 1902 Bookman was appointed biochemist (without pay) at Mt. Sinai Hospital in New York City, and in 1906 the laboratory was equipped and endowed for research, despite the skepticism of some staff physicians. With its strong connections to the New York German–Jewish community, Mt. Sinai maintained a tradition of research funded by private benefaction.[77] In the biochemistry laboratory at Johns Hopkins Hospital (1906), Carl Voegtlin, a German-trained organic chemist, worked on diagnostic techniques and the effects of diet and drugs on metabolic diseases.[78] Unlike most hospital biochemists, he was not expected to perform routine tests. At the New York Graduate Hospital, Christian Herter served as pathological chemist from 1896 to 1903 and pursued his research on bacterial intoxication in the gut. In 1897 Harvard pharmacologist Franz Pfaff was appointed part-time chemist to the new laboratory at Massachusetts General Hospital, and in 1904 a Department of Scientific Research was established with a modest endowment.

These pioneering hospitals were exceptional, of course. Folin observed in 1907 that hospitals had hardly begun to employ biochemists on a regular basis:

> Notwithstanding the present popularity of biochemical research, notwithstanding the general confession of belief in its importance, it still remains to be seen whether hospital staffs really want it.
>
> Yet the time will surely come when the medical profession will recognize in practice, as it already does in theory, that the large city hospitals should also be centers for biochemical research.[79]

Similar statements were made a few years later by William H. Warren and Abraham Flexner.[80] In retrospect, more hospitals were hiring biochemists than Folin realized. The proportion of members (or future members) of the American Society of Biological Chemists employed in hospitals rose from nil in 1895 to 9% in 1905.[81] Although the numbers are small, hospitals had clearly begun to emulate other public institutions, appointing professional scientists and providing opportunity for research. The pattern became more evident after 1910. The Montefiori Home, New York State Cancer Hospital at Buffalo, Roosevelt Hospital and St. Luke's in New York City, the Peter Bent Brigham Hospital in Boston, and the Lakeside Hospital in Cleveland were among those that reorganized their laboratories and hired biochemists around 1910. The New York Graduate Hospital organized four laboratories on the Johns Hopkins model in 1910, and under the direction of a young disciple of Chittenden, Victor Myers, became an important center of research in clinical biochemistry.[82]

The clinical diagnostic laboratory never really sustained the level of research that Folin and others thought it would in the early years. The research function was compromised by the very service role that made it possible: as the volume of routine diagnostic tests soared, laboratory staff had no time for anything else. Bookman worked as an unpaid volunteer at Mt. Sinai until 1927, while the annual number of diagnostic tests increased from a few hundred to 9,000. He was the only one of a staff of 22 who was not a physician. Franz Pfaff's successor at Massachusetts General, Dr. William Boos, pursued a narrow program of research on lead poisoning. When Folin left McLean in 1907, biochemical research ceased and was not revived until the 1920s. In 1904 Levene left the New York State Pathological Institute for the Rockefeller Institute, and Stookey left for an academic post. Voegtlin transferred after only two years to Abel's Department of Pharmacology. E. C. Kendall fled St. Luke's Hospital in 1913 for a post in the new biochemical laboratories of the Mayo Foundation. The gulf between his own ambitions and the clinicians' expectations was revealed to him when a successful clinical trial of an impure hormonal extract on patients suffering from goiter was received by attending physicians with indifference or – especially among young residents – with hostility.[83] Within five years after Victor Myers left the New York Graduate Hospital in 1924, the clinical laboratory was doing nothing but routine tests and technician training. More hospitals organized laboratory services in the 1920s, but they lost whatever advantage they may have had initially for performing research. The proportion of ASBC biochemists employed in hospitals dropped slightly around 1910 and then remained constant until 1940. Medical schools, endowed medical research institutes, and clinical laboratories proved more appropriate contexts for research in clinical biochemistry.

CLINICAL RESEARCH LABORATORIES

Within hospitals, diagnostic laboratories were overshadowed and outproduced by the research teams organized in the medical and surgical services. One of the earliest and most successful of these laboratories was organized by David Edsall at the Massachusetts General Hospital (MGH). Appointed Jackson Professor of Medicine and chief of the second medical service at MGH in 1912, Edsall immediately began to develop clinical research. He created a salaried position for a resident physician to do half-time research; by 1918 there were three such posts, and eight by 1920. To fill these positions, Edsall selected such promising young clinicians as Walter Palmer, Paul Dudley White, Joseph Aub, Carl Binger, George Minot, and James Howard Means and sent them off for a year or two of postgraduate research training in physiology or biochemistry. (Means and Aub worked with Eugene Dubois and Graham Lusk at Cornell; Palmer, with L. J. Henderson; Binger, with J. J. Abel.) Edsall fired Boos and put Folin's student, Willey Denis, in charge of the chemistry laboratory, with Folin as consulting chemist.[84] In 1918 six rooms were fitted out as a laboratory for 12 workers, who were explicitly freed from any obligation to do routine analytical work. Just before resigning his chair at MGH in 1924, Edsall persuaded several foundations to construct and endow new laboratories adjacent to a special ward of ten beds to be used for research. Known simply as "Ward 4," this laboratory became the prototype of the modern clinical research unit and its researchers won fame for their work on metabolism, nutrition, and endocrinology.[85]

Similar arrangements for clinical research were established at the new Rockefeller Institute Hospital, which opened in 1910. The director, Rufus Cole, had been head of the biology laboratory at Johns Hopkins under Lewellys Barker, and in the favorable environment of an amply endowed research hospital, Cole single-mindedly practiced Barker's ideals of clinical medicine. Biochemistry was an integral part of Cole's plans, and under the leadership of Donald D. Van Slyke, the Rockefeller Hospital became a mecca for clinical biochemists. Van Slyke's appointment was initially a makeshift one. From 1910 to 1913, the biochemistry laboratory was led by Francis H. McCrudden, who had a B.A. degree in chemistry from MIT and an M.D. degree from Harvard. Cole was not optimistic about McCrudden's promise as a researcher but hoped that he would at least get the laboratory started.[86] When McCrudden resigned in 1913 to become the director of laboratories at the Peter Bent Brigham Hospital, Flexner and.Cole decided to appoint a physiological chemist in the European style. Flexner wooed and almost won the eminent German biochemist Franz Knoop, but at the last moment was outbid by the German government.[87] Flexner then turned to Van Slyke, who was then with Phoebus Levene, as a "superior kind of stopgap." Although Van Slyke had no experience in clinical work, Flexner was impressed by his training in organic chemistry and his increasing interest in physiological problems. He also was aware that Van Slyke was beginning to chafe under Levene's one-man rule and might welcome an independent position and more scope for his ambitions:

He would readily, I think, respond to the atmosphere of the Hospital and problems would come to him or would grow out of your conferences. . . . He could not help stimulating the men and being generally helpful, and as you know, his personality is especially agreeable. He could therefore remain in the Hospital as long as it was to the best advantage all around. . . . Van Slyke is an ambitious man, and would be inclined to take up work that represented for him a wider opportunity. His understanding of medical subjects is constantly growing and becoming more effective.[88]

Levene and Cole were easily persuaded, and Van Slyke, not entirely sure that he would like hospital work, agreed to a temporary arrangement for one year.[89]

Cole put Van Slyke and his assistant, Glenn Cullen, in charge of the chemistry laboratory and hoped that their work on protein metabolism in dogs would develop along clinical lines. He gave the biochemists free access to blood and urine samples and instructed the resident staff to cooperate if special diets or other regimens were required for patients being studied. Cole also urged Van Slyke to consult and cooperate fully with the hospital physicians.[90] Cole's hopes were fully realized. Van Slyke found that ". . . the young doctors in the Hospital were all just about my age and they took me in. I began to pick up medicine pretty fast; found it fascinating. So I stayed. . . . " In 1914 Flexner sent him on the grand tour of medical institutes in London, Paris, Berlin, Strasbourg, Fribourg, and Munich to see how cooperation between biochemists and clinicians was arranged. (He was especially impressed by the arrangements between biochemist Otto Neubauer and internist Friedrich von Müller.[91]) Within a few years, Van Slyke had outgrown the old chemistry laboratory, and a new larger laboratory was outfitted for him.[92]

Cornell Medical School and Bellevue Hospital were also centers of clinical research in the 1910s. The Loomis Laboratory, endowed in 1886, included all of the medical fields, from physics and chemistry to experimental medicine. Chemists, physiologists, pathologists, and clinicians found cooperation relatively easy. Chemist Philip Shaffer later acknowledged the aid and influence of his clinical colleagues.[93] Shaffer's successor, Stanley Benedict, was also drawn into clinical research. In 1913 the Russell Sage Institute was transferred from the New York Department of Health to the Cornell Medical School (owing to a political squabble with the coroner's office). The income of the Sage endowment was devoted to the construction and maintenance of a large calorimeter and a metabolic laboratory within Cornell's teaching division at Bellevue Hospital. A fruitful partnership developed between the scientific director, physiologist Graham Lusk, and a young clinician, Eugene DuBois, who was named medical director.[94] Both were eager to develop the clinical side of physiology and biochemistry and began a program of research, using Bellevue patients, of normal nutrition requirements and basal metabolism and their changes in various diseases. The Sage group had a full-time food chemist, Frank C. Gephart, for routine analysis and relied on Benedict for advanced troubleshooting.

In 1919 Lusk and DuBois took a further step in integrating laboratory and clinic. A clinical research laboratory was established in the Cornell division of Bellevue, and DuBois was appointed medical director. He was the first full-time, salaried clinician in a municipal hospital.[95] The full-time controversy was boiling over at the time, and DuBois's first few years were troubled by criticism and harassment by practitioners. Even moderates like Simon Flexner worried about DuBois's lack of clinical experience. Most were won over; but others were actively hostile. A Dr. Meara openly ridiculed the scientific interests of DuBois, John Peters, and other young clinicians. Douglas Symmer, head of clinical pathology, insisted on controlling all research done in Bellevue laboratories and challenged the right of the Sage group to take samples of blood and urine across Twenty-sixth Street to the Loomis Laboratory for analysis. Symmer overreached himself, however: threatened with the loss of the Sage research funds, the hospital board forced him to cooperate. DuBois's group obtained full use of the excellent Bellevue laboratories and the unhindered cooperation of Stanley Benedict, Graham Lusk, and others at Cornell.[96]

From a biochemist's perspective, Lusk and DuBois's work on nutrition and metabolism was increasingly narrow and dated, with Lusk ignoring the importance of vitamins. They were most innovative, however, in the organization of research in clinical physiology and biochemistry. Doctors John Peters, William S. McCann, David P. Barr, and other clinical investigators went from Cornell–Bellevue to important positions in academic medicine. David Edsall took the Sage laboratory as a model for Ward 4.[97] Similar institutions were created in many larger hospitals in the 1920s. Francis Peabody guided a flourishing school of cooperative research on anemia in the Thorndike Laboratory of the Boston City Hospital from 1922 until his untimely death in 1927. Henry Christian created facilities for clinical and biomedical research in the Peter Bent Brigham Hospital. The Harriman Research Laboratory was endowed in 1912 at the Roosevelt Hospital.[98] In 1927 St. Margaret's Hospital in Pittsburgh established a privately endowed Medical Research Laboratory and turned to the Rockefeller Hospital for a biochemist–clinician. When Walter Palmer was appointed professor of medicine and chief of medical service at Presbyterian Hospital in 1921, he built a new chemistry laboratory and brought modern clinical research to Columbia.[99]

Some biochemists continued to see the hospital diagnostic laboratory as a kind of experiment station for medical school departments. Otto Folin wrote in 1921:

I should like to be able to go to the hospitals and say we are now prepared to do all your chemical work, and to furnish technical supervision, reagents, utensils, etc., for such work as might more advantageously be done in the hospital laboratories. In the interest of teaching and the training of men, as well as for other reasons, the employment of technicians should be almost wholly discontinued. The younger medical men together with the men getting special training in my department ought to do the work.... The financing of the plan should come wholly through this department.[100]

Evidently the diagnostic laboratories were not providing the opportunities that Folin had hoped they would. In fact, Folin's plan of linking biochemical research and training to a routine service role was already obsolete by 1920, and a new pattern of cooperation was emerging in clinical research teams. By 1930 all of his staff were involved in cooperative research projects with hospital clinicians: Yellaprageda SubbaRow helped the Ward 4 group on the biochemistry of pernicious anemia; Milan Logan worked on calcium metabolism and dental caries and was "much in demand by clinicians who get into chemical trouble."[101]

A similar pattern of events occurred at the University of Chicago when the clinical departments were organized. The original plan in 1923 called for a centralized group of clinical laboratories. Biochemist Fred Koch hoped that his department would take charge of diagnostic testing and research in clinical biochemistry. However, the new professor of medicine, Franklin McLean, had other plans. A veteran of two years with Donald Van Slyke, McLean was determined to keep clinical research within the Department of Medicine. By preventing the bacteriologists and the biochemists from taking charge of routine clinical testing, McLean also prevented them from establishing a claim on clinical research facilities. McLean's motives were both political and idealistic. Like many academic clinicians, he felt that control of research facilities was crucial to defining the role of full-time clinical scientists. He also argued that bacteriologists and biochemists were better protected from the burden of routine service, whatever they themselves desired. [102]

The center of research in clinical biochemistry was not Koch's Department of Biochemistry but the Department of Medicine. There biochemists participated in team research with clinicians, supported by the Lasker Foundation and led from 1928 to 1936 by Van Slyke's star pupil, A. Baird Hastings. Hastings described how the system worked:

In the course of making rounds with clinical members of the staff, a question has arisen which has involved the working out of a new technique. We have taken the problem to the laboratory; and if successful in working out the new technique, applied it to the clinical problem; and then after training a young clinician in the technique, turned it over to him. On other occasions it has taken the form of making the study of the clinical problem on animals. [103]

Hastings worked mainly on the role of thyroxin, a hormone of the thyroid gland, in regulating metabolism. The symbiosis between biochemistry and clinical medicine in ward laboratories produced a stimulating traffic in ideas and discovery. Problems from the clinic suggested animal experiments; experimental results were returned as useful clinical practices, which provided more grist for basic research. When Hastings succeeded Folin in 1936, he brought this mode of operation with him, routinizing practices that had evolved informally as opportunities arose.

Van Slyke operated in a similar way, but because the Rockefeller Hospital was a research hospital, he himself acted as service chief. The English clinical biochemist, Edward C. Dodds, recounted a visit in 1932:

In the Rockefeller Hospital, the research worker is the chief and the physician or surgeon is his assistant. For instance, Dr. Van Slyke, who does not possess a medical qualification, does the hospital rounds and instructs the clinicians to take careful notes of one particular aspect of the case, or to pay special attention to certain points, etc., and then to report from a clinical point of view.[104]

Van Slyke was unusually privileged. In most cases, clinicians dominated the partnership with biochemists. Without a monopoly on an essential service role, biochemists had little to bargain with. E. C. Dodds described this situation in the Columbia–Presbyterian Medical Center in 1932:

Most of the service chiefs have a laboratory of their own and they virtually do their own work. The workers in charge of these laboratories are usually pure biochemists, often young women who have a degree such as a B.A. in physiology and biochemistry. The disadvantage of this is that in the vast majority of cases the biochemist or pathologist is subservient to the clinician to such a degree that the latter cannot have a really first-class opinion from the laboratory point of view.[105]

Where clinical biochemists did not have an independent base of power in a medical school department, they were dependent upon the good will of clinicians. Their ambivalence was captured by Oliver Gaebler's description of his position in the clinical department of the Henry Ford Hospital:

Perhaps you may wonder how a clinical chemist felt in such ominous surroundings. In fact, the situation was not ominous at all. The pathologists appreciated my services, and so did the heads of clinical departments. In fact, it seemed to me that the attitude of these and other groups toward clinical chemistry was the same as that of Shakespeare's King Henry V, who protested to Kate that he was not the enemy but the friend of France, for he "loved it so dearly he would not part with a village of it."[106]

The partnership worked, but it was not always an equal partnership.

THE AMERICAN SCHOOL OF CLINICAL BIOCHEMISTRY

The strong connection between biochemistry and clinical medicine was a characteristic feature of American biochemistry in the 1920s and 1930s. By 1940, however, the founding generation of discipline builders was dying off, and a new generation of American biochemists was rejecting the clinical connection and promoting an alternative style of "general biochemistry" rooted in graduate, not medical, schools. Clinical chemistry became a separate applied-science profession, distinct from the academic discipline of biochemistry.

The principal figures in the "American school" of biochemistry were Otto Folin, Donald D. Van Slyke, Stanley Benedict, Victor Myers, and Philip Shaffer. Their students, A. Baird Hastings, Edward Doisey, Willey Denis, and a dozen or so less well-known men and women, made up a network of individuals with similar interests and a sense of community. Unlike their successors, these first-generation clinical biochemists were shaped by the marketplace rather than by their training. Folin and Van Slyke were trained as organic chemists: Folin, with Julius Steiglitz at Chicago; Van Slyke, with chemist Moses Gomberg at Michigan.[107] Benedict and Myers were both alumni of Chittenden's school.[108] Van Slyke did his first biochemical work as assistant to his father, who was chief chemist at the New York Agricultural Experiment Station. Only chance diverted him from a career in the U.S. Department of Agriculture to a career in clinical medicine. Although Folin studied physiological and pathological chemistry with Olof Hammarsten at Uppsala and with Ernst Salkowski at Berlin, he and Shaffer became clinical biochemists by working at McLean Hospital. Stanley Benedict and Victor Myers were drawn into clinical work as a result of their jobs at Cornell and the New York Postgraduate Medical School at Bellevue.

The American school of clinical biochemistry consisted of a tightly knit group, bound together by both personal and professional ties. Folin, Van Slyke, Benedict, and Myers played complementary roles. Otto Folin was the charismatic teacher. Although he was brought to Harvard as a research professor, he quickly discovered that he had the knack of inspiring students.[109] He was devoted to his graduate students, sacrificing his own research output so that many students could work in his laboratory. He denied himself the convenience of having a private research assistant so that his students could learn their craft by doing apprentice work under his supervision. Folin gave top priority to recruitment and training, rather than productivity in research.[110] Folin ran his department democratically, with an eye to developing his students and junior faculty for important posts in the discipline. He was intolerant of prima donnas. When Carl Alsberg complained that he had to clean his own test tubes, Folin snapped that he had ". . . frequently found it convenient to rinse out a few glass utensils for my own use during the past year, and I hope the time may not come very soon when I shall consider it unpleasant or beneath my dignity to do so."[111] In his professional relations, Folin was admired for his personal modesty, his courtesy to all, whatever their rank and reputation, and for his unfailing encouragement to young biochemists. Folin's students became devoted colleagues. Not perhaps in research, but as discipline builder, Folin was, as Victor Myers remarked, "the greatest biochemist of the present generation."[112]

Van Slyke stood out among the clinical biochemists for his achievements in research. Unlike many of his colleagues, Van Slyke was a master not only of analytical chemistry but of physiology and clinical medicine as well. Biochemical methods were devised and developed as an integral part of researches in physiology and pathology. Baird Hastings felt that Van Slyke represented the ideal amalgam of biochemistry and clinical medicine and the ideal leader of departments in medical schools.[113] Biochemists who were not students of Van Slyke's shared Hastings's view that he was the ideal well-rounded biochemist. L. B. Mendel, for instance: "To me he represents the type of greatest promise and progress."[114]

Van Slyke's earliest achievements were in analytical methods (e.g., a manometric assay of protein nitrogen). When he joined the Rockefeller Hospital, diabetes was the object of research there. It was known that acidosis was the cause of diabetic coma and death, but the lack of a quick and simple test for blood acidity made it impossible to predict and prevent this fatal crisis. By adapting his manometric method to measuring the carbon dioxide level in blood, Van Slyke achieved a rapid assay of acidity, and "Van Slykes" were soon in use everywhere. Van Slyke further developed the method into a general tool for clinical analysis. He taught himself kidney physiology and soon found himself in charge of a ward of patients with Bright's disease. He made major contributions to the physiology and pathology of blood, acid–base balance, respiration, and kidney and liver function.[115] Clinical problems provided opportunities to extend and improve analytical procedures; in turn, new techniques led to discoveries in the physiology of disease.

Institutional context was obviously crucial to Van Slyke's success in integrating chemistry and clinical medicine. The Rockefeller Hospital encouraged a cooperative attack on a problem from all points of view: chemical, physiological, and clinical. Van Slyke recalled that the clinicians "took us into their group and almost by force imposed their enthusiasm and their problems upon us." Van Slyke's ability to see all points of view made him an ideal leader of a research team; he was capable of pulling the work together, maintaining a balance in his team of experts, and keeping the clinical problem always in view.[116] Van Slyke's personal gifts were well suited to his role. Modest, helpful, and generous in giving credit, he encouraged his students to become independent researchers.

Van Slyke was as gifted and influential a teacher in the hospital laboratory as Folin was in the medical school. Although Folin trained more professional biochemists, Van Slyke was crucial in bridging the gap between biochemistry and internal medicine. Most of the hundred or more individuals who passed through Van Slyke's group were internists. Many went on to influential chairs of medicine or productive research careers. Representative of this type is John Peters, who became professor of clinical medicine at Yale. Peters and Van Slyke's two-volume handbook of clinical chemistry, "the bible of the iatro-chemists," embodies the symbiosis between internists and clinical biochemists.[117]

Folin's reputation rested largely on his analytical methods. Folin did try to develop a research program that combined chemistry and physiology, for example, in his work on the absorption of amino acids in the liver. But after Van Slyke disproved his theory of absorption, Folin limited his efforts to developing techniques. In 1912 he set out with his student, Hsien Wu, to devise a comprehensive scheme for blood analysis. Unlike urine, blood is a living tissue and was a challenging problem for the analyst. In the 1920s Folin's system was the standard – the "office furniture" of diagnosticians.[118] Folin was sympathetic to a broader point of view; he encouraged a young pathologist, Arthur Kendall, who could find no sympathy in his own discipline for his work on bacterial metabolism. Physicians from Henry Christian's department dropped in regularly for advice, and Folin's laboratory was filled with clinicians learning advanced techniques.[119] Folin was an effective spokesman to clinicians, as Frank Billings testified in 1919: "If Dr. Folin could command some of the patients, I am sure students taking the course in the wards would take greater interest in biochemistry."[120] But Folin himself never managed to integrate chemistry and clinical physiology as Van Slyke did.

Stanley Benedict was exclusively a methods man and made no effort to acquire a knowledge of clinical medicine. Even as an undergraduate, Benedict evinced a passion for improving analytical methods.[121] In his professional community, he was the gadfly and critic, a role he played with puckish enthusiasm. As fast as Folin invented new methods, Benedict altered and improved them. Folin was somewhat irritated by Benedict's constant criticism, but his reputation among clinicians was not diminished, and the two biochemists remained on excellent terms.[122] (Folin even invited Benedict to spend time in his laboratory working on improving his methods.) Victor Myers captured the spirit of friendly competition:

I recall very vividly the verbal tilts between Benedict and Folin. These were amusing and enjoyable, chiefly for the reason that Folin could always see their amusing side. At the Cincinnati meeting of the ASBC in 1919, Benedict picked the first Folin–Wu blood sugar method to pieces. . . . After Benedict's paper Folin got up and said "Benedict is a past master in finding flaws in perfectly good methods and if what Benedict says is so I am perfectly willing to accept it," and sat down. I whispered to Benedict, "You seem to have Folin licked." He replied, "I'll bet Folin can't get back to Boston fast enough to go over the method again." Folin gave a Harvey Lecture in February and had ironed out practically all of Benedict's criticism. Although his lecture was supposedly on another topic he could not resist coming back to his blood sugar method on several occasions. Benedict frequently got quite excited over his discussions with Folin but Folin always took them very calmly and treated Benedict somewhat as a son.

After Folin died Benedict wrote me a long letter telling me. . .how keenly he felt Folin's loss personally.[123]

Despite a shy and retiring character, Benedict was an excellent teacher. With his graduate students, he was gruff and unapproachable until he was convinced that they could deliver. He was extremely critical and unaware of the devastating effect of his criticisms; yet his fierce loyalty to his protégés inspired lasting friendships.[124]

Like Benedict, Victor Myers was primarily an analyst. Myers kept up the friendship that began when he was a student with Benedict at Yale, making a point to visit him whenever he was in New York.[125] As clinical chemistry developed into a specialized profession distinct from biochemistry, Myers took an active role in establishing professional institutions and in promoting professional identity and status: he was one of the first to focus on "the public relations problems of clinical chemistry." In the 1920s, Myers made the University of Iowa a center for training clinical chemists, primarily for hospital positions. He was also active in developing the market for clinical chemists, organizing regular demonstrations of clinical procedures for the annual meetings of the AMA. He served as examiner in charge of the Board of Clinical Pathology – a tedious, but politically important job. He was active in blocking legislation requiring clinical chemists to be physicians as well.[126]

The cohesiveness of the clinical biochemists undoubtedly contributed to their success in shaping the discipline. They helped their students into important positions, and developed a sense of collective purpose. Folin encouraged a diffident Edward Doisey to press for improvements at the St. Louis Medical School.[127] Baird Hastings recommended Van Slyke's disciple, Glenn Cullen, for Mendel's chair at Yale and wrote to Cullen: "You are my yardstick....I think that your approach to Biochemistry is exactly what medical schools should have – it is what I aim at in our department."[128] Clinical biochemistry flourished in America largely for institutional reasons – the long tradition of medical chemistry and the institutional location of the discipline in medical schools – but also because a small group of able leaders, in their different ways, made the system work.

The continuing wave of clinical reform created a booming market for clinical biochemists. Folin had turned down eight chairs by 1920. Van Slyke declined Victor Vaughan's chair and the deanship at Michigan in 1922 and refused many such offers.[129] Between 1915 and 1940, chairs of biochemistry in some 20 medical schools were filled by clinical biochemists, many of them students or former colleagues of Folin, Benedict, and Van Slyke (see Table 9.1). Most departments of biochemistry had at least one professor in clinical analysis and metabolism. Clinical biochemists set the style and held the seats of power in the discipline for a full generation.

In the 1930s, academic biochemistry and applied clinical biochemistry began to diverge. A new avant-garde felt the appeal of a "general" biochemistry dealing with general principles relevant to all the biological sciences. Leavened by the example of F. G. Hopkins's school at Cambridge and a few German institutes, American departments began to turn aside from the analytical concerns of the founding generation. At the same time, clinical chemistry evolved into a specialized occupational specialty adapted to the needs of hospital diagnostic laboratories. In the 1940s and 1950s, clinical

Table 9.1. *Selected professorial appointments of clinical biochemists*

Medical school	Date of professorship	Biochemist	Training
Marquette	1918	Joseph C. Buck	Cornell instructor, 1913–18
California	1918	Walter Bloor	Harvard Ph.D., 1911
Western Reserve	1919	J. Lucien Morris	Harvard Ph.D., 1914
Buffalo	1920	Guy E. Youngsburg	Harvard Ph.D., 1922
Illinois	1921	William Welker	Columbia Ph.D., 1907
Pittsburgh	1921	William McEllroy	Pittsburgh M.D., 1916
Tennessee	1922	Thomas P. Nash	Cornell Ph.D., 1922
Texas	1922	Byron Hendrix	Yale Ph.D., 1915
Rochester	1922	Walter Bloor	Harvard Ph.D., 1911
St. Louis	1923	Edward A. Doisey	Harvard Ph.D., 1920
Tulane	1923	Willey G. Denis	MGH (Folin), 1913–20
Oklahoma	1924	Mark R. Everett	Harvard Ph.D., 1924
Iowa	1924	Victor Myers	N.Y. Postgrad. (prof.), 1909–24
Vanderbilt	1925	Glenn Cullen	Rockefeller, 1913–21
N.Y. Postgraduate	1926	John Killian	Fordham Ph.D., 1921
Western Reserve	1927	Victor Myers	N.Y. Postgrad. (prof.), 1909–24
Tulane	1929	Sidney Bliss	Harvard Ph.D., 1925
Duke	1930	William A. Perlzweig	Columbia Ph.D., 1925
Harvard	1935	A. Baird Hastings	Rockefeller, 1921–6
Boston University	1935	Burnham S. Walker	Boston U. Ph.D., 1926
Loyola	1937	Julius Sendroy	Rockefeller, 1926–37
Cincinnati	1940	Milan Logan	Harvard Ph.D., 1928
Marquette	1944	Armand Quick	Cornell M.D., 1928

chemists acquired the familiar trappings of a profession: an association (1949), a journal (1953), regional associations, a code of ethics regarding training and licensing, and a lively concern with professional identity and the low status of the "clinical chemist" with respect to academic biochemists.[130] Clinical chemistry became a branch of applied biochemistry, with distinctive patterns of training and careers. Oliver Gaebler testified to "a growing sense of excommunication from biochemistry" in the 1930s.[131]

Gaebler attributed this growing divergence between clinical and general biochemistry not to academic snobbery but to internal developments in the discipline. The problems that had challenged the analytical skills of Folin's generation had so evolved as to require highly specialized skills. In metabolic studies, the frontier moved from experiments with whole animals to newer techniques using tissue slices or extracts to study "intermediary" metabolism (the individual chemical reactions involved in the breakdown and synthesis of compounds). Studies of tissue oxidation and enzymes were more productive and prestigious fields of research than clinical analysis. Work on the isolation and structure of vitamins and hormones required skilled organic chemists, whereas methods of clinical analysis were routinized to the point that even complex procedures could be done by technicians.

Biochemical diagnosis did not cease to develop, of course: from today's perspective, it had hardly begun. Development of clinical methods simply became the special province of clinical chemists who were not at the center of the biochemical discipline, although they adopted Folin, Benedict, and Van Slyke as their founding fathers. Medical school biochemists found their opportunities for discipline building in newer, more academically prestigious lines of research. This division of labor helped free the new generation of academic biochemists to pursue general biochemical problems without being accused of neglecting clinical applications.

In the early years of medical reform, biochemistry in America depended on its service role as an applied clinical science. Folin, Benedict, Victor Myers, Philip Hawk, and other clinical biochemists were a transitional generation, who resembled their predecessors, the medical chemists, as closely as they resembled their successors. The intellectual style of American biochemistry was shaped by its institutional basis and its service roles in the period of discipline building. By 1940 service roles in hospital laboratories were less essential for the survival of the discipline, and new intellectual opportunities beckoned in bioorganic chemistry and molecular biology. In these areas, European biochemists led the way, in part because they had not had the institutional advantages and responsibilities of an independent discipline.

CONCLUSION

The characteristics of American biochemistry define a distinctive "national style": medical school departments independent of physiology; emphasis on analytical technique and clinical application; and connection with hospital laboratories and clinical research teams. One must be cautious, however, in speaking of a national style. Americans had no monopoly on clinical biochemistry. German clinical researchers collaborated with biochemists. Such biochemists as Otto Warburg, Otto Meyerhof, Gustav Embden, Karl Thomas, and Hans Krebs were trained in medical faculties and were alert to medical themes. Britain had several outstanding centers of clinical biochemistry: E. C. Dodd's department in the Courtauld Institute at the Middlesex Hospital, Charles Harington's group at University College, and Edgar and Ellen Stedman's team at Edinburgh University. There were nonmedical styles of biochemistry in America, such as Jacques Loeb's or Russell Chittenden and L. B. Mendel's school of nutritional physiology at Yale.

In America, however, the leaders of the discipline were clinical biochemists. It was in the field of analytical methods and applied biochemistry that American biochemists equaled or surpassed their European colleagues. Because American biochemists were established in independent departments of medical schools, they were able to develop clinical biochemistry systematically, as an intellectual discipline, rather than as ad hoc responses to occasional clinical needs or in extradisciplinary contexts. In America, clinical biochemistry was accorded the intellectual prestige of an independent discipline. For almost two generations, intellectual achievements and good career prospects attracted the most able and ambitious young American biochemists to clinical problems.

In Germany, biochemical aspects of pathology and medicine were pursued outside the discipline. In Britain, chemical pathologists were a separate and lower-status professional group, mainly located in the teaching hospitals. Alternative styles of "general biochemistry" were less influential in America than in Europe. The Oxbridge school of F. G. Hopkins and Rudolph Peters dominated British biochemistry; schools of chemical physiology and bioorganic chemistry dominated German biochemistry. In America, Loeb finally fled from the clinicians to the haven of the Rockefeller Institute. Several early programs oriented toward general biology or physiology drifted toward the clinical mode. Even Mendel's group at Yale was finally absorbed by the Yale Medical School. These different tendencies are what constitute "national styles."

Disciplinary programs in biochemistry reflect the institutional contexts in which biochemists worked: their service roles, professional alliances, and the needs of their clinical clientele. Especially in the vulnerable formative years of a new discipline, intellectual priorities are shaped by the mode of production of scientific knowledge. As institutions provide a stable basis of support, disciplines may lose their distinctive style, becoming more varied and receptive to various research programs. In the late 1930s, European styles, developed in quite different institutional contexts, took root in American departments of biochemistry. By exploiting the clinical connection, biochemists created a large and stable system of institutions, and gained ready access to economic and political resources. Had biochemists tried instead to build a discipline on the basis of more highbrow programs of general biochemistry and on support from biologists and chemists, it is doubtful that they would have done as well. A conception of biochemistry as an applied science was suited to the practical ideology of the Progressive period and to the politics of medical reform. Once in place, however, the system of institutions could provide a basis for evolving programs that were less closely tied to clinical application.

10

Chemical ideals and biochemical practice

The influence of chemistry in biochemistry may seem as amorphous and boundless a theme as the influence of theology in the church. At the beginning, nearly a third of the members of the American Society of Biological Chemists had Ph.D. degrees in chemistry. Half of ASBC members who got their degrees between 1900 and 1910 joined the American Chemical Society; no fewer than 85% of the cohort with doctorates between 1930 and 1934 did so.[1] It is rare to find biochemists who did not take their undergraduate work in chemistry. Most chemists regarded biochemistry as an applied branch of their discipline, and their views enjoyed increasing deference from biochemists. How, then, to dissect such a close-woven tissue of relationships? As in the preceding chapter, we must concentrate on institutionalized roles and channels of influence. We must see what systematic opportunities there were for recruitment of chemists or for cooperative relations. We must see how adoption of chemists' theories and methods conferred strategic advantages for discipline building. We must understand how chemists' disciplinary ambitions and their role in medical school departments shaped the practice of biochemistry.

The language of "hybrid" disciplines should not mislead us into assuming that chemistry and biology or medicine had equal or symmetrical roles in the genesis and nurture of biochemistry. In fact, they did not. Biology and medicine provided problems; chemistry provided means. (Chemical means did tend, of course, to become biochemical ends.) Few biochemists came from backgrounds in biology or the biomedical sciences; chemistry was the principal source of recruits. Although medicine provided contexts for applied research, rarely was biochemistry institutionalized as a subdivision of a chemistry department. Biochemists were the middle level of a vertically integrated system: they looked to chemistry for recruits and models of methodological "rigor," and to medicine for employment and touchstones of significant research.

It seems to have been almost universally accepted that chemistry was the best basic training for biochemists. Edwin Faust wrote his mentor, J. J. Abel, that chemists and physiologists all agreed chemistry came first: "Schmiedeberg says that the man who studies medicine first and chemistry afterwards seldom 'denkt frei' and Baumann, Hoppe-Seyler, Goltz, Voit and Baeyer all express themselves to the same end."[2] Philip Shaffer set forth the strategic and intellectual advantages of long chemical training:

Much the larger number of American biochemists, teachers and investigators have been trained as chemists and not medically: and with the present great demand from clinical departments for men with training in laboratory subjects, no chemist with an M.D. is likely to remain in biochemistry. So, for our own recruits we must depend largely upon the Ph.D. men. . . . And besides, they as a class are apt to be better qualified because of the longer drill in pure science – physics, chemistry, mathematics, physical chemistry – before they go into biological work; and some of us believe that real advance in medicine is more apt to come from physics and chemistry than from medicine itself.[3]

When W. G. MacCallum sought the advice of British physiologists regarding a successor to Walter Jones, almost to a man they advised him to choose someone trained in pure chemistry. Hopkins was the sole dissenting voice, but MacCallum seems not to have taken his views seriously:

I went then to Cambridge and talked it all over with Hopkins, whose idea is quite opposite to that of Fletcher, Martin, Dudly, Robinson, Boycott, and Harington, all of whom thought the essential preliminary was the training in chemistry. Hopkins would take a biologist and train him in chemistry. He himself is no good example for he started as a public analyst's assistant and then studied medicine while lecturing at Guys. But he was strong on the idea that a regular chemist has no aptitude for biological problems and does not recognize them.[4]

Hans T. Clarke observed that biochemistry was not a fundamental chemical specialty like organic, physical, or analytical chemistry but rather an applied science in which all the basic specialties were employed.[5]

There were strategic as well as intellectual reasons why chemistry was a preferred avenue for recruitment to biochemistry. Most biologists avoided chemistry as too difficult. Individuals trained initially in medicine absorbed clinicians' ambivalence toward the biomedical sciences and found it hard to resist the opportunities of medical practice. Biology and medicine were expanding areas of professional employment for chemists – strategic resources for discipline building. Chemists were aggressive in cultivating those resources and were abetted by clinicians' deference to the ideology of "hard" science. A favored market relation with medical biochemistry was thus formed.

The potential existed around 1900 for relations of a different sort between biochemistry and chemistry. For about a decade, chemists had a real opportunity to establish biological chemistry as a subdivision analogous to organic or physical chemistry. They did not seize this opportunity, however. Only in a few special circumstances was biological chemistry included in departments of chemistry. The University of Illinois is the most important exception: though small, that group was an extremely influential source of recruits to biochemistry in the early 1920s. In most cases, however, chemistry departments offered few career opportunities for biochemists and exported recruits to a separate biochemical market. By 1910 medical schools had virtually monopolized biochemistry, with no competition from departments of chemistry.

To understand this pattern of relations, we must ask if the subdivision of chemical specialties had a strategic advantage for chemists during the critical period from 1900 to 1910. In particular, was biological chemistry important strategically for discipline builders? The answers are: subdivision was only one strategy and there were strong pressures against it; biological chemistry was not regarded as a high-status specialty until it was too late and it had become a separate biomedical discipline. This pattern can be seen in the evolving policy of the American Chemical Society (ACS) regarding specialty subgroups and in the policies of expanding university departments, like those at Illinois and Stanford.

BIOCHEMISTRY AND PROFESSIONAL POLITICS: THE ACS

The great trend in chemistry after 1900 was the explosive growth in the market for specialized professional chemists. Government bureaus like the U.S. Department of Agriculture, industrial laboratories, agricultural experiment stations, sanitary commissions, hospitals, and other institutions were demanding trained chemists for regulatory work and research. The Progressive romance with the scientific expert was in full flower, and chemists were among the first to enjoy the benefits.[6] Proliferation of specialized markets accelerated the trend toward separate professional societies and journals. As professional groups coalesced, they became aware of the need for organizations to protect their professional interests. These trends were both an opportunity and a threat to the leaders of the American Chemical Society: the promise of power and influence was challenged by separatist movements. The burning issue of the period from 1900 to 1914 for the ACS was chemical specialties and how to contain them. The debate reveals where biological chemistry stood among chemists' priorities.

The greatest threat to the society came from industrial chemists, who felt that the ACS discriminated against industrial chemistry in meetings and publications and offered inadequate political support for improving working conditions. Older specialized societies, such as the Association of Agricultural Chemists (1884) and the New York section of the British Society of Chemical Industry (1894), declined to affiliate with the ACS.[7] Even more ominous were the stirrings of separatism among academic physical and biological chemists. The large New York section of the ACS, which had led the reorganization of the 1890s, was especially alarmed by the creation of a New York branch of the Verein Deutscher Chemiker (1902), the American Electrochemical Society (1902), and W. J. Gies's group of physiological chemists.[8]

One solution to the problem of specialization was to organize semiautonomous subdivisions within the society. A committee chaired by A. A. Noyes, director of the physical chemistry laboratory at MIT, set forth such a plan in June 1903. One of the five divisions proposed was for agricultural, physiological, and sanitary chemistry. Noyes's plan was too radical for the ACS council, however. Some older chemists felt that official recognition of specialties would destroy the intellectual unity of chemistry as a whole. Ira Remsen, Edgar Fahs Smith, and J. W. Mallet strongly opposed Noyes's scheme on this ground.[9] Their vision of a general chemistry reflected their German training, their investment in a broad range of knowledge, and their privileged roles as chiefs of one-professor teaching departments.[10] A more modern version of this view was held by some of the new generation of specialists such as Wilder Bancroft, proprietor and editor of the *Journal of Physical Chemistry*. Bancroft saw physical chemistry as unifying chemistry as a whole and resisted all efforts by A. A. Noyes, his arch rival, to establish physical chemistry as a separate specialty.[11]

There was a pervasive fear that the ACS would be unable to contain the new specialties and would fission into separate societies. There were historical reasons for this fear. Only ten years earlier, American chemistry was organized into separate local societies, dominated by local chemical interests. The American Chemical Society was national in name, but in reality it was confined to New York City. In the 1890s, the New York chemists succeeded in reorganizing the ACS as a national society by incorporating local or regional societies as sections.[12] Memories of disunity and fears of secession were very much alive to the veterans of reform. Encouraging specialized journals and divisions seemed to them to be courting division and secession in a new guise. Ideology, vested interests, and historical experience all provided reasons not to recognize new chemical specialties, including biochemistry.

Moderates in the society understood that specialties would flourish whether or not the ACS acknowledged them and that they would become the real centers of professional allegiance if the ACS did not contain them. The reform group also understood the positive uses of specialization as a strategy for institutional growth and improvement. William A. Noyes, chief of the chemistry division of the National Bureau of Standards, exemplified this position. Although he opposed subdividing the ACS, he fully shared A. A. Noyes's vision of a unity of interest among chemical specialties: "Every chemist ought to feel strongly that the work done in every other field of chemistry, and indeed...in Physics and Biology as well, is likely to touch his own work at many vital points."[13] Unlike Remsen or E. F. Smith, W. A. Noyes and other moderates did not believe that one individual could encompass all of chemistry; they looked to cooperation among specialists. Unlike A. A. Noyes, they favored a cautious and gradual recognition of separate specialty interests within the ACS, to minimize the dangers of secession. As president of the society in 1904, W. A. Noyes initiated the policy of organizing meetings in specialized sections. (W. J. Gies organized a section for biological chemistry on the understanding that this was a first step toward a formal specialized division.) Noyes led the move to establish *Chemical Abstracts*, hoping that a comprehensive journal sponsored by the ACS would unite the special interests in the society.[14]

These modest efforts to accommodate specialty interests did not stem the separatist tide. In 1907 the American Institute of Chemical Engineers was organized. New journals and societies in the academic chemical specialties continued to appear. The *Journal of Biological Chemistry* (1904) and the American Society of Biological Chemists (1906) preempted ACS leadership in this growing specialty. Columbia chemist and ACS president, Marston Bogert, warned that if the ACS did not stop the trend toward separate national societies, disintegration of the ACS was only a question of time:

The society which fails to take cognizance of the growing strength of specialization and to lay its course accordingly, fails to grasp its opportunities and slowly but surely will be crowded to the wall. We should not be under the delusion that if our Society fails to recognize this tendency to specialize, specialization will therefore cease.[15]

Bogert hoped that existing specialty societies would accept affiliation as quasi-independent divisions of the ACS and that specialty journals could be attached to the ACS as parts of an omnibus journal. Gies's biochemistry section had already met jointly with the American Society of Biological Chemists, and Bogert saw such cooperation as the first step toward affiliation and merger. The *Journal of Biological Chemistry* would then become an official organ of the ACS.[16] Bogert's scheme was more or less the same as A. A. Noyes's earlier plan, but it was too little too late. In 1903 the ACS could have created new organizations; in 1908 it had to persuade established societies and journals to give up their independence. The chemists had lost the initiative.

Divisional reorganization was most successful in the industrial specialties. A division of industrial chemistry and chemical engineering, organized in 1908, was followed in 1909 and 1910 by divisions for fertilizer chemistry, agricultural and food chemistry, and pharmaceutical chemistry. A divison of biological chemistry was finally created in 1913.[17] However, the more academic divisions never fulfilled Noyes and Bogert's expectations. The society's journal did not evolve into a group of specialty journals.[18] Overtures were made to Christian Herter and J. J. Abel to absorb the *Journal of Biological Chemistry*, which Herter rejected as a threat to the independence of biochemistry.[19] Led by Abel, the pharmacologists organized their own independent journal and society. Biochemists had much less to gain than industrial chemists from an alliance with the ACS and resented the chemists' sudden shift from indifference to predatory interest once the biochemists' journal and society were going concerns. The American Society of Biological Chemists rapidly preempted the ACS as a forum for biochemical research. Gies, Abel, or Chittenden could, on occasion, recruit the best biochemists for ACS sessions, but increasingly, the biochemical section was run by applied biochemists and was devoted to agricultural or sanitary chemistry.[20]

The American Chemical Society simply moved too slowly and cautiously to capture the allegiance of academic biochemists. A letter from Frank Cameron to Wilder Bancroft reveals how ACS policies had failed to meet the needs of the academic specialties:

Neither the ACS nor its publications are useful to its members in upholding the dignity of their jobs or getting new jobs for them. The trades union idea has come in. We have seen that demonstrated already in the case of our Industrial Journal, which we were told simply had to be brought into existence to get and hold the industrial chemists. But we have a far more pronounced illustration in the *Journal of Biochemistry* [sic]. Biochemistry was not being recognized as an important subdivision of science by the institutions furnishing jobs, therefore biochemists of the better grade said: "We will make them recognize us," and they made their own society and their own journal, and the claim is made – and problably could be substantiated – that they have forced recognition from the institutions in which they were interested, especially the medical schools, and these institutions are now taking a whole crowd of men and paying better salaries for the work; opportunities are being created for the younger men to get into biochemistry, and the older men are getting more consideration and better recognition of their dignity from the institutions. . . . The attitude of those chaps is that the Chemical Society has done nothing to help them, and the Journal instead of being helpful has been rather detrimental than otherwise. Therefore the American Chemical Society can go to the devil, chase after industrial chemists and whatever it pleases. It has lost interest in. . .the scientific chemists and they will more or less rapidly drop out unless something is done to revive and hold their interest.[21]

(Cameron had just learned of Abel's resignation from the ACS and of his plans for a pharmacological society.)

DEPARTMENT POLITICS: ILLINOIS

The ambivalent policy of ACS leaders regarding biochemistry was symptomatic of the more general relation between the two professions. Chemists saw biochemistry as an important specialty to be kept within the fold of the ACS. To lose biological chemistry was bad economics and bad politics. But biological chemistry was economically much less important to chemists than industrial chemistry, or even food or pharmaceutical chemistry, and intellectually less important than the core specialties of physical or organic chemistry. These priorities are evident not only in the high politics of the American Chemical Society but in the decisions of chemistry departments to develop biological chemistry or, more frequently, to relinquish it to medical schools.

The reform of medical schools offered special opportunities for chemists to develop biochemistry. In many universities, biochemistry courses were temporarily organized in chemistry departments, until medical departments could be organized. Clinical faculties wanted the best teachers, and the best were chemists. Why then did chemistry departments offer so little competition to medical school biochemists? The answer may lie in the slight difference in the timing of medical school and university reform. Chemists adopted the strategy of specialization just about the time that biochemistry was being organized in medical schools. But chemists' first priorities were the more theoretical or economically important specialties: organic, physical, and industrial chemistry. For a few crucial years, biological chemistry was a second priority, and in those years, biological chemistry was established as a separate department in medical schools. Where there was a strong medical school, it usually prevailed; where there was no medical school, the student market did not warrant hiring a biochemist and chemists' disciplinary imperatives prevailed. The University of Illinois is a case in point.

Biological chemistry was established at Illinois in the reorganization of the Department of Chemistry following the death of A. W. Palmer in 1904. Palmer was a chemist of the old school: a generalist, a teacher, and a practical chemist, lacking in specialized research skills and out of tune with modern specialties. His department was adapted to the practical demands of one of the most populist and utilitarian state universities. (Palmer's life's work was a survey of state water resources.) The architect of reorganization was Samuel W. Parr, an industrial chemist specializing in the chemistry of Illinois coals and an academic entrepreneur of impressive vision and ability. He was supported by the new president, Edmund James, a University of Chicago man who was determined to force Eastern academic ideals upon the conservative regents and legislators.

Parr envisioned a department comprised of no fewer than eight specialized subdivisions, each headed by a full professor.[22] In addition to general, physical, and organic chemistry, Parr's plan included divisions for five applied specialties: sanitary, agricultural, pharmaceutical, metallurgical, and physiological chemistry. Parr's priorities reflected his own background in technical chemistry and his alertness to the booming market for specialized chemists. He called the dean's attention to the heavy demand for academic chemists in industry and marveled at the high salaries being offered.[23] Parr's vision combined the Midwestern tradition of practical chemistry and the Eastern academic style of specialized research. To lead the new department, Parr wooed and finally won W. A. Noyes, director of the Bureau of Standards and ACS reformer, who shared Parr's vision of a cooperative division of labor.[24]

Physiological chemistry of a sort had been practiced at Illinois for over a decade by Harry S. Grindley. A student of Wilbur Olin Atwater's, H. S. Grindley was one of the most active of the second generation of American "animal chemists." Since 1896 he had been involved in a large research project on the nutritional chemistry of meat and meat products, financed by the U.S. Department of Agriculture and the Illinois Agricultural Experiment Station.[25] Grindley's work exemplified Parr's ideal of applying basic research to the needs of regional agriculture and industry. Grindley's group was an essential part of Parr's blueprint for the new department. In early 1907, when Grindley received an offer of a chair from another university, Noyes made an emergency trip from Washington to consult with Parr and James on how to keep Grindley at Urbana.[26]

Grindley was not the only one at Illinois with an interest in physiological chemistry. Professor of Physiology George T. Kemp taught physiological chemistry, including an advanced, specialized course.[27] Kemp's department was the keystone of President James's plan to establish a medical school at the university. Kemp was appointed in 1897 when the university became affiliated with the Chicago College of Physicians and Surgeons, and a two-year program in the preclinical sciences was initiated at Urbana for students who wanted academic training before going on to professional school in Chicago. But whereas Grindley's school flourished, Kemp was beset with impediments and frustration. Development of a full preclinical program at Urbana was blocked by budget-conscious legislators. The six-year B.A.–M.D. degree program was a disaster, forcing Kemp to reduce a two-year course in physiology to one and to omit many of the lectures in physiological chemistry and all the laboratory sessions. The elementary course was flooded with students, but few returned to take the advanced course in physiological chemistry. Reasearch was almost impossible.[28] Although Kemp's style of physiological chemistry was more modern than Grindley's, it was less well adapted to the context of a state university, which was isolated from the medical school and allied mainly to agricultural and industrial interests.

Biochemistry thus became a bone of contention among Noyes and Parr in chemistry, Kemp in physiology, and the dean of the agricultural college, Eugene Davenport. Grindley played chemistry against agriculture to get the most support for his meat project. Parr courted Grindley, ignored Kemp, and tried to keep agriculture from staking a claim to biochemistry. Davenport played a waiting game, hoping to acquire Grindley but keep his project on chemistry's budget.[29] James tried to balance the contending interests.

The definition of what biochemistry was to be at Urbana was shaped by the complex political maneuvering among these various interests. In 1907, for example, Grindley was transferred from chemistry to the Department of Animal Nutrition in the College of Agriculture. Parr and Noyes agreed to this only on condition that Grindley's future role be strictly limited to animal chemistry, and that the Department of Chemistry be given a broad mandate to develop: "...this new field which is coming to be designated by bio-chemistry, that term including the smaller field of physiological chemistry."[30] Grindley's departure was an opportunity for Parr to appoint a more modern, academic biochemist, such as Elmer V. McCollum, Chittenden's prize pupil.[31] Sensitized by his encounters with cost-conscious legislators, James was loath to create competing roles. Reluctantly, he agreed to let Parr appoint a new man to Grindley's vacant chair – not necessarily a biochemist. He left the choice of a specialty to Parr and Noyes.[32] The place of biochemistry in the Department of Chemistry became an open issue.

Noyes's first priority was to develop physical chemistry as a specialty, and he wondered if the department could afford a full-time specialist in biochemistry. Because Grindley had taught general chemistry and qualitative analysis, Noyes suggested that these fields could be improved by giving Grindley's chair to a top young physical chemist, such as Gilbert N. Lewis, a colleague of A. A. Noyes's at MIT.[33] Parr made it clear that his first priority was a biochemist but left the decision to Noyes. There was no rivalry between the two.[34] Parr gave more consideration to local opportunities and was less willing to lose an established claim to biochemistry. Noyes, the outsider, was more concerned that Illinois be competitive in the growing national market for physical chemists. When G. N. Lewis declined Noyes's offer of a chair in general and analytical chemistry, Noyes backed Parr's efforts to woo McCollum and persuade the dean to develop general biochemistry within chemistry:

We should offer in the university a good course in physiological chemistry for the benefit of those students who are preparing for medicine, and someone like Professor Mathews, of Chicago, would be very suitable. . . . I feel strongly that the chemical department is the proper place for. . . work of this character and that it should be cared for in our department rather than in the department of animal husbandry.[35]

In May, however, James informed Parr and Noyes that the governor had "slaughtered" the university's appropriation and that because physiological chemistry was already taught in other departments, there could be no question of creating a competing group of biochemists.[36]

We see here, in local academic politics, the same attitudes that shaped the policies of the American Chemical Society toward biochemistry. In chemists' eyes, biochemistry was an applied chemical specialty, with potential markets in agriculture, industry, and medicine. It was important for departments that used specialization as a strategy for growth, but it was less important than such core specialties as organic, physical, or analytical chemistry. This attitude reflected the reality of student demand, which was growing very rapidly in general chemistry.[37] Chemists' attitude toward biochemistry also reflected the reality of academic politics. Unlike physical or organic chemistry, biochemistry was marginal, in the sense that other disciplines also laid claim to it. If departments of chemistry invested too heavily in plans for biochemistry, they ran the risk of getting nothing at all. Parr and Noyes wanted general biochemistry, but not at the cost of more important interests. An ambitious department had to compete in physical or organic chemistry; biochemistry was a luxury. James felt that biochemistry belonged in medicine, and economic pressures for efficiency limited the ability of chemists to establish a competing claim.

With Parr's initiative stalled by competing claims and limited resources, Grindley's program flourished in the College of Agriculture. Davenport promised Grindley an assistant professor in "physiological chemistry." Parr objected strenuously to this title, fearing that it might "serve to leave the doors wide open for occupying ground which we thought belonged to us." Davenport agreed to change the title of the new post to "animal nutrition"; however, Grindley was untroubled by Parr's semantic subtleties and, in July 1907, appointed Philip Hawk, John Marshall's assistant at Pennsylvania. Hawk had worked with Atwater on animal respiration and was a skilled analyst – just the man for Grindley's big meat project.[38] Hawk was also ambitious, a zealous researcher, author of a popular laboratory manual, and experienced in teaching biochemistry to medical students.[39] By appointing Hawk, Grindley established a de facto claim to biochemistry.

Meanwhile, the potential competition from physiology disappeared in a puff of political smoke. It is unclear how the "Kemp affair" began, but by 1908 Kemp and James were out for each other's blood. Kemp was a promising scion of the Johns Hopkins school of physiology. He was also a difficult man, combative and uncooperative, and he became increasingly embittered and defensive. According to James, Kemp was an incompetent teacher and administrator and had failed to keep up in research. Kemp, in turn, charged that James had humiliated him by denying him control of appointments and had so burdened him with teaching that it was impossible for him to do any research. Parr's failure to consult with him regarding physiological chemistry was a particularly bitter pill (although he exonerated Noyes from any share in the insult).[40] Kemp turned to politics. In 1908 he allied himself with the faction of the regents opposed to state support of medical training, and he mobilized a group of local physicians who opposed James's attempt to build a preclinical program in the university. The affair became a public confrontation. Kemp criticized James's "dictatorial" style and James attacked Kemp as incompetent. Factions of the Board of Regents exchanged angry memoranda. Kemp resigned and then repented; rebuffed and desperate, he lost control and at a meeting of the board, stole a confidential memorandum by James and had parts of it published in *Science*. It was a fatal error. Their faith in Kemp's character destroyed, the regents voted to accept his resignation, and Kemp was forced to leave.[41]

Three weeks later, Noyes stepped in to pick up the pieces:

With the resignation of Professor Kemp, there is no one...who is now competent to give instruction in this field. It appears to me that the work in this field should be cared for rather in the chemical department than anywhere else, and in view of the present call for graduate work in the field, it is necessary that we should have a man of first-class ability.[42]

James was still concerned with efficiency and pointed out that Hawk had taught medical biochemistry and was carrying out his research in Noyes's laboratory. In 1909 Hawk was appointed professor of physiological chemistry in the Department of Chemistry. Noyes then proceeded to press the dean for two junior appointments in the new division of biochemistry, to keep up with better medical schools.[43] Hawk aggressively recruited students and cranked out research:

Perhaps I may be pardoned for making a statement which may sound egotistical but which is nevertheless true.... [s]tatistics show that my laboratory HAS BEEN MORE ACTIVE IN ORIGINAL INVESTIGATION DURING THE YEARS 1909–1910 THAN HAS ANY OTHER LABORATORY OF PHYSIOLOGICAL CHEMISTRY IN THE COUNTRY....An examination of the programs of the various scientific societies in which we are interested will also show that my laboratory has TAKEN THE LEAD IN THE NUMBER OF PAPERS READ BEFORE THESE SOCIEITIES.[44]

Hawk soon felt that his efforts were not adequately rewarded, and in 1912 he accepted a chair at the Jefferson Medical College in Philadelphia. The proper location of biochemistry was once again an open issue.

James was deeply involved at the time with establishing a university medical school in Chicago; he saw the raison d'être of biochemistry as training premedical students and would have preferred to have it attached, inexpensively, to physiology.[45] Noyes, aware that possession was nine-tenths of the law, was cool and diplomatic:

On the side of an all around training in chemistry the students in physiological chemistry are very much better off when in the chemical department. Possibly on the side of physiology they would be better off in the department of physiology. . . . On the whole, however, I am inclined to think that the physiological chemists could be better cared for in affiliation with chemistry.[46]

Biochemistry stayed in chemistry, but not in grand style. Hawk's teaching duties were assigned to two young instructors, and a chair was not reestablished until William Rose came in 1922.

The period from 1912 to 1922 was one of uncertainty for the biochemists at Urbana, largely owing to the lack of a strong medical service role. James's plan for a full two-year course in the preclinical sciences at Urbana never materialized. Fewer students came to Urbana for their first two years, preferring to take four years in the medical school in Chicago. There were complaints from Chicago in 1914 that students trained at Urbana had to repeat biochemistry because they had not been taught urinalysis. Physiological chemistry at the medical school expanded as a subdivision of George Deyer's Department of Physiology, with a strong clinical bent. At Urbana, two-thirds of the students taking biochemistry in 1914 were preparing to be professional chemists or biochemists, not physicians.[47] The paths diverged.

Without a service role in medicine, biochemistry at Urbana remained a small subdivision, dependent on and overshadowed by the division of organic chemistry. Directed by Noyes's successor, Roger Adams, the Illinois school of organic chemistry flourished on the surging postwar demand for industrial chemists. William Rose was one of the best biochemists of his generation; but he was no entrepreneur. He eschewed programmatics and directed his own and his students' energies to a narrow line of research: the chemistry of amino acids. Rose's conception of biochemistry fit his role as a welcome, but minor, partner in Illinois's organic chemistry factory.[48]

The symbiosis of biochemistry and chemistry at Illinois depended on the conjunction of unusual circumstances. Most important was the presence of S. W. Parr, with his powerful vision of a multispecialty department and the administrative genius to delegate responsibility to Noyes and division heads. Grindley played an important role by establishing "animal chemistry" as a legitimate chemical specialty, but not in a way that preempted a broader program in biochemistry. Geographical separation from the medical school opened the door to the chemists, and George Kemp's blunders closed the door to a potential competitor. As President James realized, the organization of biochemistry as a subfield of chemistry went against the tide of medical reform. But circumstances prevented James from putting his policy into effect.

SCHOOLS OF BIOORGANIC CHEMISTRY

Stanford was the only major university aside from Illinois in which biochemistry was established within chemistry. Some of the same conditions obtained: geographical distance from the medical school in San Francisco and the presence of an unusual individual. Professor of Chemistry Robert E. Swain had been trained as a biochemist at Yale by Russell Chittenden and at Strasbourg and Heidelberg.[49] Like European professors of physiology, Swain had strong incentives to hang on to biochemistry but not to develop specialized roles. Murray Luck, who came to Stanford in 1926, was the first official biochemist there. Like Rose's group, Luck's enjoyed close connection with the chemists but little opportunity for discipline building, and a narrowly specialized line of research was developed.

At other universities, the first stages of the Illinois pattern were diverted by local circumstances. At Cornell, the retirement of George C. Caldwell, an agricultural chemist of Palmer's generation, occasioned the subdivision of the Department of Chemistry into specialized chairs. Organic chemist William Orndorff was made professor of organic and physiological chemistry in 1903, with a special role in the new two-year medical course.[50] But at about the same time that Kemp was self-destructing at Urbana, E. A. Schäfer was reconstituting physiology as a power at Ithaca. In 1908 Orndorff lost biochemistry to physiologist Andrew Hunter, and the chemists never got it back.

The situation at the University of Wisconsin seemed equally propitious when William J. Danelli retired in 1907. The Department of Chemistry was reorganized into specialized "tracks," almost identical with Parr's; among them was physiological chemistry. Organic chemist William Koelker was a disciple of Emil Fischer's and had strong interests in bioorganic chemistry. President Van Hise was laying plans for developing the preclinical sciences at Madison. However, Danelli's successor, physical chemist Louis

Kahlenberg, was more like Kemp than like Parr or Noyes. A tactless and opinionated man, Kahlenberg was interested only in a rather eccentric program of physical chemistry. He ran the department like a Prussian *Geheimrat*. After Koelker was killed in an accident in 1911, Kahlenberg let organic chemistry wither and showed no interest at all in biochemistry. Meanwhile, in the agricultural college, E. B. Hart was developing a large and successful school of biochemistry. By 1913 he had one associate professor, E. V. McCollum; by 1918 he had two more stars, Harry Steenbock and W. H. Peterson. By the time Kahlenberg was ousted by his colleagues in 1918, in a messy coup complete with charges of sympathizing with the German Kaiser, chemistry had long since lost any claim to biochemistry.[51]

At the University of Virginia, Joseph Kastle, an organic chemist and enzymologist, was appointed to the chair of chemistry in 1910. Kastle had worked in the U.S. Hygienic Laboratory and was interested in biochemistry. A somewhat uneasy division of labor with the physiologists, also interested in biochemistry, was worked out but ended abruptly when Kastle died in 1916.[52] Biochemistry developed at Virginia within the medical school.

It is not surprising that there were so few examples of the pattern exemplified by Illinois. Because biochemists in chemistry departments lacked regular service roles in medical teaching, discipline building depended on the efforts of exceptional individuals and was subject to all the hazards of local academic politics. In medical schools biochemists had indispensable service roles and easily preempted competition from departments of chemistry. Because of the vulnerability of the market, few American organic chemists made a serious commitment to research in bioorganic chemistry. There were fewer institutional incentives to develop a hybrid role than there were in Germany, where the absence of departments of biochemistry left room for organic chemists to fill the gap. America had few organic chemists like Emil Fischer, Heinrich Wieland, Richard Willstätter, Paul Karrer, Adolf Windaus, Adolf Butenandt, or Max Bergmann, who so profoundly influenced biochemistry in the 1920s and 1930s.

There were exceptions: at Yale, for example, organic and physiological chemists cooperated in the European style. L. B. Mendel, himself more a physiologist than a chemist, looked to organic chemists for inspiration.[53] Organic chemist Henry Wheeler and his successors, Treat B. Johnson and Rudolph Anderson, were members of the ASBC and cooperated with Chittenden and Mendel in training biochemists. Mendel had a life-long and extraordinarily productive collaboration with Thomas B. Osborne, an organic chemist at the Connecticut Agricultural Experiment Station.[54] It is no accident that a division of labor between chemical physiology and bioorganic chemistry developed in the American department that was most explicitly built on a European model. When Mendel died in 1936, one of the reasons given for not appointing a bioorganic chemist to his chair was the strength of the Johnson–Anderson school.[55]

The Department of Chemistry at Columbia was another important source of recruits to biochemistry. Organic chemist John H. Nelson did important work on enzyme chemistry and encouraged his students to pursue careers in biochemistry in the 1920s. The most famous of his recruits was John Northrop, who shared a Nobel Prize with James Sumner for his work on crystalline enzymes. The physical chemists at Columbia also had an active interest in the interface with biology and medicine. In the 1930s, Victor LaMer and Harold Urey developed methods for using heavy isotopes in biological and medical research, organized cooperative research programs, and directed their students to biological and biochemical problems.[56]

European-style bioorganic chemistry was favored in nonacademic contexts, most notably the Rockefeller Institute, whose leaders were committed to European ideals and were unconstrained by academic disciplinary politics. Phoebus Levene's department at the institute was the center of bioorganic chemistry in America. Trained in medicine, Levene gradually moved into pure organic chemistry. This tendency was reinforced by regular pilgrimages to Europe and by Simon Flexner's belief that progress in medicine would come from the basic sciences. A compulsively productive researcher, Levene was less successful as a discipline builder. Russian-born and trained in the German style, Levene ran his department autocratically. As a result, he had few disciples; only those who moved on, like Donald Van Slyke, became independent scientists.[57]

Henry Dakin was Levene's only rival in bioorganic chemistry; he too was a European, thrived in a nonacademic setting, and founded no school. Dakin began his career in organic chemistry as a student with J. B. Cohen, who directed his interest to enzymes and biochemistry. In 1904 Dakin was persuaded by Christian Herter to accept a post as his chemical assistant in his private laboratory at 819 Madison Avenue in New York. By 1910 he was virtually running the laboratory and did so officially after Herter died in 1911. In 1916 he married Herter's widow and, in 1918, moved into a new, private laboratory at the Herter estate at Scarsborough, where each year he turned out a few elegant and finely crafted research papers.[58] He was a key figure in the trans-Atlantic network centered at the Institute.

Although his work was greatly admired, Dakin had little influence on the institutions of American biochemistry. He was a pathologically shy man; his phobia of public appearance was disabling. He never gave a public lecture, refused many academic calls, and declined to attend professional meetings, even to accept honors and prizes. Dakin was the antithesis of the research managers and discipline builders who shaped institutionalized biochemistry in the 1920s. How different American biochemistry might have been if Dakin had had the organizational flair of Mendel, Gies, or Folin.

The bioorganic tradition at the Rockefeller Institute was revitalized by the arrival, in 1934, of Max Bergmann, formerly the director of the Kaiser Wilhelm Institute for Leather Research at Dresden. A disciple of Emil Fischer's, Bergmann exemplified the German style of bioorganic chemistry for American biochemists in the 1930s, and in contrast to Levene, Bergmann created a school of biochemists who had a wide influence on the discipline. Bergmann was no autocrat. He was modest and generous and gave his young colleagues the experience of an equal and intimate collaboration. Whereas Levene turned his researchers into technicians, Bergmann gave his technicians the chance to become researchers. Many young chemists and biochemists came to Bergmann's laboratory for postdoctoral study in the late 1930s and spread his style of research into departments of biochemistry in medical schools. Joseph Fruton, Emil Smith, and Carl G. Niemann became professors of biochemistry and influential department heads at Yale, Utah, and Caltech in the 1940s and 1950s.[59] Bergmann's program flourished in the disciplinary freedom of the Rockefeller Institute, in part because his research budget did not depend on medical service. It could not have flourished, however, in academic departments of chemistry.

University departments of chemistry almost never committed resources to biochemistry. They almost always preferred specialties relevant to internal disciplinary goals over those with application to other disciplines. These options were discussed in connection with Julius Stieglitz's successor at Chicago in 1935. The dean and president both favored a bioorganic chemist, who would act as a bridge to biology and medicine, such as Leopold Ruzicka and Adolph Butenandt, famous for their work on steroid hormones. The aim of the administrators was to make sure the University of Chicago was in the lead in new research fields; they saw the weakness of American universities in bioorganic chemistry as an opportunity to invest in an academic growth stock.[60] The Department of Chemistry had narrower disciplinary ambitions and favored a theoretical chemist such as Carl Ziegler. Acting Chairman H. I. Schlesinger argued that theoretical chemistry, linking chemistry to theoretical physics, was more important to the future of the discipline than the application of chemistry to biology and medicine, however trendy they might be just then: "The mine of present-day organic chemistry may become exhausted, and there must then come a period in which further theoretical veins must be opened before progress in the synthetic field can be resumed."[61] Backed up by Roger Adams and James Bryant Conant, the administration prevailed. Ruzicka was offered the chair, but he refused. Schlesinger then proposed that an Institute for the Application of Chemistry to Biology be created for Butenandt, with funds from the Rockefeller Foundation. Such an institute would, of course, have left the chemists free to use their own funds for a theoretical chemist. The dean was aware that similar schemes had attracted large foundation grants; Linus Pauling's operation at Caltech, for example. Butenandt was offered a chair, but he too declined. A theoretical physical chemist was appointed to succeed Stieglitz, and the idea of an institute for bioorganic chemistry was quietly dropped.[62] Biochemistry and medicine were important markets for chemists, but markets that chemists felt should be maintained by the disciplines that benefited from chemical experts. Their internal disciplinary goals inevitably came first when it came time to allocate limited departmental resources.

The same issue arose in the search for a successor to James B. Conant, who resigned his chair of organic chemistry to become president of Harvard in 1934. Conant had recently become interested in the bioorganic chemistry of hemoglobin and photosynthesis and hoped his successor would be someone who could cooperate with biologists – not a biochemist, however. Biochemistry, he felt, was the biologists' responsibility. Conant spelled out his ideas to Roger Adams, his choice for the chair:

We hope the new man will be in very close contact with our Department of Biology which is just being reorganized. . . . The biologists may appoint on their staff a chemist of a much more biological turn than you are. Probably this man will be younger and of a lower rank. . . . If you become somewhat more biological without in any sense becoming a biochemist, I think you would find it worth while.[63]

Adams declined, however, and the biologists dithered, leaving the chemists with the not altogether pleasing prospect of having to appoint a real biochemist.[64] They did not: Conant's successor was a pure chemist. Once again, disciplinary interest prevailed over transdisciplinary altruism.

CHEMISTS AND THE MEDICAL MARKET

Although very few departments of chemistry invested in biochemists, they were increasingly eager to provide chemists for medical departments of biochemistry. Alumni of the Illinois school were in particular demand in the early 1920s. No fewer than 17 Illinois graduates achieved important positions in medical schools; of these, 12 earned their Ph.D. degrees between 1921 and 1925 (see Table 10.1). These were the years when medical schools were expanding and reorganizing to meet the flood of students, and there was an insatiable demand for those few leading organic and physical chemists who had some interest and experience in biochemical work. Roger Adams and James Bryant Conant were offered chairs of biochemistry at Columbia, Johns Hopkins, Chicago, and other universities. William Mansfield Clark's research on the electromotive potentials of bacterial cultures at the U.S. Hygienic Laboratory made him particularly attractive to medical schools. In 1921 Clark refused an offer of Taylor's chair at Pennsylvania. In 1923 he was offered the chair of physiology at Rochester, with an initial year of leave to learn physiology, so great was the prestige of physical chemistry.[65]

Chemists' awareness of careers in biochemistry and medicine was heightened by an organized campaign by the American Chemical Society and other organizations after World War I. The principal aims of this publicity campaign were to entice chemists into

Table 10.1. *Alumni of the University of Illinois Department of Chemistry who became ASBC members and received medical school chairs*

Graduate	Year of Ph.D.	Medical school chair
Henry Mattill	1910	Rochester, Iowa
Howard B. Lewis	1915–22[a]	Michigan
John Brown	1921	Ohio State
Max Dunn	1921	UCLA
Adam Christman	1922	Michigan
Wilson Langley	1922	Buffalo
Armand Quick	1922	Marquette
Wendell Griffith	1923	St. Louis, Texas, California
Robert Hill	1923	Colorado
Walter Goebel	1923	Rockefeller Institute
Vincent Du Vigneaud	1929–32[a]	George Washington, Cornell
Ralph Corley	1924	Purdue
Richard Jackson	1925	Yale, USDA Peoria Laboratory
Clarence Berg	1929	Iowa
Wendell Stanley	1929	California
Herbert Loring	1933	Stanford
Herbert Carter	1934	Illinois

[a]Term on staff.

rapidly developing branches of chemical industry, notably pharmaceuticals and medicinals; to persuade American consumers that American drugs were just as good as German-made products; and to apply political pressure on Congress to pass protective tariffs. The need for emergency wartime production of pharmaceuticals enabled American companies to create a whole new industry, and the seizure of German chemical patents by the Alien Property Custodian gave them legal protection from competition. The Chemical Foundation was organized to hold these patents and sell licensing rights, and under the vigorous direction of Francis Garvan, it became a powerful lobby and promotional front for these nascent industries. The Chemical Foundation organized a publicity campaign to convince the public of the importance of chemists to national health and wealth.[66] Unlike the heavy chemical fields in which American industry had been concentrated, pharmaceuticals required the services of organic chemists as well as biochemists and clinical chemists to screen new drugs, design therapeutic tests, and monitor clinical trials. In the early 1920s, these new branches of chemical industry offered attractive careers for biochemists.

Demand for industrial biochemists attracted organic chemists into the field. As early as 1917, Treat B. Johnson marveled at the "enormous funds that are being provided for advanced research in the field of dyestuffs, pharmaceuticals, chemo-therapy, biochemistry and other applied lines of organic chemistry."[67] Campaigns were organized to meet the demand for trained biochemists. The Chemical Foundation gave numerous grants for medical research and fellowships. Squibb, Abbott Laboratories, Eli Lilly, Searle, Ciba, and other large pharmaceutical houses provided graduate fellowships to students working in medical chemistry. A committee of the National Research Council, chaired by Marston Bogert, patiently and systematically cultivated connections between industry, medical schools, and hospitals, "forging that friendly coalition of chemistry, pharmacy, and medicine essential to the most resultful research."[68]

Wartime service had brought many chemists into contact with biomedical scientists and biochemical problems in the Food Administration, the Gas Warfare Service, and the Sanitary Corps of the Public Health Service. Julius Stieglitz was drawn into the study of drugs as a member of the National Research Council Committee on Synthetic Drugs, and he returned to academic life alerted to the opportunities for chemists in biology and medicine. Stieglitz deployed this argument to pry new facilities for organic chemistry from the University of Chicago, trotting out Otto Folin and half a dozen of his students to demonstrate that chemistry was the nursery of biochemistry.[69] *Chemistry in Medicine*, edited by Stieglitz and paid for and distributed by the Chemical Foundation, was designed to show the beneficent effects of chemistry in medical research. Stieglitz's aim was not to promote biochemistry (biochemists as such were hardly mentioned) but to stimulate a new market for organic and physical chemists in hospitals and medical schools and to inspire young chemists to pursue these careers.[70]

The vast majority of the chemist–biochemists turned out by Stieglitz, Adams, Bogert, Nelson, and others went into industrial careers; but they constituted a pool of chemical talent available to medical schools, and the campaign of chemical boosterism certainly did not dampen the growing enthusiasm of medical school officials for pure physical or organic chemists.

The market for chemists in biochemistry was growing as fast as the supply of recruits. Departments in medical schools were expanding, fed by growing enrollments. Temporary student assistantships were being replaced by junior faculty positions, providing opportunities for specialized roles. There was more room in the 1920s for organic and physical chemists who would have been too specialized to be considered for the single chair of smaller departments. Some departments subdivided by problem areas, such as nutrition, metabolism, clinical techniques, and hormones; others followed the lines of the major subfields of chemistry. Otto Folin's plans for expansion in 1920 were a mixture of both:

> I want this department to contain three permanent experienced men. . . . One of these men should be predominantly interested in the isolation and investigation of organic products, a coming Levene or Dakin. The other. . . might be a man interested in the physico-chemical aspects of biochemistry; . . . [or] a food chemist, or again he might be a second man in organic chemistry, or a technic and metabolism man like myself. At the present time I should probably give the preference to a man who could represent the so-called colloidal chemistry. The third man. . . should be predominantly identified with metabolism work, physiological and clinical.[71]

Folin's ideal department included organic, physical, and analytical chemists. (In practice, Folin tended to appoint his favorite students, who worked in metabolism.)

A similar program seems to have guided the expansion and reorganization of biochemistry at Pennsylvania after Alonzo Taylor's resignation in 1921. Distracted by the chronic illness of his wife and his wartime service on the Food Commission, Taylor had never managed to build an important school.[72] His successor, David Wright Wilson, thus had a clean slate, and his appointments reveal the prestige of the chemical specialties. James C. Andrews came in 1922 with a Ph.D. degree in physical chemistry from Columbia and experience in industrial research. Wilson Langley and Armand Quick both had Ph.D. degrees in organic chemistry from Illinois. Two appointments were made in 1924 in nutrition and one in clinical biochemistry. Wilson and his staff emphasized fundamental chemistry in their teaching and were not enthusiasts for hospital work.[73]

Fred C. Koch, an organic chemist with experience in industrial research, led the Chicago department away from general physiology toward pure chemistry. In 1923 biochemistry was formally separated from physiology, and Koch drew his junior staff mainly from the Department of Chemistry at Chicago: Martin Hanke was a disciple of Julius Stieglitz's; Ida Kraus Ragins was an analytical chemist. In 1925 Koch proposed that two new chairs be established in biochemistry, one in physical or clinical chemistry and one in nutrition. For the first, Koch suggested either Donald Van Slyke or William Mansfield Clark, and for the second, Harry Steenbock.[74] It was a chemist's dream – chemists applying their skills to medical problems. Koch never realized his grand scheme but was active in applying physical and chemical techniques to biochemistry and collaborated with the departments of chemistry and physics.[75]

When Howard B. Lewis was called to Michigan to revitalize the moribund department of biochemistry, he brought with him a sensibility shaped by his seven years at Urbana. His first appointments were, to a man, chemists from Illinois and had closely related research interests in the chemistry of purines and amino acids, fats and proteins, sulfur compounds, and nucleic acids. In his heart, Lewis remained a chemist, and though his department was independent, relations with chemistry were very close indeed:

Our graduate students are all required to take a minor in chemistry and . . . they are given the same qualifying examinations in physical and in organic as are required for the graduate students who major in chemistry. . . . In fact, I think that many of our students take much more organic chemistry than the students in the Department of Chemistry who are majoring, say, in physical or analytical chemistry. . . . I was very happy at Illinois and had fine cooperation. Personally, if there were no Medical School in the institution with which I was connected, I believe that I would rather have the prestige of being a Division of Biochemistry in a Chemistry Department rather than to be a separate Department of Biochemistry. To be part of a big department usually means more cooperation on the part of administrative authorities. Of course, the question is influenced very largely by personal factors. I can conceive of the head of a Chemistry Department so entirely out of sympathy with biochemistry that I would prefer to be a small department and independent. . . . On the whole, if you are not attached to a Medical School, I believe that you will gain by the closer cooperation with a Department of Chemistry. . . . I miss very much here at Michigan the close cooperation I had from Roger Adams and Carl Marvel.[76]

JOHNS HOPKINS AND COLUMBIA

The proper role of pure chemists was a particularly hot issue in departments that selected as chief a physical or organic chemist (see

Table 10.2. *Appointments of chemists to chairs of biochemistry*

Medical school	Date	Professor	Chemical specialty
Columbia	1927	Hans T. Clarke	Organic
Johns Hopkins	1927	William M. Clark	Physical
New York University	1930	Keith R. Cannan	Physical
George Washington	1932	Vincent du Vigneaud	Organic
Oregon	1934	Edward S. West	Physical
Cornell	1936	Vincent Du Vigneaud	Organic

Table 10.2). Among these departments were three that had set the trend 25 years earlier and hoped to do so again in the 1930s. In some respects, the difference between generations was more a matter of research style than fundamental attitudes toward chemistry.

Johns Hopkins had always emphasized basic science, and Walter Jones had always been at heart a chemist, preferring organic chemists for his junior staff. The selection of a pure physical chemist, William Mansfield Clark, signaled a change only in research style. Jones was content to pursue a narrow range of research with the aid of a few assistants. He had no desire to have many graduate students and a large research team or to found a school. He discouraged students from becoming biochemists, and after World War I, his department simply ran down.[77] Meanwhile, the pace of university research picked up. Department heads were expected to organize broad research programs and research teams; university leaders turned to bureaus and industrial laboratories as sources of fresh talent. This was Clark's appeal: he had shown his managerial skills in managing his research team at the Hygienic Laboratory. Roger Adams, the second person on the dean's list, had organized the large graduate and research program at Illinois.[78] Clark was amazed that a medical school would want a research chemist with no experience in teaching and little knowledge of biochemistry or medicine. He made it clear that he expected to re-create at Johns Hopkins the organized research team he had at the Hygienic Laboratory. President Ames and Dean Weed made it clear that they expected no less. Reassured, Clark accepted.[79]

Clark planned a program of cooperative research on a few fundamental biological problems. Abandoning Jones's reliance on cheap student labor, Clark insisted on appointing junior faculty with specialized chemical skills to participate in team research.[80] Clark's vision took in all the major branches of pure chemistry: physical, organic, and biological, each to be represented ultimately by a full professor. On the biochemical side, Clark appointed Barnet Cohen, his co-worker at the Hygienic Laboratory, who had a Ph.D. degree in public health and specialized in bacterial biochemistry. In organic chemistry, Clark had his eye on no less a person than Morris Kharasch, a brilliant young theoretical organic chemist then at the University of Maryland. Clark had mentioned to his friend, half in jest, what a fine team they would make, not thinking he would be interested. Kharasch was interested, however, and Clark immediately wrote to Dean Weed, noting that Kharasch would bring with him four graduate students and $4,350 a year in industrial research grants, no strings attached.[81] Clark's hopes soared for a concerted attack on the mechanism of biological oxidation:

We have come to the point where we see clearly that the next step to take is to utilize the modern concepts of the electronic structure of organic molecules. No one in this country is more fertile in ideas in this field than Kharasch. Just how the junction is to be made neither of us sees clearly. If we did we could go our ways independently but in cooperation at a distance. But, as my friend Van Slyke remarked, if we can take this next step the world is ours. . . . We have our dander up for the biggest haul ever.[82]

When Kharasch accepted a call to a professorship at Chicago, Clark appointed Leslie Hellerman, a student of Stieglitz's who was an expert in the electronic theory of organic and enzyme-catalyzed reactions. Eric Ball, a young enzymologist, came as a National Research Council Fellow in 1929 and remained to develop his field, which would soon be known as "bio-energetics." However, the Depression put an abrupt end to further expansion, and Clark soon discovered that his ideal of coordinated research had to be adapted to academic traditions of laissez-faire.[83]

Clark's school remained small and select but was increasingly influential among the avant-garde of biochemists in the 1930s and, more generally, in the 1940s.[84] This occurred almost in spite of Clark, who was notoriously intolerant of biochemists who did not live up to his high standard of chemical sophistication, as few did. One biochemist expostulated to Clark's disciple, R. Keith Cannan:

Why does Clark always choose these general articles to fire off wise-cracks at benighted biochemists? He urges them to the importance of Oxidation Reduction and then blows them up when they start in a fumbling way to use it. The Lord gave and the Lord hath taken away.[85]

Cannan was amused by the reverence that the biochemists at University College had for physical chemists:

This is not because its significance is properly understood but because it is a new and strange and persuasive language. I have amongst our biochemists, a wholly fictitious reputation as a subtle mind which moves comfortably amongst erudite thermodynamic abstractions!! It is really rather amusing.[86]

Joseph and Dorothy Needham breathed a sigh of relief when their first foray into thermodynamics received Clark's approval.[87]

As a teacher, Clark was also notorious for his uncompromising insistence on sophisticated chemical theory. Clark claimed that the pleasure he took in teaching medical students made up for his disappointment in team research. Few of his students shared his delight. At the end of Clark's second year, so many of his students failed a test in basic biochemistry that the Committee on Instruction felt obliged to investigate. Clark felt the real problem was the students' lack of preparation in basic chemistry and served notice that, in future, students would be expected to be adequately prepared.[88] This conflict between chemical and clinical ideals was chronic throughout Clark's tenure. Many biochemists complained that medical students were ill-prepared in chemistry and interested only in clinical applications.[89] The structural conflict betwen the chemist's and the clinician's ideals was sharpest at Johns Hopkins because Clark and the administration deliberately pushed to the limit the idea that basic science was the engine of medical progress.

A similar policy led to the appointment of Hans T. Clarke at Columbia; but a different man in a different context gave the department a distinctive shape. Whereas Clark created a small elite research group, Hans T. Clarke's department was the largest and most influential producer of biochemists in the 1930s. Clark avoided medicine; Clarke kept his clinical fences mended and fostered a remarkable school of research in basic biochemistry.

The reorganization of biological chemistry was part of a larger plan of reorganization at P&S, which began in 1920 and dragged on for nearly a decade. Gies's department was in a sad state. When Gies took up the cause of dental reform, responsibility for running the department fell entirely on the shoulders of the junior staff. The department was ingrown and narrowly focused: Edgar Miller and Maxwell Karshan, both students of Gies's, were interested in dental biochemistry. In 1920 Abraham Flexner suggested a thorough housecleaning. Dean Darrach submitted an ambitious plan to the General Education Board calling for four new appointments and a doubling of the budget from $14,000 to $29,620. This plan bogged down in a bitter political fight over full-time clinical chairs.[90] When the smoke cleared in 1925, biochemistry was in a still worse state, despite efforts to revive Gies's Biochemical Association.[91] The old plan for reorganization was again put forward, and by 1927 large and well-equipped laboratories were ready for Gies's successor.

The medical faculty wanted to appoint a pure organic or physical chemist, either James B. Conant or Roger Adams. Adams refused, however, and after some months' delay, Conant also declined. Pressed further, Conant suggested Hans Clarke, director of the Division of Organic Chemicals at Eastman Kodak since 1914.[92] A protégé of William Ramsay's at University College, Clarke was little known outside of organic chemistry circles. He had virtually no experience in medical education; but he was a superb organizer and developer of talent.[93] Dean Darrach was quickly convinced that Clarke was the man to develop a modern research school. Clarke doubted that he was a suitable person to lead a medical department, but Conant urged him to accept, for the good of organic chemistry:

Here is a Medical Group that at last have seen the light and want a straight organic chemist to run the show. If you had suffered from the domination by physical chemists of American Chemistry and biochemistry as I have, you would appreciate the importance of the move. If you don't take the job it is a lost opportuntiy for organic chemistry. There is no one else.

May I also urge how much you owe it to yourself and above all to American science to join the very small band of reputable scientific workers in academic positions. The more I see of chemistry (and biochemistry and organic chemistry in particular) in this country the more I weep! Won't you get into a position where you can help out more directly? Every addition of a real person to the small group of scientific–academic–organic chemists is a tremendous gain for the rest of us.[94]

Clark accepted. Henry Dakin congratulated Darrach on his coup and predicted that the appointment of a chemist with industrial experience would set a trend:

I feel very confident that you have got a first rate man and stolen a march on many other institutions looking for biochemists. Of course, so many institutions feel that a biochemist must be devoted exclusively to urine and blood!...His experience at Rochester is really invaluable.[95]

Clarke's program of research leaned heavily toward organic chemistry. In addition to his personal interest in amino acids, Clarke chose to develop the field of protein and steroid hormones, then one of the hottest areas in bioorganic chemistry. A grant of $100,000 from the Chemical Foundation enabled Clarke to make ten new appointments within five years (see Table 10.3). Five were organic chemists and one was a physical chemist. Four were European-trained, and most were interested in problems like the structure of steroid hormones and the chemistry of intermediary metabolism.[96]

Clarke also cultivated the clinical faculty. Medical instruction was put into the hands of experienced teachers; joint research appointments were arranged with medicine, pathology, and ophthalmology. Clarke thus succeeded in making pure chemical research congruent with medical service roles that ensured economic security. By 1940 Clarke's department was the largest and most influential school of biochemistry in America.[97] The generation of graduate students that passed through P&S between 1934 and 1941 enjoyed a strategic position in the discipline, much as Mendel's or Gies's students had in the period from 1905 to 1914 or Roger Adams's in the early 1920s. Joseph Fruton, Earl A. Evans, Jr., Konrad Bloch, David Shemin, Dewitt Stettin, William H. Stein, James D. Dutcher, and Seymour Cohen went on to important chairs or research posts, carryng the Columbia style with them.

CONCLUSION

Johns Hopkins and Columbia testify to the enormous prestige of physical and organic chemistry among biochemists between the wars. They were the avant-garde and by definition were exceptional cases. The vast majority of medical school departments emphasized clinical biochemistry. Yet the choice between an organic or physical chemist and a clinical biochemist was a crucial issue for medical school administrators whenever an important chair became vacant. When Stanley Benedict died in 1938, the choice of a successor was between a pure chemist, like Benedict, and someone more on the clinical side. The man chosen was Vincent du Vigneaud, one of W. C. Rose's most successful converts. Du Vigneaud brought with him the outlook of an organic chemist.[98] He had already succeeded in reviving a moribund department at Georgetown Medical School, and his appointment to

Table 10.3. *Appointments to the Columbia University Department of Biological Chemistry*

Name	Date appointed	Ph.D. training	Field of Ph.D.	Research interest
Hans T. Clarke	1928	London	Organic chem.	Amino acids
Goodwin Foster	1928	Harvard	Biochemistry	Clinical methods
Michael Heidelberger	1929	Columbia	Organic chem.	Immunochemistry
Oscar Wintersteiner	1929	Graz	Organic chem.	Steroids
Crawford Failey	1930	California	Physical chem.	Biothermodynamics
Warren Sperry	1930	Rochester	Biochemistry	Lipid metabolism
Marianne Goettsch	1930	Columbia	Biochemistry	Nutrition
Irwin Brand	1931	Berlin	Organic chem.	Protein metabolism
Robert Herbst	1932	Yale	Organic chem.	Amino acid metabolism
Karl Meyer	1932	Berlin	Organic chem.	Peptide hormones
Rudolf Schoenheimer	1933	Berlin (M.D.)	Pathology	Sterol metabolism
Forrest E. Kendall	1937	Illinois	Organic chem.	Immunochemistry
Erwin Chargaff	1938	Vienna	Organic chem.	Proteins nucleic acid
David Rittenberg	1940	Columbia	Physical chem.	Isotopes

the prestigious Cornell chair enabled him to realize his ambition to found a school of bioorganic chemistry equal to those of Britain and Germany.[99] H. B. Lewis, Rose, Shaffer, Steenbock, Clarke, and Roger Adams all regarded du Vigneaud as the "real comer among the younger biochemists." The choice of an organic over a clinical chemist was a sign of the times.[100]

When E. P. Lyon retired at Minnesota in 1939, opinion was sharply divided between those who favored the "organic chemical approach" and clinicians who wanted to reverse Lyon's policy of favoring the basic sciences.[101] A. P. Mathews's retirement in 1940 from Cincinnati precipitated a similar controversy. The faculty had grown disenchanted with Mathews's efforts to teach general biochemistry and favored someone with a more utilitarian point of view.[102] Yet the chair was offered to Charles G. King, professor of chemistry at Pittsburgh, who published voluminously on the organic chemistry of vitamins and who expected to bring with him his large (and expensive) research team. The university failed to raise the necessary funds, however, and appointed Milan Logan, Folin's pupil and a star medical teacher.[103]

Baird Hastings confronted the same issue when he succeeded Folin in 1936:

One has the choice today of considering whether the teaching of biochemistry in a leading medical school should be done primarily from the standpoint of fundamental chemistry without much attention to the biological and clinical applications, or whether one should avowedly set out to teach quantitative clinical chemistry.[104]

Hastings originally planned to put the emphasis on fundamental chemistry. However, "two distinguished chemists" (Cohn? Conant?) argued that clinical applications should be ignored, and Hastings felt obliged to take a more extreme stand in favor of clinical chemistry.[105] The selection of a successor to L. B. Mendel at Yale revolved around the same issue. The biochemists at Yale and in the extended network of Sheffield alumni wanted a bioorganic chemist like Mendel. The physiologists, led by John Fulton, were determined to appoint a physiologist with clinical interests. They won: physiologist–chemist Cyril Long was appointed, amidst a chorus of lament from Mendel's friends.[106]

The issue was complicated by the emergence of university departments of general biochemistry. Hastings justified his own emphasis on clinical biochemistry by pointing to the plans for a complementary program in fundamental biochemistry in Harvard College. In 1939 he advised Cornell to select a clinical biochemist to succeed Benedict, arguing that James B. Sumner's group at Ithaca adequately represented the purely chemical side.[107] But he advised Yale to appoint a chemist like Edwin Cohn, because John Peters already represented the clinical side. Hastings argued that Cohn would stimulate his best students to obtain additional training in pure physics and chemistry and that departments led by pure chemists should be the principal suppliers of professors of biochemistry for medical schools.[108]

The enthusiasm for appointing organic or physical chemists to medical school chairs reflected a widespread perception that the future of biochemistry lay in pure chemistry. Yet no medical school department chief would willingly relinquish the training of future leaders to university chemists.

Intellectual and institutional imperatives conflicted. For first-generation biochemists, clinical application ensured both intellectual influence and financial stability. For their successors, the choice was more complex: clinical application ensured stable markets, but intellectual leadership entailed breaking loose from service roles into more theoretical lines of chemical research. The imperatives of chemical research and medical teaching diverged. Ambitious department chiefs had to strike a balance between influence in medicine and influence in their discipline, as H. B. Lewis observed:

There seems to be a diversity of opinion as to the proper direction of physiological chemistry to go in the United States – shall it become essentially clinical or is it to be a branch of pure science with clinical applications as far as students are concerned?[109]

In practice, the balance struck between general and clinical biochemistry, between chemists and clinicians, varied from school to school and shifted with changes in the system of medical education and research.

The issue itself was constant, because it reflected the basic political economy of the discipline. Biochemistry received recruits from chemistry and fed biochemists into a predominantly medical market. The vast majority of departments depended financially and politically on service roles in training clinicians and cooperating in clinical research teams. Few had independent sources of support, and chemistry departments offered no opportunities for programs in general biochemistry. Biochemists looked to basic chemistry for their methods and ideals but to clinical medicine for legitimation and support. Their disciplinary values were strategies for adapting to market realities. Biochemists' deferring to pure chemists while clinging to old clinical ways reflects the particular relations that developed historically between the two disciplines.

II

Biological programs

Although the realities of biochemists' careers were shaped by medical service roles, their aspirations were less bound to the quotidian. From time to time, biochemists have claimed that biochemistry is not limited to medicine but comprises the chemical aspects of all the biological and medical disciplines. This conception of biochemistry as a basic biological discipline had its roots less in useful applications than in reductionist ideologies; it looked less to the present than to the future. Russell Chittenden's 1908 presidential address to the American Society of Biological Chemists exemplifies this biological program:

It is well understood today that all the phenomena of life are to be explained on the basis of chemical and physical laws, and it is partly because of a clear recognition of this fact that biological chemistry has finally attained the eminence it has now reached as a division of biology: a branch of study that promises much in the ultimate explanation of the most intricate...problems of life....As a result, physiological chemistry has developed by leaps and bounds, until today special laboratories and journals devoted to this subject are to be found on all sides....Under the broad term of biological chemistry, we are dealing with a subject which...concerns itself with the chemical processes of living organisms, and...these are as many and varied as the organisms themselves.[1]

Heredity and variation, growth and morphogenesis, energy transformations and regulation, all would yield to the biochemist's skills. Zoology, botany, bacteriology, physiology, pharmacology, pathology – in all of these disciplines, the biochemist could stake his claim.

This biological program is both an intellectual design and a political platform for establishing territorial rights and boundaries with neighboring disciplines. Programmatic statements of this sort have characterized periods of active discipline building or changes in the ecology of the biomedical disciplines: the mid-nineteenth century in Germany; the years of medical reform in Britain and the United States, from 1900 to 1915; and the 1960s, when biochemists were challenged by the achievements and claims of the molecular biologists.

The actual content of programmatic statements changed with time, as biochemists drew upon the most current and dramatic discoveries in chemical biology. In his 1870 lecture "On the origin and sources of life forces," Felix Hoppe-Seyler drew upon the great conceptions of the mechanistic physiologists: the transformations of energy from sunlight through photosynthesis and metabolism to animal heat and muscular force. The origin of living protoplasm and the unity of living forms were compelling themes, reflecting the popularity of the cell and protoplasm theories and the discovery of *Urschleim* – "Bathybius Haeckelii" – in deep-sea ooze.[2] In his preface to the first volume of his journal in 1887, Hoppe-Seyler claimed for physiological chemistry the chemical aspects of all biological disciplines.[3]

The programmatic statements of the early 1900s likewise reflected recent discoveries in chemical biology. The intracellular enzymes that catalyzed simple oxidations and syntheses were heralded as models of complex physiological processes like respiration and growth.[4] Eduard Buchner's discovery of cell-free fermentation in yeast extracts was celebrated as a victory of mechanistic biology.[5] In 1901 Franz Hofmeister depicted the living cell as a biological machine shop, with enzymes arranged on colloidal structures like machine tools on an assembly line.[6] The spectacular discoveries of bacterial toxins, antitoxins, agglutinins, hemolysins, precipitins, and other chemical entities convinced many that all the phenomena of infection and resistance belonged in the realm of the biochemists. Paul Ehrlich's side-chain theory of antibody formation was received as a general theory of biochemical synthesis.[7] Discoveries of small molecules, "hormones," that had dramatic physiological effects gave confidence to far-sighted biochemists like F. G. Hopkins that the study of small molecules could illuminate fundamental biological processes.[8]

Jacques Loeb's work on the chemical mechanism of tropisms, fertilization and cell division, and parthenogenesis was frequently cited in programmatic statements. Chemical biologists emulated Loeb's attempts to reveal that growth followed the simple kinetic laws of autocatalytic chemical reactions. Loeb's own work was motivated by his militantly materialistic beliefs, and books like *The Dynamics of Living Matter* (1907) brought Loeb's mechanistic views to a wide audience of chemists and biologists.[9]

Forty years later, a generation of biochemists who witnessed the discovery of the double helix, the genetic code, and the one-gene–one-enzyme concept formulated their own characteristic program. Behind this variety of subject matter, however, is a constancy of purpose: to establish biochemistry as a discipline with intellectual rights to the chemical aspects of all the biological and biomedical disciplines. The biological program was a political platform, put forward in periods when opportunities for discipline building were greatest. Theories had strategic as well as intellectual significance.

In the 1900s, the biological program provided a rationale for the transformation of medical to biological chemistry. It justified biochemists' desire to consolidate their outposts in various disciplines into separate university departments and professional organizations. It reflected biochemists' efforts to escape the confines of clinical medicine and responded to medical reformers' hopes of infusing the biomedical disciplines with the ideals of basic biological science. The biochemists' program implied a greater role in research and graduate training and in a broad range of professional employment. Intellectual ambitions and institutional opportunities were for a time closely congruent in the period of reform.

Programmatic ambitions are not always realized, of course, and ideological weather is notoriously fickle. Enthusiasm for university-style biomedical science was at its height for only about a decade. As the partnership between biochemists and clinicians was reestablished, biochemists' intellectual ideals were shaped by their roles and the realities of medical politics. Medical schools offered little encouragement to a broadly biological program. Combined departments of physiology and biochemistry were no more hospitable to the biological ideal, because physiologists themselves were busily cultivating a partnership with clinical medicine. Broad intellectual ambitions were of little use in discipline building.

In theory, departments of biology might have been contexts in which institutional goals and service roles reinforced rather than diverted the biological program of biochemistry. In practice, there were few such opportunities. Despite the influence of Loeb, T. H. Morgan, F. R. Lillie, and other experimental biologists, most departments of biology prior to World War I were still dominated by morphology and evolutionary biology and offered no roles for biochemists. In the mid-1920s, there was a movement in leading universities to develop physicochemical biology and to encourage cooperative research with physicists and chemists. "General physiology" was often seen as the cornerstone of reform, and in some cases, roles for biophysicists and biochemists were planned. Few positions for biochemists were actually created in biology departments, however. Experimental biologists preferred to collaborate with chemists than to appoint biochemists to positions that might go to real biologists. Where biochemistry lacked indispensable service roles in medicine, its ecological space was claimed and occupied by its better-established neighbors in chemistry and biology, just as had happened in German universities 50 years before. In somewhat different ways, the departments at Yale, Columbia, Chicago, and California illustrate these general trends.

THE YALE SCHOOL

The premier American school of biochemistry developed as a university department in close connection with physiology and organic chemistry. Chittenden had no competition from the Yale Medical School and trained his students for a broad variety of academic and professional jobs, including medicine. The Sheffield School was a context in which a broadly biological style of biochemistry might flourish, and Chittenden offered some of the clearest formulations of the biological program. He pointed to the work of Loeb and Mathews on the chemistry of growth and to the recent discoveries in genetics as signs that morphogenesis, heredity, and the Mendelian "factors" would soon be explained in terms of the chemistry of nucleic acids and proteins. He shared the growing belief in the physiological importance of small molecules, speculating that the dibasic amino acids, lysine and arginine, might hold the key to fertilization and cell division. Chittenden had an unusually clear conception of the importance of intracellular enzymes and how intermediary metabolism was carried out in successive, orderly steps by specific enzymes. Plants, microorganisms, invertebrate and vertebrate animals, as well as man, Chittenden claimed as proper materials for the exercise of the biochemist's skills.[10]

This expansive vision reflected actual practice at Yale, at least between 1900 and 1910. In the 1890s, Chittenden's research was limited to work begun with Kühne on the degradation products of proteins. After 1900 a much broader range of problems was under investigation: intermediary metabolism of proteins, purines, and fats; nutrition; enzymes in invertebrates and fungi; hormones and immunoproteins; and biological oxidations and reductions. L. B. Mendel's early papers on nutrition were really aimed at the fundamental process of growth. Mendel's work was characteristic of the broad biological outlook of the early 1900s. A decade later, Mendel was using growth as a quantitative measure of the role of amino acids and vitamins in nutrition.[11] By the 1920s, most of the papers from the Yale school concerned the chemistry of amino acids and nutrition. This shift from a varied program of research to one concentrated in nutritional physiology reflects a more general decline of enthusiasm among biochemists for the big biological problems, as well as the increasing dominance of medical biochemistry.

Chittenden's expansive program was a tactical response to his changing political situation at Yale in the period of medical reform. From 1900 on, the Sheffield School was faced with increasingly powerful rivals in the biomedical sciences, both from the medical school and from Yale College. Bringing the experimental sciences into the orbit of Yale College was the linchpin of President Arthur T. Hadley's plan to make Yale a modern university. For the medical reformers at Yale, physiology, bacteriology, and physiological chemistry were the key to their planning for a complete medical school, begun in earnest in 1906. Chittenden's claim that biological chemistry encompassed the chemical parts of biology, physiology, bacteriology, and pathology was the key strategy in his 20-year-long, two-front campaign to preserve the independence of the Sheffield Scientific School. The intellectual and political meanings of his program are indistinguishable.

Hadley's determination to welcome the sciences into Yale College was given urgency by the success of the Sheffield programs. Between 1899 and 1906, enrollment in Yale College increased from 1224 to 1351 (10%), while enrollment in Sheffield increased 80%, from 495 to 896. Most alarming, it was not the engineering and professional courses that were growing most rapidly but the academic courses in biology and chemistry that were organized specifically for Yale College students. In 1905 Chittenden inaugurated a course in general biology and physiology, emphasizing its value as a liberal study. Hadley was determined to reclaim biology, at least, from the Scientific School. In 1906 Yale College terminated the 1888 contract under which Sheffield taught biology to Yale undergraduates, and Hadley undertook to raise endowment for a university biology laboratory. The Sheffield board responded with their own plan for a new biology laboratory. Chittenden's position as director of the Scientific School was simple and uncompromising: Sheffield had nurtured experimental biology during a time when Yale had disdained it, and Sheffield was entitled to the fruits of its vision and labors.[12]

Hadley's position was more complicated. He felt the moral justice of Chittenden's claims and was counting on the prestige and accomplishments of the Sheffield faculty to attract endowment and scientific talent to Yale. Hadley also saw Chittenden, with his strong liberal ideals, as a strategically placed ally in his plan to domesticate the medical sciences. Hadley wanted Yale College to accept professional schools as equal partners in the university, but he feared giving these schools, with their utilitarian ideals, too much influence. The movement for home rule in the biomedical disciplines was especially strong in the 1900s: Hadley noted uneasily "the growing cry of *medical subjects in the medical school*."[13] He was not unhappy to have the biomedical sciences under Chittenden's control, for the time being.

However, the Sheffield School was also the main impediment to Hadley's ambition for a university dominated by Yale College and the graduate school. A school of professional science was an institutional anachronism in 1905, and Chittenden's determination to preserve its autonomy ran counter to Hadley's efforts to bring the professional schools under central control. Hadley's treatment of the Sheffield School reflected these conflicting aims. He supported Chittenden's claims in the more applied fields, notably physiological chemistry, but pressed Chittenden gently but unrelentingly in zoology and general biology, which he felt belonged in Yale College.

Chittenden's broad biological conception of biochemistry appealed to Hadley as a means of uniting academic and practical ideals, and from 1897 on, his annual reports were vehicles for Chittenden's views. Hadley saw physiological chemistry as a bridge uniting Yale College and Yale Medical School: "May we not hope that physiological or biological chemistry will not be divided between pseudo-antagonistic interests, but rather be unified under one roof to serve biology and medicine, science and art?"[14] Chittenden's biological program served Hadley's intellectual and political interests, and Hadley joined Chittenden in combating the growing tendency to regard biochemistry as a technical premedical subject rather than as a broadly biological discipline:

A new biological chemistry is arising to contribute its explanations in the study of the dynamics of living matter. Botany, Zoology, Bacteriology are creating new fields for chemical research, which in turn find unexpected practical applications....Biological chemistry can serve in manifold functions; its identity should be maintained and suitably recognized.[15]

While supporting Chittenden's ambitions for biochemistry, Hadley also pressed forward with his plans to make biology a university subject. In 1907 a new professor of comparative anatomy, Ross Harrison, was appointed in both the university and the Sheffield School, and three years later, ground was broken for a university zoological laboratory.[16] Chittenden was obliged to make a strategic retreat. In 1912 the Sheffield biology course was reorganized as a premedical course (without physiological chemistry), and a new preprofessional course was organized in biology with emphasis on physiological chemistry, bacteriology, and hygiene, aimed at the public health market.[17] Chittenden's reliance on a more explicitly professional style narrowed the institutional basis in the Sheffield School for "pure" biology and also, perhaps, for a broad biological style of biochemistry.

Physiology and physiological chemistry were the bones of contention in Chittenden's skirmishes with the medical school. Chittenden had taught both subjects for the medical school since the 1880s and was determined to keep his grip on these strategic service roles.[18] As separate roles developed in the medical school, however, pressures for medical "home rule" grew more intense. Chittenden's chief competition arose from within his own family. In 1902 his protégé, Yandell Henderson, was appointed assistant professor of physiology in the medical school and almost at once took up the cause of medical home rule. As a graduate student, he had already begun to challenge Chittenden. Walter Jones was in Albrecht Kossel's laboratory when Henderson burst upon the scene in 1899:

Henderson came along about a week ago and is now revolutionizing the science. He has "The Yale" but otherwise seems a very well behaved young fellow. I have heard him trying to tell Kutscher (after 10 minutes acquaintance) something like this: "Man sagt in Amerika, es giebt nur ein Chemiker auf der ganzen Welt und er heisst Kossel. Und ist Chittenden auf der ganzen Welt? Nein, nein er ist nur gegen die ganze Welt." Henderson has broken loose from Yale and is over here for at least a year.[19]

Henderson was bright, ambitious, opinionated, aggressive, and tactlessly outspoken, and he chafed as Chittenden and Mendel continued to teach the medical course in physiology themselves.[20] Henderson's ardent promotion of clinical physiology reflected his desire for independence from his mentor.

Chittenden also was careful to keep control of medical biochemistry. Around 1903, Chittenden delegated responsibility for this course to Frank P. Underhill, one of his most talented protégés (Ph.B. 1900, Ph.D. 1903). Underhill took up clinical work and quickly made a reputation by his research on diabetes and carbohydrate metabolism, kidney disorders resulting from diabetic acidosis, and the effects of diet on the composition of urine. By 1910 Underhill's clinical work equaled Mendel's in volume and quality. The medical faculty liked Underhill's style of biochemistry and tried to detach Underhill from the Sheffield School to head a clinically oriented department in the medical school. However, Chittenden continued to pay Underhill's salary and refused to transfer him to the medical school.

It was not Underhill but Henderson who led the struggle to pry physiological chemistry loose from Chittenden's grasp. Underhill was modest and tended to suffer quietly; not so Henderson: in the debate over the disposition of biology in the period from 1905 to 1906, he lobbied strongly for the university side against Sheffield. He pressed Chittenden to share control of physiological chemistry with the medical school and then tried to organize a rival department, a move that earned him a reproach from Hadley and the disagreeable task of explaining his actions to Chittenden.[21] Chittenden won: in 1906 the medical and scientific schools signed a contract providing that the Sheffield Scientific School teach the preclinical courses to medical students (Mendel taught physiology, and Underhill physiological chemistry).

The decision to go ahead with a complete medical school in 1909 encouraged the medical faculty to press Hadley once more to transfer the preclinical sciences to the medical school. Chittenden again refused. In 1912 Underhill was appointed professor of pathological chemistry in the medical school in the expectation that a full department of physiological and pathological chemistry would be created as soon as endowment could be found. Endowment was not forthcoming, however, and because five-sixths of Underhill's salary still came from the Sheffield School, Chittenden was able to prevent the medical faculty from staking out an independent claim. The medical dean, George Blumer, was unwilling, for both sentimental and political reasons, to cross Chittenden:

> While there is no question that this faculty believes that the proper place for a Department of Physiological Chemistry is in a Medical School, the fact remains that in this University the Department of Physiological Chemistry has not so developed. It is an indisputable fact that under Professor Chittenden a Department of Physiological Chemistry has been built up which enjoys a world wide reputation....From the University standpoint it is difficult to see the necessity for the Medical School undertaking to teach Physiological Chemistry.[22]

Blumer pointed out that Chittenden's department served other, nonmedical, disciplines, which might be offended if the medical school tried to monopolize physiological chemistry. Chittenden's strategy of a broad biological program and multiple alliances was paying off.

Whereas Underhill bore his frustrations quietly, refusing several outside offers, Henderson pressed Underhill's cause with increasing zeal.[23] In 1914 Henderson challenged Blumer to press Chittenden harder:

> What you speak of as your "detachment" of standpoint as to physiological chemistry is deserving of a simpler name. It's really funny. You go to Chittenden to get him to contribute something [for a joint position] and you come away without this, leaving behind you a promise that we will never have any physiological chemistry, and yet pleased with the way you "handle Chittenden," and consider it in part due to his "gratitude." He is as grateful as a fox is to a goose.[24]

If Underhill resigned from Sheffield, his course in physiological chemistry would be taken over by Mendel. Dean Blumer stuck to his view that rival departments were inefficient, unfair to Chittenden, and inconsistent with university policy of central university departments serving all the professional schools.[25] Chittenden's reputation, his strategy of multiple alliances, and the political vitality of the one-university idea made it impossible to develop a rival department of biochemistry, at least while Chittenden was in charge.

Underhill gave up on physiological chemistry. In 1917 he was installed temporarily in pathology and then in the new Department of Experimental Medicine. Finally, in 1920 he was put in charge of the new Department of Pharmacology. Thus one of the few Americans who might have equaled Van Slyke was squeezed out of the profession. Underhill died in 1932, never having realized his full potential as a pioneer in clinical biochemistry.

In 1920 Chittenden retired, and the Sheffield School was finally dispersed as a separate faculty. Physiological chemistry was transferred to the medical school, with L. B. Mendel as professor and director.[26] Despite the change in venue, Mendel's department continued as a virtually autonomous school of nutritional physiology. Mendel kept the clinical sciences at arm's length and took less interest in teaching medical biochemistry than in maintaining his large graduate program in biochemical nutrition. Although Mendel prided himself on his breadth of view as a biochemist, to the medical faculty his department seemed increasingly narrow and isolated from modern trends in physiology and medicine.[27] By the 1930s, Mendel was also isolated from new trends in general biochemistry. Encysted in the Yale Medical School, Mendel's school did not enjoy the benefits of connections with either clinical medicine or basic biology.

Seen in the context of institutional change, Chittenden's programmatic statements have a clearly political purpose. His broad biological conception of biochemistry was a response both to recent discoveries in chemical biology and to the competitive challenges that he faced from the collegiate and medical faculties at Yale. For a decade, the congruence of intellectual and institutional imperatives resulted in creative innovation in research and teaching. For another decade, Chittenden's strategy enabled him to fight a successful rearguard fight against the tide of medical reform. But institutional realities made it less and less likely that the ideal of a truly *biological* chemistry could be realized: Underhill's drift into the orbit of the medical school; Ross Harrison's dominance of experimental biology; the anachronistic position of the Sheffield School; the encysting of Mendel's group in the medical school. An expansive, exemplary program gradually contracted to an anomalous ingrown school.

COLUMBIA P&S

The history of the Columbia department is a variation on the same theme. At Yale, a university context favorable to a broad biological style of biochemistry was eroded by growing medical competition. In Columbia's College of Physicians and Surgeons, William J. Gies found that the medical context made it impossible to develop the kind of university connections that he had enjoyed as a student at Yale. Gies consciously imitated Chittenden and Mendel's program and strategies of institution building; but without a reputation or allies, he had none of Chittenden's advantages in academic politics. Gies's efforts illuminate the difficulties of trying to realize the promise of the biological program.

Gies always intended that biochemistry would become a university subject, and he seized every occasion to assert that biochemistry was a basic biological science. When President Butler proposed in 1903 to unite similar departments in P&S and Columbia College into university divisions of physical and biological sciences, Gies made a strong claim that his department belonged in both divisions: "...development of our department will depend upon intimate relations of cooperation with the departments of chemistry and biology."[28] The plan was dropped, however, and Gies had to improvise connections whenever opportunities arose. Gies aggressively sought connections with nonacademic, civic institutions – a strategy developed to a fine art by Presidents Low and Butler.[29] Gies cultivated every possible alliance:

I am building up my department here to include a laboratory at the Zoological Park, one at the Botanical Garden, one at the *Aquarium*, one in connection with the laboratories of *Zoology* and of *Physics*, also in connection with our *maternity* hospital and our *clinics*, to say nothing of the more obvious relationships with other [medical] departments...such as the bacteriological. At least a dozen men of *diversified* biological interests are or will be involved in this scheme of advancing biological chemistry here at Columbia.[30]

What Gies needed was an indispensable service role outside P&S. However, his plan to teach biological chemistry in Columbia College was thwarted by the pure scientists, who were suspicious of alliances with P&S. In 1899 and again in 1904, Gies offered to teach physiological chemistry to students of chemistry and biology, but he was rebuffed. In 1906 he was still hoping to give the "long contemplated course of lectures and demonstrations in biological chemistry at Columbia College as a pure science elective." These rebuffs only made him more determined to prove himself to the chemists and biologists.[31]

Although he failed to establish biochemistry as a university subject, Gies did succeed in building informal cooperative relationships with other departments around specific research projects. The biologists were more receptive than the chemists, especially those with extraacademic ties. In 1902 Gies initiated cooperative research on plant chemistry at the New York Botanical Garden and, as consulting chemist, offered a laboratory course in plant physiology. In 1905 he arranged with Edmund B. Wilson, Thomas Hunt Morgan, and Gary Calkins in the Department of Biology to carry out cooperative research in the biology laboratory and to teach the chemical half of the physiology course for science students. While consulting weekly with the zoologists, Gies directed student research on the effects of chemicals on hydra and, at Morgan's suggestion, investigated the chemical reactions in regenerating tissues and growing leaves.[32] Gies also made contact with zoologist Henry Fairfield Osborn and proposed to carry out cooperative research in the new laboratory being planning at the New York Zoo. Gies persuaded Osborn to add a large room for joint researches on material from zoo animals. A working relationship with the new Rockefeller Institute was also established when two institute fellows, Nellis Foster and William Salant, cooperated in research on protein and carbohydrate metabolism. Gies's early collaborators included S. J. Meltzer, Phoebus Levene, and Christian Herter from the institute and others from Roosevelt Hospital and the Cornell Medical School.[33]

Gies also tried to co-opt a group of chemists working with Henry Sherman in Teachers' College on nutrition, food chemistry, and home economics. In 1908 he agreed to organize a laboratory of physiological chemistry there and to give the basic lectures in Sherman's course on nutrition. In the same year, a laboratory of dietetics was created for Chittenden's disciple, Mary Swartz. Gies saw his chance: appealing to Butler's desire for efficiency and centralized university departments, Gies proposed that Sherman and Swartz be transferred to biological chemistry and that his expanded department be recognized as a university subject on a par with chemistry and biology.[34] In this way, he hoped finally to breach the political wall between the medical and academic sciences:

It seems to me that the Department of Biological Chemistry should include all those teachers of the chemistry of biological materials and conditions, whose instruction is primarily biological and especially physiological in purpose. Instruction in the chemistry of dietetics and nutrition cannot amount to much if it is not broadly biological.[35]

Sherman and Swartz agreed to Gies's plan but anticipated that the Department of Chemistry might feel possessive about food chemistry. They were right, and ideals of intellectual affinity did not prevail over the realities of departmental power. Sherman was transferred to chemistry, where he developed a premier school of food chemistry.[36] Biological chemistry remained a medical discipline at P&S.

In some respects, Columbia was as likely a context as Yale for a biological style of biochemistry. Columbia too was absorbing its affiliated professional schools as operating divisions. President Butler and the reformers at P&S favored a more academic style in the preclinical sciences and more intimate connections with the basic sciences. But Chittenden and Mendel enjoyed a position in a collegiate graduate faculty, whereas Gies's only strength was his role in medical teaching. Chittenden had only to parry challenges from a weak medical school; Gies had to sell his services to indifferent or suspicious chemists and biologists.

Institutional realities shaped the practice of biochemistry at P&S more than Gies's programmatic ideals. Gies was a chemist, not a physiologist like Mendel, and was not much concerned with biological processes. The department's research up to 1903 was about evenly divided between isolation of constituents from animal and plant tissues and urinalysis.[37] A medical student who took Gies's course in 1916 reported that "he spoke...very little of theoretical chemistry but much of the application of the subject at hand to clinical medicine."[38] The careers of the 54 graduates of the Ph.D. program between 1906 and 1929 reveal a strong connection with medical education and clinical medicine (see Table 11.1). The most successful were professors in second-ranked medical schools.[39]

Gies's strategy of cooperation with biologists and chemists did not result in a distinctive research style. Projects were undertaken opportunistically and did not, as a rule, lead to lasting institutional roles. The most telling point made against Gies by his critics on the medical faculty in 1911 was the lack of a coherent research program. After 1911 his interest in discipline building slowly but steadily declined; rather, it was diverted to reforming dental education.

Gies's interest in dental medicine grew out of one of his many cooperative research projects, this one initiated in 1909 by the New

Table 11.1. *Career patterns of Columbia University graduates in biochemistry*

Ph.D. cohort	Number of Ph.D.s	Major institutional affiliation						Major research interest		
		Med. educ.	Indus. & USDA	Clin. med.	Univ.	Res. inst.	No info.	Nutrit.	Clin. chem.	Bio-med.
1906–10	8	2	2	2	1		1	2	2	2
1911–15	16	9	3	3	1			3	4	3
1916–20	12	3	4		1		4	1	2	
1921–5	10	2	1	1	1	3	2	1	4	1
1926–9	8	2	1	3			2	3	2	3

York Institute of Stomatology. A collaborative research project in dental biochemistry developed into a major program. Gies was appointed to the dental faculty, founded the *Journal of Dental Medicine* in 1919, and became involved in the movement to reorganize proprietary dental schools on a university basis. In the early 1920s, he headed the Carnegie Foundation Commission on Dental Education. The "Gies Report" of 1926 did for the dental profession what the Flexner Report did for medicine.[40]

In his professional activities, Gies increasingly adopted the role of an outsider and gadfly. In 1917, for example, he attempted to set up a counterorganization to the American Society of Biological Chemists, to recognize achievement in teaching rather than in research.[41] He did almost no research after about 1912 and left the running of the department increasingly to his junior staff. After World War I, few graduate students were attracted to Gies's school. The department became a convenience for locally employed physicians or biochemists to acquire an academic credential. No fewer than eight alumni of the Rockefeller Institute got their formal degrees at P&S; however, the department did not benefit from contact with the biologists and chemists at the Institute.[42] By 1920 Gies had become the chief impediment to the reforms he had tried to bring about 20 years before.

JACQUES LOEB'S DISCIPLES

Prospects for the biological program seemed brightest in the two departments founded by Jacques Loeb, at Chicago and Berkeley. These departments were led by able individuals, Albert P. Mathews and Thorburn Robertson, who shared Loeb's vision of a "general" physiology in which biochemistry had a central role. Yet by 1920 both departments had reverted to the standard medical type. As Loeb had feared, American institutional realities ran counter to his intellectual ideals.

Albert Mathews was one of the few American biochemists who was trained as a biologist. He studied zoology with E. B. Wilson and Henry F. Osborne, physiological chemistry with Albrecht Kossel, and in 1898 he acquired a Ph.D. degree in zoology and physiology with John G. Curtis at Columbia.[43] During his years at Chicago, Mathews's work followed Loeb's closely – too closely for Loeb's comfort. Mathews resembled W. J. Gies in style and temperament: an enthusiast, whose faith in biochemical ideas often outran his sober judgment. John Curtis wrote that Mathews "suffers from an ardor of temperament such as many artists, notably musicians, display; and...this works so strongly upon his intellectual processes as to make him an uncertain judge of scientific results, and probably, an unsafe guide for students of science...."[44] Henry Bowditch shared Curtis's view, and J. J. Abel considered Mathews "a highly gifted, mercurial man, who is liable to make big mistakes and perhaps big finds in his scientific work."[45] Mathews's ardor was by no means a liability in a period that was optimistic about reform and biomedical discovery. Not unlike the molecular biologists of a later time, Mathews was regarded by more sober citizens with a mixture of awe and alarm. He was an influential, if controversial, member of the founding generation of American biochemists, active in professional organizations such as the JBC, the ASBC, and the AMA Council on Medical Education. He was an influential teacher, department chief, and author.

In 1902 a breach between master and disciple occurred when Mathews and his brother, a journalist, published a popularized article on a theory of nerve action then being investigated in Loeb's group. Loeb was outraged and, characteristically, saw an innocent peccadillo as scientific original sin:

Mr. Mathews has shown an unusual, not to say brutal disregard of the code of scientific ethics by utilizing my partly imperfect ideas and publishing them, before I had time to publish them myself. He has moreover laid claim to ideas on which my students had been at work before he came here....[It] is obvious that the presence of such a character in a laboratory must have a demoralizing effect, in as much as the free expression of ideas in Seminar and otherwise must cease....I consider Mr. Mathews' work unsound and of such a character as to sooner or later injure the reputation of the University. I am afraid the men at Harvard had come to the same conclusion when they recommended him to us. There can be but little doubt that they wished to get rid of him.[46]

Loeb henceforth regarded Mathews as a renegade. It was a common pattern with Loeb's more ambitious and assertive disciples.

Despite Loeb's ill will, Mathews was well placed to build a school of chemical biology at Chicago when Loeb left in 1902. Loeb's successor, George N. Stewart, was an electrophysiologist and gave Mathews a free hand to develop the chemical side of physiology and biology. Stewart's departure in 1903 and Mathews's promotion to full professor in 1905 left him the senior member in physiology, and the department became strongly oriented toward chemical biology. (A separate Department of Biochemistry was established in 1916.[47]) Yet there was an increasing gap between Mathews's intellectual program and the actual practice of biochemistry at Chicago, which drifted toward a clinical style. Mathews continued to theorize in Loeb's grand reductionist style about the physicochemical nature of intracellular oxidation, growth, and pharmacological action, not always with success. Abel and Arthur Cushney dismissed his theory of drug action;[48] Loeb castigated his colloidal theory of adsorption as "vitalistic."[49] Mathews preached a broad vision of biochemistry and appealed to many constituencies: "The science...stands in a close and complementary relation with zoology, botany, anatomy, pathology, physical physiology, and bacteriology on the one hand, and with chemistry on the other."[50] Yet his textbook, based on his own teaching, had no sections on general biological processes as distinct from human physiology and pathology and gave little coverage of current research on biological oxidation. A long appendix was devoted to clinical analysis. Mathews's role in the university was to teach medical students, and his audience shaped his disciplinary ideals. In practice, biochemistry at Chicago reflected the increasing presence of the new medical school far more than it did Loeb's program of chemical biology. Mathews left in 1919 to organize a program in clinical biochemistry at the University of Cincinnati Medical School.

Biochemistry at the University of California followed a similar pattern. When Loeb left Berkeley in 1910,he was succeeded by T. Brailsford Robertson, perhaps the most talented of Loeb's disciples. As a student at the University of Adelaide, he had excelled in both physiology and physics. Robertson was Loeb's ideal experimental biologist, equally adept in physics, chemistry, and biology. Loeb's militantly reductionist beliefs shaped Robertson's career as a biochemist. Together they developed a theory that the growth of cells and organisms was an autocatalytic process, following the same laws as simple chemical reactions.[51] Robertson's biochemical theory of higher nervous functions bears the same ideological stamp, and his empirical work on the physical biochemistry of proteins grew directly out of his concern with fundamental biological processes. His book, *Principles of Biochemistry* (1920), was written for students of agriculture, general biology, and applied chemistry as well as medicine. Robertson announced that he made no distinction between biochemistry and experimental biology. Whereas Loeb had warned medical students away from his course, Robertson sought to entice them in.[52] Unlike most authors who made such claims, Robertson delivered. His book included chapters on the physical chemistry of protoplasm, intracellular oxidation, bioluminescence, fertilization and development, growth, and higher nervous functions. It was the only biochemical text prior to the 1950s that actually integrated general biochemistry and biology; it is the most coherent formulation of the biological program for biochemistry.

Robertson had the energy and entrepreneurial skills to realize this program at Berkeley. Like his mentor, Robertson had a sharp tongue and confidence in his superior gifts; unlike Loeb, he was willing to do battle with a negligent administration and hostile medical colleagues. Owing to Loeb's disdain of academic politics, the department was small and chronically undernourished. While the number of students increased tenfold between 1910 and 1915, the faculty shrank by 25% in size and by 50% in salaries. Advanced students wanting to do research had to be turned away. Robertson and his colleague in physical physiology were only associate professors and had the help of only a single instructor. Comparison with similar departments elsewhere bore out Robertson's complaints (see Table 11.2).[53] Robertson succeeded in reversing these trends. He threatened to resign, warning Dr. Moffit that his successor would be certain to make far greater demands; he bullied his dean to increase the budget to prevent his closing down the department in midterm. In 1915 Robertson was promoted to professor and head of an independent and expanded Department of Biochemistry and Pharmacology.[54]

It is clear, however, that Robertson was running against the tide. The medical faculty grew in influence as reform succeeded. Hard-pressed administrators allocated resources to indispensable services, and Robertson's main service role was teaching medical students. Biochemistry attracted far fewer students from the basic sciences than did physiology (Table 11.3).[55] Robertson did not have the clientele to support a program in general biochemistry. His book was not a commercial success: Mathews's went through six editions; the second edition of Robertson's (1925) was the last. The market was for medical biochemistry, and the institutional basis of biochemistry was the medical school not general biology. Robertson

Table 11.2. *Comparison of various university departments of biochemistry, 1915*

Department	Staff	Assistants	Salaries (in dollars)	Expenses (in dollars)	Undergraduate students	Graduate students
Harvard	6	2½	10,800	4,700	85	10
Yale	5	1	11,000	?	30	12
Pennsylvania	3	2	9,800	2,700	90	5
Chicago	6	5	9,060	3,000	150	7
California	2	1	4,940	1,750	88	0
California (proposed)	5	2	10,400	3,900		

Table 11.3. *Enrollments in the University of California, 1914/15*

Field	Biochemistry Undergraduates	Research	Physiology Undergraduates	Research
Medical	31	1	31	8
Nonmedical	28	5	154	30

left Berkeley for Toronto in 1918 and in 1920 returned to Australia, where he became involved in nutrition work. His influence on American biochemistry had ceased well before his death in 1930 at the age of 46.

The biological program did not long survive the departure of Loeb's disciples from Chicago and California. Mathews was succeeded by his understudy, Fred C. Koch, a student of Julius Stieglitz's who had spent seven years as an industrial chemist in the Armour Packing Co. before getting his Ph.D. degree with Mathews in 1912.[56] Koch's eclectic research interests dealt mainly with the isolation and purification of hormones and vitamins and the improvement of analytical methods. His style of biochemistry fit perfectly the needs of the new University Hospital and Medical School, which opened in 1924. Robertson was succeeded by Walter Bloor, a disciple of Folin's, and then by Carl Schmidt,[57] who had been a professional chemist with the San Francisco Power Co. and the Berkeley Board of Health before getting his Ph.D. degree with Robertson in 1915. Schmidt acquired Robertson's interest in the physical chemistry of proteins but not his mentor's broad vision or his concern with biological processes. Schmidt was a chemist in the Department of Pathology when he was called to the chair, and under his guidance, the department found its raison d'être in medical biochemistry.[58] Koch and Schmidt exemplified the applied chemistry style that dominated American biochemistry in the 1920s.

There are many reasons why the biological program for biochemistry was not realized even in contexts as favorable as Yale, Columbia, Chicago, or Berkeley. Intellectual ideals, drawing upon the rhetoric of medical reform and reductionist ideology, proved less important than the bread-and-butter service roles biochemists played in medical schools. Connections with clinical departments were more rewarding, intellectually and strategically, after 1910 than connections with biologists. The grandiose theories that characterized chemical biology in the 1900s gave way to technical research on the chemistry of cellular constituents, especially vitamins and hormones. Such work was less risky, more productive of publishable papers, and more relevant to pathology and medicine; in short, better suited to the reward system of a preclinical discipline.

Another reason for the failure of the biological program was its advocates. The dynamic of Loeb's circle was highly centrifugal. Sooner or later, Loeb quarreled with most of his disciples, usually over intellectual property rights, as in Mathews's case. Martin Fischer, who accompanied him to California in 1910, fell from grace when he adopted a colloidal theory of proteins. In 1913 Loeb exhorted Isidor Traube not to include Fischer on the editorial board of a new journal of physicochemical biology:

Fischer...is one of the most unscientific men it has been my good pleasure to meet. He and Wolfgang Ostwald were at my laboratory simultaneously and became friends. If it were not for that, nobody would ever have heard of Fischer. Leaving aside the plagiaristic feature of his work, I do not think that any man of standing and who knows him has any respect for him left.[59]

Wolfgang Ostwald eventually earned Loeb's wrath for espousing what Loeb regarded as "vitalistic" theories of colloidal chemistry. Loeb wrote to Otto Meyerhof in 1923: "I can't get over being surprised that German chemists would let themselves be hoodwinked by so incompetent and silly a man as Ostwald."[60] Loeb's correspondence is laced with similar attacks on the opinions and morals of his former disciples. Even his relation with Robertson, whom he tried to get to the Rockefeller Institute in 1914, seems to have cooled.[61] Loeb was uneasy about putting his reputation on the line for others. For example, after exerting himself to find positions for Selig Hecht and Leonor Michaelis, Loeb panicked and wrote to Simon Flexner that they were unpleasant men and second-rate scientists.[62] Loeb's science was his religion, and he saw disagreement as apostasy and apostasy as wickedness. He dominated or ignored his less-able students and disinherited his best students when they disagreed with him.

The contrast between Loeb's school and the tightly knit, supportive, and cooperative network of clinical biochemists who had worked with Folin, Van Slyke, and Benedict is striking and significant. Had Loeb been more able to subdivide chemical biology for systematic development by a network of student–colleagues, his influence on American biochemistry might have been much greater than in fact it was.

If prospects for the biological program were dimming in departments of biochemistry, what about university departments of physiology or biology? General physiology, consisting of biochemistry and biophysics, was a potentially viable context for biochemists, yet few biochemists were employed in general physiology. Only a few general physiologists, like Frank Lillie and E. Newton Harvey, ever qualified for election to the American Society of Biological Chemists. General physiology itself remained a minor current in American physiology, which was dominated by medical concerns. Perhaps Loeb was right that medical schools could never be congenial settings for general physiology. After 1910 departments of physiology were increasingly oriented to human physiology and gave little encouragement to chemical biology. After World War I, Loeb made concerted efforts to revive general physiology in America by importing European stars. He tried to entice Otto Warburg to emigrate and was eventually successful in finding a job for Leonor Michaelis. Isolation, political turmoil, and financial chaos made research difficult in postwar Germany.[63] Warburg felt that the setback of the war had given Americans a clear lead in physicochemical biology.[64] Germans were more willing to consider emigrating, and American universities were more willing to risk appointing European prima donnas. Following his Nobel Prize and an American lecture tour in 1923, Otto Meyerhof was considered for positions at Rochester, Pennsylvania, and Chicago.[65] A. V. Hill was offered a chair of general physiology at Johns Hopkins in 1923.[66] However, few German physiologists actually came to America. Inflation was stabilized in Germany, and many Americans concluded that German scientists were more trouble as teachers and colleagues than they were worth as scholars.[67] General physiology remained a minor academic specialty.

Even the best young general physiologists found it hard to find jobs. They were too specialized to qualify for chairs of physiology in medical schools, and the existence of strong medical departments made it difficult to create competing university departments. Max Morse, a Columbia-trained chemical biologist, lamented in 1915 that he could not find a position in general physiology and was "...about to throw up the sponge and take the plunge into a career of pure medical biochemistry." He noted that half a dozen of Loeb's most able disciples had to do likewise to survive:

Mathews, Lyon, Eyster, ..., Gortner, McClendon, Ralph Lillie and many others who would have gone into general physiology if there had been any sort of openings have gone into soil survey work, general biology, medical physiology, etc.[68]

Morse had turned down several positions in medical schools, including the headship of the Department of Biochemistry at Oregon. Loeb advised him to take a medical job and try to continue his own research.[69] In the next 15 years, Morse taught biochemistry in four medical schools and then turned to industrial research.

Austrian-born Selig Hecht was caught in the same bind: he was neither a traditional medical physiologist nor an academic zoologist.[70] Hecht was trained in mathematics, zoology, and physiology, yet he found himself teaching for four years at Creighton Medical College in Omaha, Nebraska. After five years of research as a fellow of the National Research Council and the International Education Board, he still had trouble finding an academic post. So too did the young biophysicist Ralph Lillie when his job with the National Electric Light Association Research Laboratory was eliminated in 1924. A student of Loeb's (Ph.D. 1901), Lillie had had a distinguished career at Harvard, Pennsylvania, and Clark.[71]

In the mid-1920s, a number of universities created programs in general physiology. These programs often consisted of positions in biophysics and biochemistry and were designed to serve a nonmedical clientele. In 1926 T. H. Morgan saw a general trend to institutionalize Loeb's style of general physiology.[72] Ralph Lillie was appointed to a special chair at Chicago in 1924.[73] A gift of $10,000 from the General Education Board enabled Morgan to create a position in biophysics for Selig Hecht in Columbia's Department of Zoology.[74] Positions or programs in general physiology were established at Harvard, Princeton, Johns Hopkins, Stanford, and Cornell.

This sudden interest in general physiology was part of a larger reform movement in academic biology. For several decades, Loeb,

Morgan, F. R. Lillie, Raymond Pearl, and others had been saying that experimental biology was a better basis upon which to subdivide biology than zoology and botany. As long as traditional zoologists and botanists controlled departments of biology, this intellectual program was not an effective platform for reform. In the mid-1920s, however, research-oriented universities began to reorganize their departments of biology by function rather than by subject matter. This change reflected the growth of graduate instruction and problem-oriented group research and the increasing role of foundation support for projects. Specialties like genetics and general physiology, which dealt with processes common to animals, plants, and microorganisms and used physicochemical methods, became strategically important to university leaders looking for a competitive edge in the production of research. Reformers like the Flexners and Wycliffe Rose, head of the General and International Education Boards, saw these same specialties as strategic areas for research that was theoretically fundamental and ultimately useful for scientific medicine.

The movement for general physiology had limited success even in the elite research schools. Departmental jealousies often confined general physiology to informal programs, blocking the establishment of new departments. Although biologists and chemists learned new habits of cooperation in interdisciplinary research, in only a few cases were specialized positions created for biochemists. Without the service roles of medical teaching and clinical research, biochemistry as a collective, institutionalized activity did not flourish. The limits to roles for general biochemists are revealed by the experiences of Princeton and Stanford.

The Department of Biology at Princeton was a particularly promising context for chemical biology. Professor of Biology E. Newton Harvey had fallen early under Loeb's spell, and as Morgan's student, he began biochemical and physiological work on bioluminescence, to which he devoted his whole career.[75] In 1919 Harvey converted a wartime training course in sanitary chemistry into an undergraduate course in general biochemistry, which he continued to teach until a specialized position was created for a biochemist in the late 1930s.[76] In 1921 he moved from makeshift facilities to a new biochemical laboratory.

Harvey's interest in bioluminescence brought him to the attention of physical chemist Hugh Taylor, who was an expert in radiation and chemical activation. They served together on a National Research Council Committee on the Relations between Physics and Biology, and in 1925 they planned a cooperative research program on photosynthesis.[77] The absence of strong professional schools at Princeton seems to have encouraged horizontal linkages between basic sciences, in contrast to the vertical linkages between basic and clinical sciences typical of medical schools. Halston J. Thorkelson of the General Education Board (GEB) felt that a strong spirit of cooperation between the Princeton chemists and biologists was an "unusual opportunity for innovative research."[78] The absence of medical biochemistry at Princeton (one of the few major research universities without a medical school) left the way clear for a style of biochemistry linked to basic biology.

A plan to establish separate departments of biochemistry and biophysics was considered in 1925, in connection with an application to the GEB for endowment of scientific research. The planning committee was aware of the GEB's interest in interdisciplinary research and felt that departments of biophysics and biochemistry would be bridges between chemistry and biology. In the end, however, they decided to utilize existing departmental structures and asked for support for research on radiation in the departments of astronomy, physics, chemistry, and biology.[79]

The decision not to establish departments of biochemistry and biophysics reveals just how great an advantage established departments had over new ones in competing for research funds. The science departments were desperate for new research endowments. Princeton alumni were far more forthcoming for undergraduate activities than they were for scientific research, and the drive to raise $5.5 million for the natural sciences was flagging.[80] Moreover, foundations were more interested in strengthening existing capabilities for research than in underwriting whole new academic departments. Karl Compton emphasized to the GEB the efficiency of multidisciplinary projects using existing department strengths.[81] Princeton received $1 million from the GEB toward a $3 million endowment fund for the departments of biology, chemistry, and physics.[82]

Without an indispensable service role in medical teaching, biochemistry survived at Princeton only as a part of Harvey's personal research program. In 1926 Princeton refused Harvey's request for a junior appointment in physiology and biochemistry.[83] This was the European pattern: intellectual achievement in a context that offered little chance for institutional independence or growth.

Similar steps were taken at Stanford in 1926, when President Ray Lyman Wilbur approached the General Education Board with a proposal to support a group of physicists, chemists, and biologists in applying physics and chemistry to biological problems.[84] There was already considerable activity in chemophysical biology at Stanford. Zoologist Charles V. Taylor was noted for his biophysical studies of subcellular structures. Lawrence Irving, a young instructor in biology, was studying muscle biochemistry with Gustav Embden on an NRC fellowship. Chairman of Chemistry Robert E. Swain, a student of Chittenden's (Ph.D., 1904), had taught physiological chemistry since Stanford's affiliation with Cooper Medical College and had a proprietary interest in the border area between chemistry and biology. Carl Alsberg, in the Food Research Institute, participated in Swain's graduate program, and Murray Luck had just been appointed instructor in biochemistry in the Department of Chemistry.[85]

President Wilbur's concern for biochemistry and biophysics was strategic as well as intellectual. He aspired to make Stanford a leader in research and graduate training. University leaders were deeply concerned in the mid-1920s that universities would lose out to specialized research institutes in the competition for foundation funds. Wilbur and others recognized that universities could best compete by organizing cross-departmental research groups. Stanford harbored a number of autonomous research institutes, such as the Hoover Food Research Institute and the Carnegie Laboratory, and Wilbur proposed to organize department research in the same fashion.

Wilbur also believed that the clinical reform movement had resulted in an unhealthy shift of influence and power from the pure science faculties to medical schools:

At the present time anatomy, . . . neurology and embryology, physiology, physiologic chemistry and bacteriology are included in some degree in all medical schools. In fact, there has been a steady insistence on the part of the medical profession that these basic sciences belong in the medical curriculum and nowhere else. This attitude has been a definite obstacle to the advance of physiology and anatomy in America. . . . These basic sciences need to be set free from the limited claims of the medical curriculum.[86]

Wilbur hoped that a program of interdisciplinary research in biophysics and biochemistry would redress the balance of power between Stanford and its medical school. The biologists welcomed the research institute idea and asserted the strategic role of biology in project research:

The day of cooperative effort is at hand in this field of research, and the great advances of the future will come from the bringing closer together of highly trained workers in physics, biology and chemistry for a more concerted attack upon the mysteries of living protoplasm.[87]

The rapid growth in graduate studies after 1918 gave Wilbur confidence that the new programs could survive financially without depending on service roles in medical instruction.[88]

Biochemistry as such was not part of the original 1927–8 plan. The GEB pledged $750,000 toward a new research building, and Wilbur had his eye on endowment for existing science departments.[89] Funds for a new building were not forthcoming, however, and to get research started, Charles V. Taylor initiated a modest project on the effects of x rays on the structure of living cells.[90] Taylor, Murray Luck, and physicist Harry Clark, recently arrived from the Rockefeller Institute, began work together in 1929. Meanwhile, Wilbur revived an earlier plan to regroup the science departments into divisions, in part to encourage more interdisciplinary team research. As part of this reorganization, he proposed to create an independent Department of Biochemistry in the Division of Biological Sciences.[91] The biologists again expressed eager interest in expanding the chemical side of biology, which hitherto had been the territory of the medical school.[92] By 1930, however, the planning committee was less enthusiastic about a separate department, and in the end, biochemistry remained within chemistry.[93] Why?

Swain was not in favor of creating a Department of Biochemistry within the biology division, and his views were shared, surprisingly, by Charles Taylor, the most vocal promoter of chemical methods among the biologists. Taylor felt that biophysics and biochemistry belonged in physics and chemistry because, as new fields, they needed academic respectability:

The real, and to me rather serious problem concerns not biophysics, but biophysicists. The newness of the field...offers temporary haven for ne'er-do-wells who are neither biologists nor physicists. I am told that there is a prominent biophysicist in a leading American university who never has had a single course in physics. As a biophysicist that is worse than it would be had he never had a course in biology. And this suggests a growing conviction of mine with which you as a biochemist will, I feel sure quite agree, viz., that just as the biochemist approaches biological problems by way of chemistry, so also must the biophysicist approach basic problems in biology by way of physics....I recall clearly your statement to me once that the biochemist should officially maintain his primary affiliations with chemists rather than with biologists. That is a sound policy. Precisely the same should hold for the biophysicist. I am deeply anxious to see biophysics established here at Stanford. And our fine opportunity is to make it bio-*physics* rather than...physical biology. The latter rightly belongs in the biological group, but the former in the physical group of the sciences. There is an essential difference here, both in emphasis of training and in point of view.[94]

Although few put it quite so crisply, Swain and Taylor's view seems to have been widely held by chemists and biologists. Both were suspicious of new specialty groups, with their unfamiliar standards of achievement, and were anxious not to upset established disciplinary interests. Chemists and biologists who were most interested in biochemistry or biophysics were precisely those who had the greatest professional interest in preserving their grip on these specialties. Separate departments were simply competitors for important problems and scarce university resources. At Princeton, Stanford, and wherever biochemistry did not have a role in medical teaching, it was cultivated not in departments but by ad hoc groups of chemists and biologists.

HARVARD: STYLES OF GENERAL BIOCHEMISTRY

A program in general physiology and biochemistry also developed at the Harvard Medical School, not in Folin's department, though, but in the Physical Chemistry Laboratory created by David Edsall in 1920 as a refuge for Folin's old rival, L. J. Henderson. Since his break with Folin ten years earlier, Henderson had detached himself from the medical school. He pursued his research on acid–base balance in blood at the Massachusetts General Hospital and taught his course in general biochemistry in Harvard College. But he felt the lack of institutional roots in the medical school. In 1920 he was offered a new chair of general physiology at Johns Hopkins. Henderson intimated to Dean David Edsall that he would welcome a closer connection with the medical school and that he would never have detached himself had Folin not made it impossible for him to stay. With the backing of clinicians J. H. Means, George Minot, and Reginald Fitz, Edsall created an endowed research laboratory for Henderson. Thus protected from Folin, physiologists, and unsympathetic clinicians, Henderson turned out his theoretical works on blood as a physicochemical system.[95]

The research program of Henderson's laboratory was largely shaped by his student and lieutenant, Edwin Cohn. Cohn was a product of the Rockefeller Institute circle. The younger brother of the clinician Alfred Cohn, Edwin knew Loeb and Henderson as family friends. He studied chemistry with Julius Stieglitz and did his dissertation with biologist F. R. Lillie and Henderson at Woods Hole. Henderson then packed Cohn off to learn organic chemistry from Thomas B. Osborne and physical chemistry from Søren Sørensen, Svante Arrhenius, and William Hardy.[96] Cohn was no orthodox biochemist but a chemist–biologist.

Cohn's talents complemented Henderson's. The romantic intellectual, Henderson delighted in new ideas, as long as they were avant-garde; a brilliant teacher and thinker, Henderson was an indifferent administrator. Cohn exemplified the American style of research manager: ambitious, organized, and eager to shape a large research program. As Henderson's restless intellect carried him first into industrial physiology and then into sociology, Cohn mobilized the resources of the Physical Chemistry Laboratory for a systematic investigation of the physical basis of physiologically active proteins.

The hallmark of Cohn's research style was his combination of chemical means and biological ends. He made use of the most advanced physicochemical theories and the most novel and sophisticated technical equipment to understand such basic biological processes as secretion, respiration, excitation, and muscle contraction. Physiologist Alexander Muralt, who worked with him in the late 1920s, believed that Cohn was laying the basis for a "theoretical biology."[97] Cohn was influenced by Henderson's conception of blood as a physiological system that obeyed simple laws of physical chemistry, but he was more interested than Henderson in explaining the physiological behavior of complex molecules in the body. This interest drew him into sophisticated theoretical chemistry. In 1925 Cohn attended a series of lectures at MIT by the theoretical chemist Peter Debye and realized that the Debye–Hückel theory of dipolar ions might be the key to understanding the physiological behavior of multicharged proteins. A close working relation developed between Cohn and a theoretical physical chemist at MIT, George Scatchard. Scatchard became a regular participant in Cohn's research seminar, making important contributions to the theory of the proteins in solution.[98] At about the same time, Cohn's interest shifted from the chemical individuality of proteins (an interest he had acquired from T. B. Osborne and L. B. Mendel) to the behavior of small, physiologically active proteins, such as insulin, thyroxin, or secretin.[99] His idea was that the physiological activity of these and other functional proteins must have to do with their solubility and dielectric properties in the tissues or body fluids. Cohn's aim was to measure these properties, explain them theoretically, and thus ultimately give a physicochemical account of physiological actions. In the 1930s, Cohn's group systematically worked out this program, using almost every conceivable physical technique.[100]

Cohn did tend to lose the biological ends in the pursuit of more and better chemical means. Linus Pauling, for example, wondered what all that painstaking accumulation of data really added up to.[101] However, Cohn continued to enjoy the admiration and respect of physiologists and biochemists alike.[102] Cohn's work was one of the showpieces of the Rockefeller Foundation's program in experimental or molecular biology.[103] Cohn's was one of the ten groups selected by Harvard President James B. Conant in 1937 for development as interdisciplinary research institutes, on the model of the departments of chemistry, physics, and biology at Caltech.[104] The Physical Chemistry Laboratory represented an alternative style of biochemistry that was more chemical and more biological than Folin's and the medical biochemists'. Cohn actually integrated chemistry and biology, and his work was extremely influential among biochemists in the 1930s. Cohn's success depended, however, on the independence provided by endowment and on privileged access to foundation funds. Like F. G. Hopkins, Cohn was an anomaly in a system dependent on the clinical connection; he could not have achieved so much had he been less insulated from the political economy of his discipline.

A program in biochemistry was also established at Harvard College in the 1920s, based not on research but on undergraduate teaching. Its success depended on unique local circumstances, however, and it had no imitators. Attempts to create a real department of biochemistry in the 1930s failed, for many of the same reasons that similar initiatives failed at Princeton, Stanford, and elsewhere.

The Tutors Program in Biochemical Sciences began as another of David Edsall's experiments in "correlation."[105] As dean of the medical school, Edsall was troubled by the disjunction of collegiate and professional training. Students who took the basic sciences as freshmen or sophomores forgot all they learned by the time they entered medical school. Those who majored in science forfeited the benefits of a liberal education. Edsall's solution was to organize courses in general physiology and biochemistry for juniors and seniors. Edsall hoped to achieve the integration of the European six-year medical course without losing the advantage of the American eight-year course.[106] Edsall did not want to extend professional studies back into the college years but, rather, to teach the first preclinical sciences in a collegiate context as liberal studies.[107] General physiology and biochemistry were the strategic links between college and medical school. Edsall's scheme fit President Lowell's plan to revitalize liberal humanistic studies at Harvard College by creating a tutorial system modeled on Oxford and Cambridge.[108] Lowell approved of Edsall's plan. The departments of biology, chemistry, and physics saw no threat to their interests and welcomed support for the sciences at a time when the humanities were in the ascendency at Harvard.[109]

The Tutors Program was initially organized around physiology, building upon the success of L. J. Henderson's university program in general physiology.[110] (The first head tutor, Hallowell Davis, was a neurophysiologist and protégé of Walter B. Cannon's.) Within a few years, however, the Tutors Program took a more chemical bent and was renamed "Biomedical Sciences." Davis was succeeded in 1928 by Ronald M. Ferry, a biochemist and disciple of Henderson and Cohn. He was joined in 1929 by John T. Edsall (David's son), who, like Henderson, had come from physical chemistry to medicine. After two years with F. G. Hopkins's group at Cambridge, Edsall became associated with Henderson and Cohn's Physical Chemistry Laboratory at the medical school. Davis urged students to minor in chemistry (provoking complaints of discrimination from the other departments), and by 1928 the curriculum included three courses in chemistry and one each in physics and biology.[111] By 1932 seven of the ten tutors were biochemists, some from Folin's staff, but most from the Henderson–Cohn group.

The Tutors Program was a toehold in the university for general biochemistry, with links to chemistry and biology rather than to clinical medicine. As a teaching program it was a great success; however, it had no institutional basis, being wholly dependent on the goodwill of established departments for staff and student research facilities. Tutors had no official role in research or graduate training. In 1932 Ferry and John Edsall drew up a proposal to establish a university department of biochemistry.[112] Henderson and Cohn had been talking for years about such a department, and their accomplishments at the Physical Chemistry Laboratory suggested to Dean Edsall that a similar department of biochemistry would be no less successful.[113] Nothing came of Ferry and Edsall's scheme, however, mainly because of opposition from the departments of chemistry and biology.

The opposition of the chemists and biologists reflected their departmental interests. The Tutors Program brought them students, resources, and visibility; a separate department of biochemistry would have deprived them of valuable intellectual territory. The chemists saw biochemistry as bioorganic or natural products chemistry and felt it belonged in their bailiwick. Louis Fieser was becoming a leader in the field of natural products chemistry. James B. Conant had been moving his research toward biology for some years and had published a theory of photosynthesis (which amused his biologist friends).[114] The chemists' interest in bioorganic chemistry increased their desire not to let it slip out of their domain. Elected to succeed President Lowell in 1933, Conant deferred to his former colleagues and declined to support Ferry and Edsall's plan for a separate department.[115] The biologists agreed with the chemists. Professor of General Physiology William J. Crozier argued that if a department of biochemistry were established, it should be part of chemistry:

Obviously, the relations between what I may call "Functional Biochemistry" and Physiology are close. But I presume that if Biochemistry is to attain there the status desired for it, its most fruitful development would be in rather close communion with Physical and Organic Chemistry.[116]

Like C. V. Taylor, Crozier felt that attachment to chemistry would ensure status and respectability for border sciences.

The Harvard chemists and biologists made desultory efforts to develop biochemistry. In 1934 Roger Adams was offered Conant's chair to develop a bioorganic school, but Adams declined.[117] The biologists also considered appointing a junior biochemist, of a more biological sort, in connection with the reorganization of zoology, botany, and physiology into the Division of Biology.[118] George Wald, a young protégé of Selig Hecht's, was appointed in 1934 to build up physicochemical biology. Wald had a strong interest in the biochemistry of color vision and, by 1940, was teaching a biochemistry course much as Harvey was at Princeton. In both chemistry and biology, however, biochemistry was pursued by individuals; there was no real support for an organized program analogous to Cohn's group at the medical school. Entrenched interests were too strong.

CALTECH

A modest but successful program in biochemistry and biophysics was established at the California Institute of Technology in T. H. Morgan's Division of Biology. Biochemist Henry Borsook, a student of Hardolph Wasteneys's and a second-generation Loebian, was appointed in 1929. A year later, Kenneth Thimann was appointed in plant physiology and biochemistry, and Robert Emerson in biophysics.[119] It was an able and energetic group; Borsook's work on thermochemistry and the chemical dynamics of biological oxidation and biosynthesis exemplified the latest trend in chemical biology and attracted a small but influential group of postdoctoral fellows in the 1930s. At Caltech, Loeb's ideal of general physiology was partly realized, but only partly.

In many ways Caltech was an ideal context for this style of biochemistry. It was an elite school of science and engineering, with virtually no connections with medical teaching and a strong commitment to basic research. The institute was also deeply committed to interdisciplinary research in such fields as astrophysics and chemical physics.[120] Morgan's Division of Biology was established specifically to develop a program of physicochemical biology. Chemist Arthur A. Noyes and physicist Robert A. Millikan, the architects of institute policy, strongly supported cooperative research in the border areas between biology and the physical sciences. The promise of interdisciplinary cooperation was one of the main attractions of the proposal they made to Morgan. Noyes was especially taken with the potential of chemical biology, and the Caltech leaders were well connected with foundations that aimed to promote inter-disciplinary areas like biochemistry and biophysics.

Yet at the same time, Borsook's operation suffered from some of the same constraints that hampered similar programs elsewhere.

Morgan was clearly much more interested in genetics than in general physiology and much more successful in marshaling resources for genetics. There was also competition from chemistry; by 1940 the real center of "molecular biology" at Caltech was not biology but Linus Pauling's group in bioorganic chemistry. Whereas Pauling got big foundation grants, Borsook was increasingly involved in extramural medical work on nutrition. Without a built-in service role in medicine, chemical biology tended to be divided between its more powerful neighbors at Caltech no less than at Princeton, Stanford, and Harvard.

The earliest schemes for developing biology at Caltech were connected with plans for a new medical school in Southern California. The core of these schemes were departments of biochemistry and biophysics – natural links between the physical sciences and medicine. Arthur Noyes was the most persistent advocate of this plan. The other two members of the Caltech troika, George Ellery Hale and Robert Millikan, were much less eager to plunge into medical research. Millikan toyed with the idea of a research hospital and a small research-oriented medical school, which might provide the same leaven to medicine that Caltech was already providing in engineering. Hale feared that a medical connection would swallow up science and engineering and compromise Caltech's reputation as a research institution.[121] Wycliffe Rose encouraged Hale's misgivings, and the plans fell through.

Meanwhile, Noyes seized an opportunity to get biochemical research started in a small way. In 1922 a local physician offered Noyes $12,000 a year for research on insulin, and a makeshift research laboratory was soon in operation.[122] Noyes saw this project as the potential basis for a full department of biochemistry. With this plan in mind, he brought J. J. Abel to Pasadena in the spring of 1924 to pursue research on crystallizing insulin. Noyes hoped that Abel would stay at Caltech as head of a new department of biochemistry and biophysics, which ultimately would become the core of a Division of Biology.[123] In 1925 Noyes laid his plan before the General Education Board:

It is . . . desirable to introduce as soon as possible those branches of biology which have close relations with physics and chemistry. . . . Thus it would be highly advantageous to provide at once for research laboratories of biochemistry (including chemical pharmacology) and of biophysics (including general physical physiology).[124]

Noyes's plans for a biology division included chairs of biochemistry, biophysics, general biology, and chemical bacteriology and provision for research on hormones and enzymes, radiation biology, photochemistry, and applications of physical chemistry to biology. It provided for medical research in special wards of the Pasadena Hospital and for training of selected medical students and physicians in research.[125]

The GEB did not buy Noyes's plan, but Noyes continued to encourage local initiatives. In 1925 Dr. Lorena Breed offered to raise the funds for a metabolic research laboratory. Noyes responded with enthusiasm. Millikan and Hale were skeptical but could not resist the prospect of opening channels to wealthy medical patrons. They agreed to establish a "Biological Research Fund" on the condition that the metabolic laboratory would become part of the future department of biochemistry.[126] The expected benefactions did not materialize, however, and in 1927 Noyes's plans for biochemistry were swept up in a more ambitious program for biology.

In the spring of 1925, Hale finally discovered the man he wanted to create a Division of Biology. He and Millikan approached Morgan with a plan for a school devoted to physicochemical biology, and Morgan accepted. Nearly $3 million was raised, mainly from Trustees William Kerckhoff and A. C. Balch and the GEB. The Division of Biology was launched in the same grand style that chemistry and physics had been in 1920 and 1921.[127] Dr. Breed still talked of large donations, but Hale and Millikan were glad to be rid of medical projects. Morgan's presence diminished the financial and intellectual appeal of a connection to medicine through biochemistry.

Noyes was loath to abandon his hopes for biochemistry and suggested that it might be affiliated with his own division.[128] He was just then trying to entice James B. Conant to Pasadena to lead a new group in organic and bioorganic chemistry, and he saw biochemistry as a crucial link to Morgan's group.[129] Morgan encouraged Noyes and wrote Trustee Arthur Fleming: "Organic chemistry will always be...the rallying point for physiological work."[130] When Conant declined, however, the whole scheme fell through.

Biochemistry was included in Morgan's plan for the new Division of Biology, but not so grandly. Morgan envisioned a core of three departments: genetics and evolution, general physiology, and developmental mechanics, with biochemistry and biophysics to be added later.[131] Noyes, Hale, and Millikan had envisioned a division centered on general physiology (biophysics and biochemistry) with close connections to chemistry and physics.[132] Biochemistry was far less important to Morgan. He sincerely believed in the promise of chemical biology and often said that the future of genetics lay in the physiology and biochemistry of gene expression.[133] But Morgan just did not know how to practice what he preached. He had devoted most of his career to genetics and evolution, fields in which chemistry and physics were not of immediate use. He was unfamiliar with physiology and was less energetic and effective in locating the best physiologists and enticing them to Caltech. Trained in the old school, he had little real sense of how exactly physiology or biochemistry might apply to genetics. Inevitably, Morgan succeeded best in what was closest to his own heart.

Morgan's priorities became apparent as soon as he began to translate his grand scheme into specific appointments. By August 1927, he was writing Hale in a more cautious vein: "While I am anxious to emphasize the dynamic physiological character of the work, I shall try to avoid the criticism that we are leaving the older and less important sides of biology in the background." In his search for the best men, Morgan seized opportunities as he found them, and he found them where he knew to look:

The time is not far off when individual names will have to be considered. In the genetic field, where I know my ground, this will not be difficult; but when it comes to the physiologists, I shall have to go more slowly, and perhaps hold up the situation until I go abroad next spring.[134]

Morgan quickly assembled an outstanding group of geneticists. However, his search for a general physiologist and biochemist was a story of unreasonably high hopes and lost opportunities. Morgan made an offer to William J. Crozier, knowing that Crozier was dissatisfied with the support he was getting from Harvard. Crozier declined when he got a large grant from the GEB. Morgan also tried to pry Selig Hecht loose from Columbia and John Northrop from the Rockefeller Institute, with no success.[135] But Morgan did not snap up Leonor Michaelis, a top general physiologist who was being let go by Johns Hopkins, for fear that Michaelis, a Jew, might bring his group of young Jewish co-workers with him.[136] He did not make an offer to Albert Raymond, Abel's former assistant in the insulin work because he did not want to part him from Phoebus

Levene.[137] Five years after it was founded, Morgan's division still had no full professor of physiology and, with no powerful leader to push it, the physiological group remained undeveloped. Despite the appointments of Borsook, Emerson, and Thimann, the original plan for biochemistry and biophysics was only partly realized.[138]

Biochemistry at Caltech remained a minor specialty within biology, dependent on informal cooperation for support and drawn increasingly to medicine. In 1931 Emerson complained of the parochial interests of the biologists, all "milk-bottle-molasses and beef-hash-muscle in outlook.... The biochemistry section is highly medical in outlook and seems to me very narrow."[139] Morgan tended to retreat to his own interests in genetics and did not push vigorously for physiology and biochemistry.[140] Borsook pursued opportunities in medical research outside Morgan's school. External events also pushed him away from biology. Medical research was one of few areas of research that appealed to philanthropists in the depth of the Depression. A large portion of Morgan's endowment had been wiped out in the Crash, and he went along with medical schemes, more out of desperation than real enthusiasm. Borsook proposed to hire the British neurophysiologist J. H. Gaddum, "A man who Morgan half-jokingly calls a 'medical' physiologist that Borsook has put over on him – though he heartily approves of him."[141] However, the timely award of a Nobel Prize to Morgan secured a large gift to biology and obviated the need to develop a line of medical research.[142]

Borsook continued work along medical lines. By 1935 his research had shifted from free-energy measurements to nitrogen metabolism, and in the late 1930s and 1940s, he devoted a great deal of time to vitamins, nutrition, and public health.[143] In areas related to biology and physical chemistry, Borsook was increasingly overshadowed by Linus Pauling. With lavish assistance from the Rockefeller Foundation, Pauling realized Noyes's old dream of cooperative research in the border areas between chemistry and biology.

CONCLUSION

The story was always the same where biochemistry was situated outside a medical school. Without service roles in medicine, biochemists were no match for well-established biologists and chemists who were alert to the benefits of entrepreneurship in cooperative research. Institutional contexts that favored research on basic biological problems did not enable biochemists to institutionalize roles and mobilize resources. Biologists who saw chemistry as the key to progress in biology looked to collaboration with organic or physical chemists; it was too important an area to give over to biochemists. Because biochemistry was a separate medical discipline, most biologists saw it either as irrelevant to their own disciplinary goals or as direct competition.

The decline of the biological program between 1910 and 1940 was neither a failure of scientific imagination nor a failure of chemical biologists to produce important discoveries. It was a consequence of the political economy of academic science. Conditions that favor intellectual innovation do not necessarily facilitate institutional consolidation and growth, and vice versa. Departments of biology provided few roles for biochemists. Medical biochemists were rewarded for discovering a new vitamin or hormone, not for tackling large biological problems. There was no congruence between intellectual programs and strategies for discipline building.

The biological program of biochemistry was adapted to a different kind of political economy. It required large graduate programs, a diverse clientele in the basic university sciences, and outside patronage for research not tied to clinical goals. What support there was for general biochemistry in the 1920s and 1930s came from contexts in which these conditions were met. Graduate programs were expanding to meet the demand for teachers in a booming collegiate market. Some foundations, like the General Education Board and the Rockefeller Foundation, shifted their goals from medicine to biomedical research. The interdisciplinary style of research institutes was transplanted into those university departments able to attract foundation grants. These conditions enabled a few exceptional individuals to cultivate general biochemistry within departments of chemistry or biology or in independent research institutes. But opportunities for growth were limited in such contexts by lack of essential service roles and by disciplinary rivalries. The presence of a medical school made it difficult to create competing departments; without a clinical connection, it was hard to justify having biochemistry at all.

12

Epilogue: Toward a molecular biology?

Particular scientific styles flourish only where intellectual priorities are congruent with institutional structures and goals. That is the central theme of Chapters 9-11. This process of accommodation is clearest in the case of clinical biochemistry. True, the time was ripe for discoveries in clinical analysis, metabolism, and nutrition; but biochemists' concentration on these problems reflects an institutionalized system of service roles, markets, and professional alliances. Because human and material resources were readily mobilized for clinical biochemistry, this style dominated the discipline for a generation or more. Meanwhile, equally attractive opportunities for discovery in chemical biology did not become fashionable, except in a few marginal contexts where intellectual opportunities were also vehicles for marshaling institutional support. Contexts that provided intellectual support for chemical biology generally also had built-in limits to growth. This was the case in most departments of chemistry and biology and in nonmedical programs of general physiology. Because bioorganic chemistry or chemical biology conferred little strategic or political advantage, these programs did not attract large numbers of biochemists.

This argument assumes a stringent process of selection: intellectual styles that do not fit institutional goals will not survive. This may be a realistic assumption for periods of rapid institutional innovation. Institution builders must be aware of the strategic uses and limitations of disciplinary programs; entrepreneurs must accommodate their ideals to market conditions. Once established, however, institutions are neither fixed nor inflexible; fixed structures can usually be adapted to a wide variety of uses. Institutions shape behavior but do not determine it. In a period when graduate programs are expanding, as they did after 1945, internal disciplinary ideals gain over routine service roles. Diversity arises as researchers avoid competition by seeking new problems, and new problems create new markets and new relations among disciplines. There is a tendency in disciplines akin to genetic drift in species. The increasing influence of physical and organic chemists in the 1920s and 1930s was facilitated by the steady drift of chemists into biochemistry but was limited by pure chemists' tendency to internalize the benefits and externalize the costs of this market relation. The relation between biochemistry and biology was likewise altered by a gradual drift in biochemists' research interests.

The late 1930s saw the beginning of a remarkable expansion in biochemists' interests in biological oxidation, intermediary metabolism, biosynthesis, and macromolecules. Aided by new laboratory technologies, biochemists mapped metabolic pathways and began to think of large molecules in terms of their functions in the cell. In the 1950s, the first revelations began in molecular genetics, gene replication, and the genetic control of enzyme synthesis. Most of these stunning discoveries in "molecular biology" were not made by biochemists, however. George Beadle and Edward Tatum's one-gene–one-enzyme concept; Jacques Monod and Francois Jacob's operon and central dogma of gene expression; Linus Pauling's alpha helix; and Watson and Crick's double helix were all the work of biologists, chemists, and physicists, who made it clear that they regarded biochemists as plodders. This pattern is not mere chance. Biochemists' institutions provided some opportunities and material support for their expanding interests in cell physiology but also set limits to their vision and to the pace of change. These limits were dramatized by the unexpected discoveries of the molecular biologists. The pace of change in biochemistry was determined – and limited – by institutionalized habits, roles and values.

The topics that held biochemists' attention in the late 1930s and 1940s were extensions of traditional biochemical concerns. They were not imported from biology, unlike the problems of molecular genetics. Such problems as bioenergetics, intermediary metabolism, and the behavior of macromolecules were well suited to the medical school contexts in which they were developed. The study of metabolic pathways and cycles was an ideal compromise for a generation of biochemists who were making a gradual transition from clinical to more biological concerns. Metabolism was obviously relevant to human physiology and pathology; it was easy to justify its claim upon medical school resources. Intermediary metabolism was ideally suited to new physical techniques like isotopic tracers. The high productivity of researchers in this area was a great competitive advantage. Freed from clumsy and laborious animal feeding techniques, biochemists rapidly unraveled the individual steps of biosynthetic pathways and the citric acid and other cycles. Rudolf Schoenheimer and Hans Krebs, the two leaders in this area, were both trained as pathologists and were unusually alert to new laboratory methods; both made a smooth transition from pathology to biochemistry in the mid-1930s.[1] Their careers were exemplary of the times.

A second problem connecting old and new in biochemistry was biological oxidation. Long a subject for model building by chemists and enzymologists, this problem was opened to experimental study when it was recognized that some well-known vitamins and coenzymes were components of the chain of active compounds that transferred electrons from glucose to oxygen with the production of usable energy. Otto Warburg, David Keilin, and others developed spectroscopic techniques to identify the intermediate steps of the respiratory chain and opened this area to research by a standing army of enzymologists.

The study of macromolecules showed a similar pattern of development. Proteins and nucleic acids had long been familiar objects of biochemical research, but in the 1930s they began to be studied in a new way, not as passive structures, but as functional agents. The ultracentrifuge, another new laboratory technology, revealed these substances to be long polymeric chains, with functional specificity that depended on their molecular shape. The sequence of subunits began to be understood as a kind of biological information, translated from genes during development. This outlook was first applied to proteins, with their diverse array of subunits and, in the 1940s, was extended to the nucleic acids, the substance of the genes.

Biochemists also began to concern themselves with a group of problems that had not traditionally been regarded as their intellectual territory. Bacteriophage and viruses began to attract biochemists' interest to the grey area between dead chemicals and living organisms. Here again, however, there are clear links to traditional biochemical interests. Biochemists regarded viruses as a special kind of self-replicating enzyme. The crystallization of enzymes by James Sumner and John Northrop was followed by the crystallization of viruses by Northrop and Wendell Stanley, a chemist recruited by Simon Flexner to virology.[2] The chemical study of viruses used the same techniques that had been applied to physiologically active proteins and enzymes.

There are now good technical accounts of these developments.[3] The point here is simply that they exemplify the increasing interest of biochemists in the molecular basis of biological phenomena, growing out of but going beyond an immediate relevance to human physiology and pathology. Biochemists were much less involved in cell physiology and biochemical genetics, where there were fewer points of contact with traditional biochemical interests.[4] Moreover, many of these new developments occurred outside the disciplinary reward system of biochemistry departments. Loeb, Northrop, Stanley, and Oswald Avery at the Rockefeller Institute; Warburg at the Kaiser Wilhelm and Keilin at the Molteno Institute; the Carlsberg Institute, Cambridge, and Caltech – these contexts permitted a greater range of biochemical research than traditional departments of biochemistry, but only for a select few.

How then did these new ideas take root in large medical school departments of biochemistry, which had the resources to develop them on a large scale? What limits did traditional, service-oriented departments place on the development there of molecular biology? These questions may not be answerable in a systematic way. Introduction of new techniques, problems, and perspectives depended on particular individuals and local resources. There was no reform movement and no effort to standardize department policy. Innovations frequently occurred not by imposition of new research priorities from the top but through evolution of ongoing research by department rank and file. A few unsystematic examples will illustrate this point.

At Columbia, pathologist Rudolf Schoenheimer was led to develop the isotope tracer technique by a fortuitous encounter with physical chemist Harold Urey and his student, David Rittenberg. These chemists were eager to investigate the biological applications of heavy isotopes, in part to secure foundation support for their chemical work on isotopes. Schoenheimer quickly recognized the promise of isotopes for the study of metabolic pathways, and his work on the pathology of lipid metabolism, to which he had first applied the new technique, was soon overshadowed by a large program of research on fundamental biochemistry, supported by grants from the Rockefeller and Macy foundations. The success of

Schoenheimer's work radically affected the department's research program in the bioorganic chemistry of steroid and protein hormones. In 1934, when Schoenheimer was accommodated as a refugee from Hitler's Germany, the hormone chemists were the stars. Five years later, Schoenheimer was getting the best graduate students and the lion's share of research funds.[5]

Similar developments took place in other leading departments. Baird Hastings came to Harvard Medical School in 1935 intending to develop the department's strength in clinical biochemistry. By 1940 his research program was dominated by work on bioenergetics, intermediary metabolism, and biosynthesis, including pioneering work using the radioisotope carbon-11. Although Hastings encouraged these initiatives, they came from the grass roots. For example, Yellapragada SubbaRow's work on nutrition and the pathology of vitamin deficiency was transformed when it became clear that the vitamin, nicotinic acid, was a key factor in biological oxidation and reduction. Benjamin Alexander, a young physician working with SubbaRow, was sent to Cambridge to get some training with Hopkins in bioenergetics, and he quickly realized that the Harvard group had stumbled into one of the hottest areas of basic research: "With each new paper published I become more and more convinced of the fundamental nature of our problem."[6] What the clinical biochemists at Harvard discovered was a new programmatic rationale for their ongoing research. Other young biochemists also made new initiatives, with Hastings's encouragement. Birgit Vennesland, trained at Chicago in bacteriology and physical chemistry, came to Harvard to work with Hastings on the chemical physiology of potassium and calcium metabolism, using radioactive isotopes from the new Harvard cyclotron. Within a year, however, Vennesland was working on the fixation of CO_2 in plant and animal tissues using carbon-11. (Vennesland had learned isotope techniques and intermediary metabolism with Earl A. Evans, a student of Schoenheimer's.) Another young biochemist, Jack Buchanan, persuaded Hastings to let him work on the fixation of CO_2 in fatty acids, an idea suggested by Schoenheimer's Dunham lectures.[7]

Hastings played the role of facilitator, encouraging initiatives in his young postdoctoral workers. Immediately after the war, a major project in isotope research was mounted, including work on intermediary metabolism, with a large grant from the Office of

Naval Research. The number of graduate students increased from 2 in 1945/6 to 20 in 1949/50. In 1950 three private foundations and two government agencies provided $18,120 for research by 15 postdoctoral fellows supported by the National Institutes of Health, the National Research Council, and several private foundations. In 1946 Eric Ball, a veteran of Warburg's laboratory, was appointed to a special professorship in charge of graduate studies. By 1949 clinical biochemistry was only one of half a dozen subspecialties that included cell physiology, intermediary metabolism, enzymology, nucleic acids and cell division, and regulation of cellular functions.[8]

In each university, innovation reflected local personalities and contingencies, but the changes were always in the same direction. In 1930 David Greenberg returned to Berkeley from a year of study with F. G. Hopkins inspired to initiate programs of research in enzymology, metabolism, and protein synthesis. In the late 1930s, Greenberg's interest in mineral metabolism led him to the new isotope technology and collaboration with one of Ernest Lawrence's assistants at the Radiation Laboratory. From there, he and Carl Schmidt were led to research on intermediary metabolism using radioactive isotopes of nitrogen and sulfur produced by Lawrence's cyclotron, with support from the Rockefeller Foundation.[9]

Traditional research also began to change in Howard Lewis's department at Michigan. In the late 1930s, a new generation of postdoctoral fellows and instructors were hired, with a range of experience and interests quite different from those of Lewis's generation. Lila Miller came from a year at the Carlsberg Institute at Copenhagen; Adam Christman from a year with David Keilin. Michigan was a large teaching department, and Lewis was occupied with lecturing and administration. Like his counterparts elsewhere, he was a facilitator, making sure that his younger staff had the equipment they needed, such as spectrophotometers and a Warburg apparatus.[10] In 1947 Lewis sought an appointment in chemical microbiology, and in 1948 he initiated a graduate course in general biochemistry aimed at students of biology, zoology, and plant physiology. The text was Ernest Baldwin's *Dynamic Aspects of Biochemistry*, a how-to guide to Hopkins's school. Lewis wrote his friend Henry Mattill: "...the point of view of the book has so impressed me that I feel that all of our students should be entirely exposed to it.[11] Mattill had already organized such a course at the University of Iowa Medical School, where the new trends were also being felt.[12]

Lewis was somewhat less alert than Clarke and Hastings to new opportunities for large-scale biomedical research. He was astonished by the large sums of government money available for the asking after World War II. He resisted organizing large team research projects, clinging to the ideal of individual research; he did not exploit his connection with Project Phoenix, a large government-sponsored project in nuclear biology and medicine that grew out of the Manhattan Project. Because of heavy teaching loads, the fine new equipment in the department was unused much of the time. A report of departmental research on the eve of Lewis's retirement in 1954 is a picture of a traditional medical department in transition, with work on clinical biochemistry still predominating but mixed with research on viruses, nucleic acids, and intermediary metabolism.[13]

To a greater or lesser extent, every medical school department was adapting to new intellectual opportunities and competitive challenges. New fashions in research problems; laboratory technologies and increased laboratory productivity; dependence on the new patrons of basic biomedical research; expanding audiences in the biological sciences; rapidly expanding graduate programs – these were indicators of the accelerating pace of change in the style and social relations of biochemistry. A whole new generation of textbooks appeared in the mid-1950s, replacing those oriented toward basic chemistry or clinical applications. The new texts in *general* biochemistry were aimed at a broader audience and did not cater to the special needs of medical students. They concentrated on theoretical developments since the 1930s.[14] An informal survey of medical school departments in 1954 reveals how many were catering to graduate and postdoctoral students. (see Table 12.1).[15]

Biochemists in the late 1930s had a sense that they were witnessing the coming of age of their discipline, yet few biochemists ever recovered that coherent programmatic vision of biochemistry as a biological discipline that some in the early 1900s had glimpsed and lost. Few biochemists were interested in the great unsolved problems of biology, and fewer still had any sympathy with the swashbuckling molecular biologists who swept down in the 1950s and carried off the richest prizes in molecular genetics, protein synthesis (a field tilled by biochemists) and cell physiology. As chemists, biologists, bacteriologists, and others began to intrude on their turf, biochemists began to act like embattled defenders of a conservative faith.

Table 12.1. *Comparative sizes of major medical school departments of biochemistry, 1954*

School	Staff			Students	
	Professors, associate professors	Assistant professors, instructors	Post Ph.D., associate Ph.D. candidates	Medical	Nonmedical
California	3	2	35	76	16
UCLA	4	3	6	50	6
Chicago	13	19	46	72	30
Columbia	13	7	29	120	21
Cornell	3	1	13	85	6
Duke	5	1	17	78	14
Harvard	2	8½	11	130	15
Illinois	3	5	8	167	15
Iowa	6	3	18	118	2
Johns Hopkins	2	3	7	75	5
Michigan	5	5	17	200	20
Oregon	4	2½	17	72	3
Stanford	3	0	35	62	15
USC	3	3	40	68	2
Tufts	2	4	12	115	8
Utah	5	9	13	54	18
Vanderbilt	2	4	11	52	2
U. Washington	4	4	14	75	0
Washington U.	3	5	6	86	8
Western Reserve	5	4	17	82	8
Wisconsin	3	2	14	85	15
Yale	3	6	24	80	0

Many biochemists felt their sense of collective identity slipping away. One wrote to Hans Clarke:

I don't know how you define biochemistry these days. . . . The distinction between biochemistry and biophysics becomes less and less clear. . . . Even journals are having difficulty in keeping their titles meaningful: Journal of Physical Chemistry; of Chemical Physics; of Biophysics; of Biophysical Chemistry; of Theoretical Biology – and so on. The neat classifications just don't fit any more.[16]

Another marveled at the "increasing use of hyphenated words, which has perhaps reached its most significant apex in molecular biophysics."[17] Just as a profusion of names had heralded the competition between medical chemistry and biochemistry around 1900, so too were new hyphenated hybrids symptomatic of the competition between biochemistry and molecular biology in the 1950s. The increasing sense of conflict with molecular biologists reflects the limits set on biochemists' imaginations by the historical development and social relations of their discipline.

Many biochemists feared that these new names were strategies to detach new areas of research from biochemistry and make them separate disciplines. Official pronouncements urged biochemists to take the most catholic view of their discipline, in order to co-opt poachers. Philip Handler exhorted the American Society of Biological Chemists to be tolerant and receptive:

Although various of these problems are now viewed by some as the especial province of alleged disciplines other than biochemistry, such as molecular biology, cell biology, biophysics, molecular biophysics, etc., since each is concerned with molecular structure and molecular interactions, I prefer to view them as facets of biochemistry. . . .

[If] we continue to welcome into our Society those who practice biochemistry even though, for the moment, they be self-identified as biophysicists, molecular biologists, or geneticists, if we never lose sight of the hyphenated nature of our discipline and the necessity for adequate training in the areas on both sides of the hyphen, then we can assure the continued vigorous growth of biochemistry.[18]

Other biochemists, such as Erwin Chargaff, were no less jealous guardians of biochemists' turf but were less tolerant of intrusions from outsiders. Molecular biology, he quipped, was simply the practice of biochemistry without a license.[19]

British biochemists were no less anxious than Americans about competition from molecular biologists. At a meeting of the Biochemical Society in 1964, Rudolf Peters complained that the term "molecular biology" was simply a new ploy to get grant money. R. A. Morton counseled vigilance and flexibility to maintain the unity of a discipline spread over biology, chemistry, microbiology, neurology, pharmacology, and genetics: "The sharp boundaries between sciences have gone; trespassing involves only a shrug and territories are 'invaded' without apology.... This calls for psychological readjustment and reconstruction of teaching, organization, and administration."[20] J. N. Davidson observed that departments of chemistry and biology were casting predatory eyes at biochemists' turf and warned that biochemists might become mere assistants to "big brother biologist."[21] John C. Kendrew sympathized with biochemists' distaste for "molecular biology":

The term is resented by many biochemists who feel that in the eyes of the world they have no part in currently fashionable fields which in reality are their own territory and which in a sense they were the first to explore.[22]

Kendrew proposed substituting the expression "biology at the molecular level." Hans Krebs, chairing an official committee of the Biochemical Society, had a simpler solution: "Since the expression 'biology at the molecular level' is uncomfortably long-winded, we will instead use the term 'biochemistry.' "[23] Biochemists laid claim to the chemical aspects of all the biological and biomedical sciences.

Competition with molecular biologists was a distinctive feature of the history of biochemistry after 1950. Biologists and chemists regarded biochemists as narrow-minded specialists, who were neither proper chemists nor biologists and who were interested only in the petty details of metabolic pathways. A. V. Hill wrote: "The trouble with so many biochemists or physiological chemists, or whatever one calls them, is that they either know no chemistry or no physiology or no biology."[24] To biochemists, molecular biologists were addicts to grandiose theories based on scant knowledge of basic biochemistry. It seemed like cheating when their leaps of imagination were spectacular successes.

These conflicting perceptions were partial and complementary visions of a more complex reality. It is true that some biochemists were moving toward a more broadly biological range of research interests. Biochemistry in 1953, the annus mirabilis of the double helix, was more expansive and diverse than it had ever been. It is also true, however, that this expansiveness and diversity were sharply limited. The shift to more broadly biological disciplinary programs was tentative and evolutionary at a time when the pace of discovery in molecular biology was fevered and revolutionary. Biologists and chemists made the big discoveries in part because they were not hindered by biochemists' traditions and burdened by the weight of biochemists' knowledge. Biochemists felt that they would soon have made the same discoveries in a more orthodox way, by patiently assembling solid facts, had they not been one-upped by cocksure opportunists. Biochemists were slowly redirecting their disciplinary priorities toward biology, but the political economy of medical departments and the traditional core problems, which served to unify the discipline, limited the pace and scope of change.

This pattern of limited innovation reflects institutional relations that had developed between 1910 and 1930. Chemical biology was adapted to institutional contexts that did not reward biochemists with specialized roles. Biochemists who flourished on medical service roles were not drawn to work in chemical biology. Medical school biochemists had to balance conflicting goals: if they left general biochemistry to the graduate schools, they forfeited their future influence in the discipline. If they abandoned clinical biochemistry, they risked losing the clientele on which their prosperity depended. Accustomed to adapting their research to service roles, many biochemists were not alert to external sources of funds for basic biological research. Philip Shaffer, for example, saw himself as a "poor getter" of foundation funds.[25] Warren Weaver saw biochemistry as the centerpiece of his program in molecular biology (a term he helped popularize), yet almost all of the foundation's projects were carried out by chemists and biologists, almost none by biochemists.[26] Because molecular biologists were free of medical service roles, they were better able to exploit new opportunities and resources for cooperative research in the untilled border areas between biology and chemistry. They were not tied to utilitarian goals of nutrition or clinical medicine; they were not obliged to maintain and defend disciplinary turf and thus could afford a more freewheeling style.

In the 1940s and 1950s, leading medical school departments of biochemistry expanded their graduate programs; served more students in general microbiology, genetics, and cell physiology; created new roles; and equipped laboratories for research on macromolecules, protein synthesis, and the regulation of enzyme action. They established a symbiotic relationship with patrons of basic research, like the Office of Naval Research, the National Institutes of Health, and the Atomic Energy Commission. But these innovations did not fundamentally change the institutional structures and relations that had been created in the early 1900s. The momentum (or inertia) of medical service roles and the heavy investment in traditional research programs set limits to radical change. Biochemistry expanded tremendously and spawned diverse new subspecialties, but always within a basically fixed institutional structure.

Location of archival sources and abbreviations

The letter and number codes following names of archives or collections (e.g., Hopkins Papers, ADD 7620AA; MRC, PF 106; UCLonA AM/D/194) designate particular record groups within the larger collection. The number codes following RF and GEB refer to record series.

Institutional archives

CornMedA	Cornell University Medical School Archives, New York, New York
GEB	General Education Board, Rockefeller Archives Center, North Tarrytown, New York
HarvMedA	Harvard University Medical School Archives, Countway Medical Library, Boston, Massachusetts
JHUMedA	Johns Hopkins University Medical School Archives, Baltimore, Maryland. Medical Deans' files are in the Welch Medical Library, Baltimore, Maryland
MRC	Medical Research Council, 20 Park Crescent, London, England
NYUCP	New York University Council Papers, New York University Archives, New York, New York
RF	Rockefeller Foundation, Rockefeller Archives Center, North Tarrytown, New York
UCalA	University of California Archives, Bancroft Library, Berkeley, California
UCalPP	University of California Presidents' Papers, Bancroft Library, Berkeley, California
UCamA	Cambridge University Archives, Cambridge, England
UChicA	University of Chicago Archives, Regenstein Library, Chicago, Illinois
UChicPP	University of Chicago Presidents' Papers, Regenstein Library, Chicago, Illinois
UCLonA	University College London Archives, London, England
UCLonRO	University College London Record Office, London, England
UColA	Columbia University Archives, Butler Library, New York, New York
UColCF	Columbia University Central Files, Low Library, New York, New York
UEdinA	Edinburgh University Archives, Edinburgh, Scotland
UIllCS	University of Illinois College of Science, University of Illinois Archives, Urbana, Illinois
ULeedsA	Leeds University Archives, Leeds, England
ULivA	Liverpool University Archives, Liverpool, England
UMichA	University of Michigan Archives, Bentley Library, Ann Arbor, Michigan
UMinnPP	University of Minnesota Presidents' Papers, University of Minnesota Archives, Minneapolis, Minnesota
UOxA	Oxford University Archives, Oxford, England
UPennA	University of Pennsylvania Archives, Philadelphia, Pennsylvania
UVaA	University of Virginia Archives, Charlottesville, Virginia
WashUMedA	Washington University Medical School Archives, St. Louis, Missouri

YaUA   Yale University Archives, Sterling Library, New Haven, Connecticut
YaUMedA   Yale University Medical School Archives, New Haven, Connecticut

Individual archives

Abel, John J.	Welch Medical Library, Baltimore, Maryland
Adams, Roger	University of Illinois Archives, Urbana, Illinois
Alderman, Edwin A.	University of Virginia Archives, Charlottesville, Virginia
Bancroft, Wilder	Cornell University Archives, Ithaca, New York
Burton, Marion L.	University of Michigan Archives, Bentley Library, Ann Arbor, Michigan
Chittenden, Russell H.	Yale University Archives, Sterling Library, New Haven, Connecticut
Clark, William M.	American Philosophical Society Library, Philadelphia, Pennsylvania
Clarke, Hans T.	American Philosophical Society Library, Philadelphia, Pennsylvania
Cole, Rufus	American Philosophical Society Library, Philadelphia, Pennsylvania
Conklin, Edwin G.	Princeton University Archives, Firestone Library, Princeton, New Jersey
Crozier, William J.	Harvard University Archives, Pusey Library, Cambridge, Massachusetts
Edsall, David T.	Harvard Medical School Archives, Countway Medical Library, Boston, Massachusetts
Eliot, Charles W.	Harvard University Archives, Pusey Library, Cambridge, Massachusetts
Erlanger, Joseph	Washington University Medical School Archives, St. Louis, Missouri
Flexner, Simon	American Philosophical Society Library, Philadelphia, Pennsylvania
Folin, Otto K.	Harvard Medical School Archives, Countway Medical Library, Boston, Massachusetts
Garvan, Francis P.	University of Wyoming Archives, Laramie, Wyoming
Gates, Frederick T.	Rockefeller Archive Center, North Tarrytown, New York
Hadley, Arthur T.	Yale University Archives, Sterling Library, New Haven, Connecticut
Hale, George E.	California Institute of Technology Archives, Pasadena, California
Harper, William R.	University of Chicago Archives, Regenstein Library, Chicago, Illinois
Hastings, A. Baird,	Harvard Medical School Archives, Countway Medical Library, Boston, Massachusetts
Hecht, Selig	Columbia University Archives, Butler Library, New York, New York
Henderson, Lawrence J.	Harvard University Archives, Pusey Library, Cambridge, Massachusetts
Hopkins, Frederick G.	Cambridge University Archives, Cambridge, England
James, Edmund	University of Illinois Archives, Urbana, Illinois
Lewis, Howard B.	University of Michigan Archives, Bentley Library, Ann Arbor, Michigan
Lillie, Frank R.	University of Chicago Archives, Regenstein Library, Chicago, Illinois
Loeb, Jacques	Manuscript Division, Library of Congress, Washington, D.C.

Long, Cyril N. H.	American Philosophical Society Library, Philadelphia, Pennsylvania
Luck, Murray	Stanford University Archives, Palo Alto, California
Mendel, Lafayette B.	Yale Medical School Archives, New Haven, Connecticut
Millikan, Robert A.	California Institute of Technology Archives, Pasadena, California
Morgan, Thomas H.	California Institute of Technology Archives, Pasadena, California
Noyes, Arthur A.	California Institute of Technology Archives, Pasadena, California
Opie, Eugene	American Philosophical Society Library, Philadelphia, Pennsylvania
Shaffer, Philip A.	Washington University Medical School Archives, St. Louis, Missouri
Swain, Robert E.	Stanford University Archives, Palo Alto, California
Terry, Robert J.	Washington University Medical School Archives, St. Louis, Missouri
Trimble, Harry	Harvard Medical School Archives, Countway Medical Library, Boston, Massachusetts
Underhill, Frank	Yale University Archives, Sterling Library, New Haven, Connecticut
Welch, William H.	Welch Medical Library, Baltimore, Maryland
Wilbur, Ray L.	Stanford University Archives, Palo Alto, California

Miscellaneous collections

E. F. Smith Collection, University of Pennsylvania Library, Philadelphia, Pennsylvania

College of Physicians Library, Philadelphia, Pennsylvania

National Library of Medicine, Bethesda, Maryland

Survey of Sources for the History of Biochemistry and Molecular Biology, American Philosophical Society Library, Philadelphia, Pennsylvania

Notes

CHAPTER 1 Introduction: On discipline history

1 Fritz Lieben, *Geschichte der physiologischen Chemie* (Hildesheim, W. Germany: G. Olms Verlag, 1970); Joseph S. Fruton, *Molecules and Life: Essays in the History of Biochemistry* (New York: Wiley, 1973); Marcel Florkin, *A History of Biochemistry*, 3 vols., (Amsterdam: Elsevier, 1972–9).

2 C. E. Rosenberg, "On the study of American biology and medicine: some justifications," *Bull. Hist. Med.* 38 (1964): 364–76; R. H. McCormmach, "Editor's foreword," *Hist. Stud. Phys. Sci.* 3 (1971): ix–xxiv.

3 C. E. Rosenberg, "Toward an ecology of knowledge: on discipline, context and history," in Alexandra Oleson and John Voss, eds., *The Organization of Knowledge in Modern America 1860–1920* (Baltimore, Md.: Johns Hopkins University Press, 1979), pp. 440–55 (quotation is from p. 443).

4 C. E. Rosenberg, "Factors in the development of genetics in the United States: some suggestions," *J. Hist. Med.* 22 (1967): 27–46.

5 For example, see R. E. Kohler, "The reception of Eduard Buchner's discovery of cell-free fermentation," *J. Hist. Biol.* 5 (1972): 327–53; R. E. Kohler, "The Lewis – Langmuir theory of valence and the chemical community, 1920–1928," *Hist. Stud. Phys. Sci.* 6 (1975): 431–68.

6 Gerald L. Geison, *Michael Foster and the Cambridge School of Physiology* (Princeton University Press, 1978).

7 Gerard Lemaine, Roy Macleod, Michael Mulkay, and Peter Weingart, eds., *Perspectives on the Emergence of Scientific Disciplines* (The Hague: Mouton, 1976); M. J. Mulkay, G. N. Gilbert, and S. Woolgar, "Problem areas and research networks in science," *Sociology* 9 (1975): 187–203; Darryl Chubin, "The conceptualization of scientific specialties," *Sociol. Quar.* 17 (1976): 448–76; David O. Edge and Michael J. Mulkay, *Astronomy Transformed* (New York: Wiley, 1976), ch. 10.

8 John Servos, "Physical chemistry in America, 1890–1933: origins, growth and definition" (Ph.D. diss., Johns Hopkins University, 1979); P. Thomas Carroll, "Perspectives on academic chemistry in America" (Ph.D. diss., University of Pennsylvania, in progress); John O'Donnell, "The origins of behaviorism: American psychology, 1870–1920" (Ph.D. diss., University of Pennsylvania, 1979). Dorothy Ross, "The development of the social sciences" in Oleson and Voss, eds., *Organization of Knowledge*, pp. 107–38; Margaret W. Rossiter, "The organization of the agricultural sciences," in Oleson and Voss, eds., *Organization of Knowledge*, pp. 211–48.

9 Daniel J. Kevles, *The Physicists* (New York: Knopf, 1977).

10 R. E. Kohler, "The enzyme theory and the origins of biochemistry," *Isis* 64 (1973): 181–96.

11 Joseph Ben-David and Avraham Zloczower, "Universities and academic systems in modern societies," *Eur. J. Sociol.* 3 (1962): 45–84; J. Ben-David, *The Scientist's Role in Society* (Englewood Cliffs, N.J.: Prentice-Hall, 1971); J. Ben-David and R. Collins, "Social factors in the origins of a new science: the case of psychology," *Am. Sociol. Rev.* 31 (1966): 451–65.

12   Avraham Zloczower, "Career opportunities and the growth of scientific discovery in 19th century Germany" (M. A. diss., Hebrew University, Jerusalem, 1966); Joseph Ben-David, "Scientific productivity and academic organization in nineteenth century medicine," *Am. Sociol. Rev.* 25 (1966), 451–65.

13   Joseph Ben-David, *Fundamental Research and the Universities* (Paris: Organization for Economic Cooperation and Development, 1968); see also Charles E. McClelland, *State, Society, and University in Germany 1700–1914* (Cambridge University Press, 1980).

14   C. E. Rosenberg, "Science, technology, and economic growth" (1971); reprinted in *No Other Gods,* (Baltimore, Md.: Johns Hopkins University Press, 1976), pp. 153–72.

15   See the essays in Oleson and Voss, eds., *Organization of Knowledge.*

16   Yaron Ezrahi, "The political resources of American science," *Sci. Stud.* 1 (1971): 117–33; Yaron Ezrahi, "The authority of science in politics," in Arnold Thackray and Everett Mendelsohn, eds., *Science and Values* (New York: Humanities Press, 1974), pp. 215–51.

17   Ezrahi, "Political resources," p. 118.

18   Rosenberg, "Toward an ecology of knowledge," pp. 440–55.

CHAPTER 2 *Physiological chemistry in Germany, 1840–1900*

1   Allbutt and Langley to Vice Chancellor, 22 February 1905, UCamA, CUR 39.44.

2   Hans-Heinz Eulner, *Die Entwicklung der medizinischen Spezialfächer an den Universitäten des deutschen Sprachgebiets* (Stuttgart: Ferdinand Enke, 1970).

3   F. G. Hopkins, "On current views concerning the mechanisms of biological oxidation (with a foreword on the institutional needs of biochemistry)," *Skand. Archiv. Physiol.* 49 (1926): 35–59.

4   Eulner, *Spezialfächer,* appendixes.

5   Christian v. Ferber, *Die Entwicklung des Lehrkörpers der deutschen Universitäten und Hochschulen, 1864–1954* (Göttingen: Vandenhoeck & Ruprecht, 1956), pp. 197–209. I have lumped honorary, but not emeritus, professors with *ordinarius* professors.

6   Joseph Ben-David, "Scientific productivity and academic organization in 19th century medicine," *Am. Sociol. Rev.* 25 (1960): 828–43; Avraham Zloczower, "*Career Opportunities and the growth of scientific discovery in 19th century Germany*" (M.A. diss., Hebrew University, Jerusalem: 1966.)

7   Zloczower, *Career Opportunities,* pp. 114–21.

8   Justus v. Liebig, *Reden und Abhandlungen* (Leipzig: Winter, 1874), pp. 7–36; Jack B. Morrell, "The chemist breeders: the research schools of Liebig and Thomas Thomson," *Ambix* 19 (1972): 1–58.

9   Johannes Conrad, *The German Universities for the Last Fifty Years,* trans. John Hutchinson (Glasgow: D. Bryce, 1885), pp. 154–68.

10   Theodore Billroth, *The Medical Sciences in the German Universities* (originally published in 1876; New York: Macmillan, 1924).

11   F. G. Holmes, "Introduction," in Justus Liebig, *Animal Chemistry,* reprint ed. (New York: Johnson Reprint, 1964), pp. vii–cxvi.

12   Bernard Gustin, "The emergence of the German chemical profession, 1790–1867" (Ph.D. diss., University of Chicago, 1975).

13   Hans Simmer, "Aus den Anfängen der physiologischen Chemie in Deutschland," *Sudhoffs Arch.* 39 (1955): 216–36; Fritz Hesse, *Julius Eugen Schlossberger...Begründer der physiologischen Chemie in Tübingen* (Düsseldorf: Triltsch, 1976); Gustav Hüfner, "Das physiologische-chemische Institut," in *Festgabe zum 25 Jährigen Regierung...König Karl* (Tübingen: H. Laupp, 1889), pp. 55–7; Julius Schlossberger, *Lehrbuch der organischen Chemie* (Stuttgart: J. B. Müller, 1850).

14   R. Wagner, "Adolph Strecker (1822–1871)," *Ber. dtsch. chem. Ges.* 5 (1872): 125–31.

15   E. T. Nauck, *Zur Vorgeschichte der Wissenschaftlich-Mathematischen Facultät der Albert-Ludwigs-Universität Freiburg i. Br.* (Fribourg: E. Albert, 1954), pp. 41–7.

16 Ibid., pp. 47–9. Latschenberger narrowly missed being appointed to succeed Otto Funke in the chair of physiology.

17 Albrecht Kossel, "Zur Errinerung an Eugen Baumann," Z. physiol. Chem. 23 (1897): 1–22. Marion Spaude, Eugen Albert Baumann (Zurich: Juris Verlag, 1973); Eugen Baumann, Die synthetischen Prozesse im Thierkorper (Berlin: Hirschwald, 1878).

18 Nauck, Vorgeschichte, pp. 48–50; Walter Hückel, "Heinrich Kiliani," Ber. dtsch. chem. Ges. 82 (1949): i–ix.

19 Arthur Hantsch, "Das chemische Laboratorium," in Festschrift zur des 500 Jährigen Bestehens der Universität Leipzig, 4 vols. (Leipzig: Hirzel, 1909), vol. 4, pp. 70–89 (see pp. 70–1). Carl G. Lehman, Lehrbuch der physiologischen Chemie, 2nd ed. (Leipzig: Engleman, 1853).

20 Hantsch, "Chemische Laboratorium," p. 71; E. von Meyer, "Zur Errinerung an Hermann Kolbe," J. prakt. Chem. 30 (1884): 417–66.

21 Theodore Curtius, Robert Bunsen als Lehrer in Heidelberg (Heidelberg: J. Hörnung, 1906), pp. 6–9. Liebig was called first, but after a year of wooing and dithering, he declined, because he no longer cared to be a gehetzen Schulmeister.

22 E. Stubler, Geschichte der medizinische Fakultät der Universität Heidelberg (Heidelberg: Winter, 1926), pp. 288, 296; Curtius, Robert Bunsen, pp. 6–9.

23 Eulner, Spezialfächer, pp. 88–9; A. Hilger, "Eugen Freiherr Gorup v. Besanez," Ber. dtsch. chem. Ges. 12 (1879): 1029–35. Gorup-Besanez was in the philosophical faculty from 1855 and was one of the last professors of chemistry trained in medicine.

24 Marie Reindel, Lehre und Forschung in Mathematik und Naturwissenschaften insbesondere Astronomie, an der Universität Würzburg von der Gründung bis zum Begin des 20. Jahrhundert (Neustadt: Begener, 1966), pp. 100–1, 117–19, 128.

25 G. Sticker, "Entwicklungsgeschichte der medizinische Fakultät," in Max Buchner, ed., Aus der Vergangenheit der Universität Würzburg (Berlin: Springer, 1932), pp. 383–790 (see pp. 616–17).

26 Holmes, "Introduction," pp. cii–ciii; E. Beckmann, "Johannes Wisclicenus (1835–1902)," Ber. dtsch. chem. Ges. 37 (1904): 4861–946; Sticker, "Entwicklungsgeschichte," pp. 663, 672–5.

27 Heinrick Weiland, "Das chemische Laboratorium des Staates," in Karl A. Müller, ed., Die Wissenschaftlichen Anstalten . . . München (Munich: Oldenbourg, 1926), pp. 266–71.

28 Karl Kisskalt, Max von Pettenkoffer (Stuttgart: Wissenschaftlichen Verlag, 1948), p. 26. The Medical Faculty of Munich was unusually conservative and slow to adopt the ideals of scientific medicine; see Heinz Goerke, "Die medizinische Fakultät von 1472 bis zum Gegenwart," in Laetitia Boehm and Johannes Spörl, eds., Die Ludwig-Maximillians-Universität in ihrer Fakultäten (Berlin: Dunckert & Humblodt, 1972), vol. 1, pp. 185–280.

29 Weiland, "Chemische Laboratorium," p. 267; Laetitia Boehm and Johannes Spörl, eds., Die Ludwig-Maximillians-Universität: Ingolstadt, Landshut, München 1472–1972 (Berlin: Dunckert & Humblodt, 1972), pp. 280–1; Karl Kisskalt, "Das hygienische Institut," in Müller, Wissenschaftlichen Anstalten, pp. 72–9.

30 Otto Frank, "Nachruf Carl Voit gewidmet," Z. Biol. (Munich) 51 (1908): i–xxiv; Holmes, "Introduction," pp. xcv–cix; Otto Frank, "Das physiologische Institut," in Müller, Wissenschaftlichen Anstalten, pp. 233–7.

31 Gustav Anrich, Die Kaiser-Wilhelms-Universitäts Strassburg und ihrer Bedeutung für die Wissenschaft 1872–1921 (Berlin: W. de Gruyter, 1923). This and other histories were written after World War I as obituaries for the university.

32 Eugen Baumann and Albrecht Kossel, "Zur Errinerung an Felix Hoppe-Seyler," Z. physiol. Chem. 21 (1895): i–lxi.

33 Kossel, "Eugen Baumann," p. 4; R. H. Chittenden, The Development of Physiological Chemistry in the United States (New York: Chemical Catalogue, 1930), pp 29–31.

34 Richard V. Zeynek, "Zur Errinerung an Gustav v. Hüfner," *Z. physiol. Chem.* 58 (1908): 1–38.

35 Baumann and Kossel, "Felix Hoppe-Seyler," p. xi

36 Zeynek, "Gustav Hüfner," p. 19. Quotation is from Hüfner, "Physiologische –chemische Institut," p. 55.

37 Felix Hoppe-Seyler, *Ueber der Entwicklung der physiologische Chemie und ihre Bedeutung für die Medicin* (Strasbourg: Trübner, 1884), pp. 27–32.

38 Ibid; Felix Hoppe-Seyler, *Quellen der Lebsenskrafte* (Berlin: Carl Habel, 1871); Felix Hoppe-Seyler, *Physiologische Chemie* (Berlin: Hirschwald, 1877).

39 Faust to J. J. Abel, 17 July 1895, Abel Papers.

40 Zeynek, "Gustav Hüfner," p. 19.

41 Drechsel to Abel, 16 April 1896, Abel Papers.

42 Drechsel to Abel, 28 December 1896, Abel Papers.

43 Faust to Abel, 30 April 1897, Abel Papers.

44 Reid Hunt to Abel, 10 November 1902, Abel Papers.

45 Franz Hofmeister, *Die chemische Organization der Zelle* (Brunswick: Vieweg, 1902). *Beiträge zur chemischen Physiologie und Pathologie: Zeitschrift für die gesammte Biochemie* was initiated in 1902.

46 Karl Auwers, "Heinrich Limpricht," *Ber. dtsch. chem. Ges.* 42 (1909); 5001–36 (see pp. 5011–12); Werner Rothmaler et al., *Festschrift zur 500-Jahrfeier der Universität Greifswald*, 2 vols. (Greifswald: at the University Press, 1956), vol. 2, pp. 310–2.

47 Nauck, *Vorgeschichte*, pp. 51–2; Walter Hückel, "Heinrich Kiliani," *Ber. dtsch. chem. Ges.* 82 (1949): i–ix (see p. vi) Karl Thomas, "Franz Knoop," *Z. physiol. Chem.* 283 (1948): 1–8. A plan to include physiological chemistry in physiology was rejected in 1915.

48 Everett Mendelsohn, "The biological sciences in the nineteenth century: some problems and sources," *Hist. Sci.* 3 (1964): 39–59; Everett Mendelsohn, "Physical models and physiological concepts: explanation in nineteenth century biology," *Br. J. Hist. Sci.* 2 (1965): 201–19; Charles Culotta, "German biophysics, objective knowledge and romanticism," *Hist. Stud. Phys. Sci.* 4 (1975): 3–38.

49 Carl Hürthle, "Das physiologisches Institut," in Georg Kaufmann, ed., *Festschrift zur Feier des 150-Jährigen Bestehens der Universität Breslau*, 2 vols. (Breslau: F. Hirt, 1911), vol. 2, pp. 274–81 (see p. 277).

50 Eulner, *Spezialfächer*, p. 81; P. Grützner, "Zum Andenken an Rudolf Heidenhain," *Arch. gesammte Physiol.* 72 (1898): 221–65; Hürthle, "Physiologisches Institut," pp. 277–82. A formal position of *Abteilung-Vorsteher* was created for Franz Röhman; see Anon., "Franz Röhman," *Ber. dtsch. chem. Ges.* 52A (1919): 114.

51 Ewald Hering, "Das physiologische Institut," in *Die Institute der medizinischen Fakultät an der Universität Leipzig* (Leipzig: Hirzel, 1909), pp. 21–38 (see pp. 21–3); Heinz Schröer, *Carl Ludwig* (Stuttgart: Wissenschaftliche Verlag, 1967); Zeynek, "Gustav Hüfner," p. 12; S. Garten, "Ewald Hering," *Arch. gesammte Physiol.* 170 (1918): 501–22.

52 Emil Du Bois-Reymond, *Reden* (Leipzig: Voit, 1886–7), vol. 2, pp. 369–83 (quotation is from pp. 372–73).

53 Gustav Fritsch, "Das physiologische Institut," in Max Lenz, ed., *Geschichte der Königliche Friedrich-Wilhelm-Universität zu Berlin*, 4 vols. (Halle, E. Germany: Waisenhaus, 1910–18), vol. 3, pp. 154–64 (see pp. 157–8). Rubner's specialty was respiration and nutrition; see Max Rubner, *Kraft und Stoff in Haushalte der Natur* (Leipzig: Akademische Verlag, 1909).

54 Kossel, "Eugen Baumann," pp. 1–22; W. Will, "Carl Schotten," *Ber. dtsch. chem. Ges.* 43 (1910): 3703–14. (Schotten was assistant from 1881 to 1891 and taught clinical chemistry.)

55 Eulner, *Spezialfächer*, p. 85. Ernst Giese and Benno v. Hagen, *Geschichte der medizinischen Fakultät der Friedrich-Schiller-Universität Jena* (Jena, E. Germany: G. Fischer, 1958).

56 On Erlangen, see Eulner, *Spezialfächer*, pp. 88–9.

57 F. Suter et al., "Friedrich Miescher, 1844–1895," *Helv. Physiol. Pharmacol. Acta*, Suppl. 2 (2) (1944): 5–43; Marcel Mommier, "Physiologie," in Ernst Staehlin, ed.,

Lehre und Forschung an der Universität Basel. . .(Basel, Switzerland: Birknanser, 1960), pp. 100–3; Karl Bernhard, "Physiologische Chemie," in *Lehre und Forschung*, pp. 103–6; Gerhard Schmidt, *Das geistige Vermächtnis von Gustav v. Bunge* (Zurich: Juris Verlag, 1974). Bunge was succeeded by physiologist–biochemist Karl Spiro.

58 Felix Hoppe-Seyler, "Vorwort," *Z. physiol. Chem.* 1 (1877): i–iii.

59 The six new institutes were at Innsbruck (1869), Prague (1872), Königsberg (1873), Vienna (1874), Rostock (1875), and Bern (1877). The Austrian institutes were in "medical chemistry" and combined elementary, physiological, and clinical chemistry.

60 Eduard Pflüger, "Die Physiologie und ihre Zukunft," *Arch. gesammte Physiol.* 15 (1877): 361–5; Billroth, *Medical Sciences*, pp. 60–1.

61 Billroth, *Medical Sciences*, pp. 49–50.

62 Giese and Hagen, *Medizinischen Fakultät*, pp. 503–6. Schulz spent the rest of his career in a frustrating battle for an independent institute.

63 Frank, "Physiologische Institut," pp. 236–7.

64 Simmer, "Anfängen der physiologischen Chemie," p. 225.

65 Felix Marchand, "Das pathologische Institut," in Max Lenz, ed., *Universität Berlin*, pp. 165–77; Russell C. Maulitz, "Rudolf Virchow, Julius Cohnheim and the program of pathology," *Bull. Hist. Med.* 52 (1978): 162–82; Erwin H. Ackerknecht, *Rudolf Virchow* (Madison: University of Wisconsin Press, 1953).

66 Marchand, "Pathologische Institut," pp. 166–7; Carl Neuberg, "Ernst Salkowski zum 70. Geburtstag,"*Dtsch. med. Wochenschr.* 40 (1914): 1870–71.

67 Because Ludwig's initial plan for his institute had only one *Abteilung* (histology), it is possible that he added chemistry to preempt the pathologists; see Hering, "Physiologische Institut," pp. 21–2.

68 Eulner, *Spezialfächer* pp. 112–38.

69 Ibid., p. 82; O. Langendorff, "Otto Nasse," *Arch. gesammte Physiol.* 101 (1904): 1–22; Hans-Heinz Eulner, "Die Einrichtung der medizinischen Fakultät und ihre Geschichte,"in *450 Jahre Martin-Luther-Universität Halle-Wittenberg*, 3 vols. (n.d., n.p., circa 1953), vol. 2, pp. 485– 92; Oswald Schmiedeberg, "Erich Harnack," *Arch. exp. Path. Pharmakol.* 79 (1915): i–vii.

70 Otto Schlüter, Emil von Skramlik, and Ellsabeth Schoen, "Emil Abderhalden zum Gedächtnis," *Nova Acta Leopold* 14 (1952): 143–89; H. Hanson, "Emil Abderhalden (1877 bis 1950)," *Nova Acta Leopold. 36 (1970): 257–317.*

71 *Alexander Ellinger, "Max Jaffé,"* Ber. dtsch. chem. Ges. 46 (1911): 831–47.

72 Franz Hofmann, "Das hygienisch Institut," in *Festschrift Universität Leipzig*, vol. 3, pp. 93–120.

73 Martin Hahn, "Karl Georg Flügge," *Dtsch. Biogr. Jahrb.* 5 (1923): 69–73.

74 Richard Feller, *Die Universität Bern 1834–1934* (Bern: P. Haupt, 1935), pp. 224, 261–2, 403–4. Nencki's laboratory was physically located in the Institute of Pathology; see Marcel H. Bickel, *Marcell Nencki, 1847–1901* (Bern: Huber, 1972) and Martin Hahn, "Marcell Nencki," *Ber. dtsch. chem. Ges.* 35 (1902): 4503–21.

75 Drechsel nearly succeeded to a second chair of chemistry in the Tübingen–Fribourg style in 1897, when the unpopular professor of inorganic and technical chemistry was forced to resign. Both the medical and philosophical faculties wanted Drechsel, but because they could not agree in which Drechsel would be, the authorities gave the chair to the second candidate, an inorganic chemist; see Feller, *Universität Bern*, pp. 215–16, 425.

76 T. Leber, "Willy Kühne," in K. Friedrich, ed., *Heidelberger Professoren aus dem 19. Jahrhundert* (Heidelberg: at the University Press, 1903), pp. 207–20; Gerhard Denecke, "Die medizinische Fakultät zu Marburg von 1866–1927 und ihre Institut," in Kurt Goldammer, comp., *Marburg die Phillipps-Universität und ihre Stadt* (Marburg, W. Germany: Elwert, 1952), pp. 594–620. For example, see Walter Jones to Abel, 16 July 1899, Abel Papers.

77 Richard Willstätter, *From My Life* (New York: Benjamin, 1965); Paul Karrer, "Heinrich Wieland," *Biogr. Mem. Fellows R. Soc.* 4 (1958): 341–52; Emil Fischer, *Aus meinem Leben* (Berlin: Springer, 1922); Carl Harries et al., "Emil Fischer,"

Naturwissenschaften 7 (1919): 843–82; Emil Fischer, "Bedeutung der Stereochemie für die Physiologie," *Z. physiol. Chem.* 26 (1898): 60–87; Emil Fischer, "Synthetical chemistry in its relation to biology," *J. Chem. Soc.* 91 (1907): 1749–65.

78 Richard Willstätter, *Problems and Methods in Enzyme Research* (Ithaca, N.Y.: Cornell University Press, 1927).

79 Joseph S. Fruton, *Molecules and Life* (New York: Wiley, 1972), pp. 131–40, 204–14; John T. Edsall, "Proteins as macromolecules: an essay on the development of the macromolecular concept and some of its vicissitudes," *Arch. Bochem. Biophys. Suppl.* 1 (1962): 12–20. There is no adequate treatment of the colloid craze, but see Marcel Florkin, *A History of Biochemistry* (Amsterdam: Elsevier, 1972), pp. 284–94 and B. Helfrich, "Max Bergmann, 1886–1944," *Ber. dtsch. chem. Ges.* 102 (1969): i–xxvi.

80 In the 1930s, organic and physical chemists led biochemists out of the theoretical thickets they had planted in the preceding decades. Hermann Staudinger and The Svedberg, for example, played crucial roles in the revival of macromolecular theories. Adolf Butenandt, Paul Karrer, Leopold Ruzicka, and other bioorganic chemists were heroes of the biochemical avant-garde; see Hermann Staudinger, *From Organic Chemistry to Macromolecules: A Scientific Autobiography* (New York: Wiley, 1970); The Svedberg, "The ultracentrifuge and the study of high-molecular weight compounds," *Nature* 139 (1937): 1051–62; A. Butenandt, "Adolf Windaus," *Proc. Chem. Soc.* (1961): 131–8; A. Wettstein, "Paul Karrer 1889–1971," *Helv. Chim. Acta* 55 (1972): 313–28; Leopold Ruzicka, "In the borderland between bio-organic chemistry and biochemistry," *Annu. Rev. biochem.* 42 (1973): 1–20.

81 Graham Lusk to Robert Lambert, 16 September 1929, RF, 717A, box 12.

82 "Proposal for aid for research fellowships," undated [1929], R. M. Pearce to Alan Gregg, 24 September and 24 October 1929, Gregg to S. M. Gunn, 28 February 1930, Thomas to D. O'Brien, 26 July 1932, 16 August 1934, "Appraisal, July 1938," RF 717A, box 12.

83 H. J. Deuticke, "Gustav Embden," *Ergeb. Physiol.* 35 (1933): 32–49.

84 David Nachmansohn et al., "Otto Meyerhof (1884–1951)," *Biogr. Mem. Natl. Acad. Sci.* 34 (1960): 153–82; Rudolf Peters, "Otto Meyerhof," *Obit. Not. Fellows R. Soc.* 9 (1954): 175–200; Alexander v. Muralt, "Otto Meyerhof," *Ergeb. Physiol.* 47 (1952): i–xx; Otto Meyerhof, *Chemical Dynamics of Life Phenomena* (Philadelphia: Lippincott, 1924).

85 Hans Krebs, "Otto Heinrich Warburg, 1883–1970," *Biogr. Mem. Fellows R. Soc.* 18 (1972): 629–99; Hans Krebs, *Otto Warburg: Zellphysiologe, Biochemiker, 1883–1970* (Stuttgart: Wissenschaftliche Verlag, 1979); Robert E. Kohler, "The background to Otto Warburg's conception of the *Atmungsferment*," *J. Hist. Biol.* 6 (1973): 171–92.

86 Selig Hecht to William Crozier, 24 November 1924, Crozier Papers.

87 Wald to Hecht, 1 October 1932 and 1 April 1933, Hecht Papers; Ball to W. M. Clark, 13 March 1938, Clark Papers.

CHAPTER 3 *Physiology and British biochemists, 1890–1920*

1 Data were gathered from the annual *Commonwealth Universities Yearbook*.

2 Manchester University *Calendar* (1909/10–1913/14). "Biochemistry" meant fermentation chemistry to many at the time.

3 E. C. Dodds, "Fifty years of the Bland–Sutton Institute," *Middlesex Hosp. J.* (1964): 112–19; F. Dickens, "Edward Charles Dodds (1899–1973)," *Biogr. Mem. Fellows R. Soc.* 21 (1975): 227–67; Richard Pearce, "Medical Education in England," pp. 139–42, RF, 401, box 22; E. C. Dodds, "The teaching of chemistry," *Br. Med. J.* (1949II): 505–8; J. Lowndes, "Robert H. Adders Plimmer," *Biochem. J.* 62 (1956): 353–7; G. W. Ellis, "John Addyman Gardner," *Biochem. J.* 41 (1947): 321–4.

4 Gerald L. Geison, *Michael Foster and the Cambridge School of Physiology* (Princeton University Press, 1978); R. D. French, "Some problems and sources in the foundation of modern physiology in Great Britain," *Hist. Sci.* 10 (1972): 28–55.

5 Sherrington to Vice Chancellor Monsarrat, 7 January 1914, ULivA 5/3/9. Sherrington noted that American and Canadian universities were ahead of British in providing for separate chairs of physical and chemical physiology.

6 Ibid. Wilmot Herringham and Walter Fletcher, "Memorandum presented to the University Grants Committee...May 1921" (London: H.M. Stationery Office, 1921).

7 University College *Calendar* (1887/8–1900/1). The assistant professorship rotated every three years or so. Osborne was at Tübingen from 1897 to 1899; see "Report of a committee of the senate on the claim of W. A. Osborne to title of assistant professor," 15 November 1901, UCLonA, AM/D/194.

8 Ernest H. Starling, "The Department of Physiology," unpublished typescript, (circa 1927), UCLonA, Mem II B/B; Arthur Harden, "Samuel B. Schryver, 1869–1929," *Biochem. J.* 24 (1930): 229–32; V. H. B., "Samuel B. Schryver," *Proc. R. Soc. London, Ser. B* 110 (1932): xxii–xxiv; "Report of the claims of Dr. S. B. Schryver to the post of lecturer," 4 July 1904, UCLonA, AM/D/278b.

9 Starling, "Department of Physiology," pp. 7–8.

10 H. Hale Bellot, *University College London, 1826–1926* (London University Press, 1929), pp. 379–404, 406–410; Royal Commission on University Education in London, *Final Report* (London: H.M. Stationery Office, 1913); William H. Allchin, *Account of the Reconstruction of the University of London*, 4 vols. (London: H.K. Lewis, 1905–8); see also documents in the minute books of the faculty of medical sciences, vol. I and "Letter book," vol. 31, UCLonRO; Anon., "A new institute of physiology in London," *Br. Med. J.* 1909 (I): 1436–44.

11 E. A. Schäfer, Untitled historical sketch of the Department of Physiology (circa 1930), p. 1, UEdinA, Gen 2007/5; Senate minute, 28 July 1899, in "College minutes," vol. 11, p. 456, UEdinA; Anon, "William Rutherford," *Nature* 59 (1899): 590–1.

12 Schäfer, Sketch, pp. 2–3; Senate minutes, 26 July and 2 November 1901 and attached report "Requirements of the various departments" (draft C), 23 November 1901, 18 October 1902 in "College Minutes," vol 12, pp. 242–49, 270–5, 280, 417, UEdinA. Minute, 16 October 1902 in "Medical faculty minutes," UEdinA.

13 Rudolph Peters, "The Department of Biochemistry, University of Oxford," *Methods Probl. Med. Educ.* 18 (1930): 109–18.

14 Francis Gotch, "The urgent necessity for the extension of the physiological laboratory," 27 April 1907, in *Hebdomadal Council Papers*, vol. 77, pp. 27–30, UOxA.

15 Minute, 3 February 1914, in "Natural science faculty board minutes," vol. 3, p. 25; "Memorandum concerning the annual grant to the Department of Physiology," 14 March 1914, in *Hebdomadal Council Papers, vol. 97*, pp. 293–5, UOxA.

16 Hudson Hoagland to W. J. Crozier, 12 September 1930, Crozier Papers. Haldane had expected to succeed Gotch and resigned when Sherrington was appointed in 1913. I have found no official record of a plan for a second chair.

17 H. W. Lyle, *King's and Some King's Men, Being a Record of the Medical Department of King's College from 1830 to 1909* (Oxford University Press, 1935), pp. 243–57; H. King, "Otto S. Rosenheim (1871–1955)," *Biogr. Mem. Fellows R. Soc.* 2 (1956): 257–67. Rosenheim was promoted to reader in 1915.

18 Glasgow University *Calendar* (1905/6 and 1906/7).

19 A. N. Shimmin, *The University of Leeds. The First Half-Century* (Leeds University Press, 1954), pp. 25–35; Arthur Chapman, *The Story of a Modern University. A History of the University of Sheffield* (Oxford University Press, 1955), pp. 120–58, 274–5; Rudolph Peters, "John B. Leathes," *Biogr. Mem. Fellows R. Soc.* 4 (1958): 185–91.

20 H. B. Charlton, *Portrait of a University, 1851–1951* (Manchester University Press, 1951), p. 179. Manchester University *Calendar* (1920/1).

21 Geison, *Michael Foster*, pp. 370–7.

22 T. R. Elliott, "Walter Morley Fletcher," *Obit. Not. Fellows R. Soc.* 1 (1934): 162; W. M. Fletcher and F. G. Hopkins, "The respiratory process in muscle and the nature of muscular motion," *Proc. R. Soc. London, Ser. B* 89 (1917): 444–67.

23 J. Needham, "Frederick Gowland Hopkins," *Notes Rec. R. Soc. London* 17 (1962): 117–62.
24 Z. M. Bacq, *Chemical Transmission of Nerve Impulses. A Historical Sketch* (London: Pergamon, 1975); John Parascandola and Ronald Jasensky, "Origins of the receptor theory of drug action," *Bull. Hist. Med.* 48 (1974): 199–220.
25 J. N. Langley, "Arthur Sheridan Lea (1853–1915)," *Proc. R. Soc. London, Ser. B* 89 (1915): xxv–xxvi; Michael Foster, *A Text-Book of Physiology* (Philadelphia: Lea, 1895), p. 865.
26 "Report of the General Board of Studies on a university lectureship in chemical physiology," 18 May 1898, *Reporter* (Cambridge), 1898, p. 837.
27 H. H. Dale, "Frederick Gowland Hopkins," *Obit. Not. Fellows R. Soc.* 6 (1948): 115–45 (see p. 127); F. G. Hopkins, "Autobiography," in Joseph Needham and Ernest Baldwin, eds., *Hopkins and Biochemistry* (Cambridge: Heffer, 1949), p. 20; J. Needham, "Frederick Gowland Hopkins," *Perspect. Biol. Med.*, 6 (1962): 2–46; *Reporter*, (Cambridge) 1899, p. 510.
28 S. H. V., "Joseph Reynolds Green, 1848–1914," *Proc. R. Soc. London, Ser. B* (1915): xxxvi–xxxviii.
29 Arthur Croft Hill, "Reversible zymohydrolysis," *J. Chem. Soc.* 73 (1898): 634–58; R. E. Kohler, "The enzyme theory and the origin of biochemistry," Isis 64 (1973): 181–96.
30 "Report of the General Board," 18 May 1898, *Reporter* (Cambridge), 1898, pp. 837, 951.
31 Hopkins, "Autobiography," pp. 7–12, 16–19. Dale, "Hopkins," pp. 126–8.
32 Hopkins, "Autobiography," pp. 21–3.
33 Hopkins to Norman Pirie, 30 October 1942, Hopkins Papers, ADD 7620 AA; Needham, "Hopkins," p. 26.
34 Denys A. Winstanley, *Later Victorian Cambridge* (Cambridge University Press, 1947); A. J. Tillyard, *A History of University Reform from 1800 to the Present Time...* (Cambridge: Heffer, 1913).
35 "Amended report of the special board for medicine," 23 January 1914, *Reporter* (Cambridge), 1913, pp. 564–71, 682–95.
36 Geison, *Michael Foster*, p. 327; Anon, "John Newport Langley in memoriam," *J. Physiol.* 61 (1926): 1–15; Selig Hecht to W. J. Crozier, 8 October and 8 November 1925, Crozier Papers. Langley personally owned the *Journal of Physiology* and exercised his proprietary rights freely. He prevented W. H. Gaskell, who had Foster's broad vision, from being an active influence in departmental policy.
37 Walter Fletcher, "Professorial fellowships and the needs of the university," 20 May 1910, Trinity College Council *Reports* (1910). I wish to thank the master of Trinity College for making this document available.
38 Memorandum from Langley, in "Report of the General Board of Studies on a readership in chemical physiology," 16 May 1902, *Reporter* (Cambridge), pp. 905–6.
39 Fletcher, "Professorial Fellowships," pp. 1–3.
40 "Discussion of the report of the General Board of Studies," 21 May 1902, *Reporter* (Cambridge), 1902, pp. 994–5, 1049.
41 A. C. Chibnall, "The road to Cambridge," *Annu. Rev. Biochem.* 35 (1966): 1–22 (see p. 11).
42 Allbutt and Langley to the Vice Chancellor, 22 February 1905, UCamA, CUR 39.44.
43 Correspondence between the Vice Chancellor and Fletcher, Gaskell, Darwin, and others, February 1905, UCamA, CUR 39.44.
44 "Report of the Council of the Senate on the Quick bequest," 12 March 1906, *Reporter* (Cambridge), 1906, pp. 577–81, 778–81; Trustees to the Vice Chancellor, 5 October 1906 and Vice Chancellor to Eagleton, 2 November 1906, UCamA, CUR 39.44. The professors of zoology and botany backed protozoology; the professor of agriculture backed genetics; G. O. Liveing, professor of chemistry, put bacteriology and forestry first.

45 Fletcher, "Professorial Fellowships," pp. 1–3.
46 J. N. Dalton to J. N. Clark, 19 July 1909, E. H. Pooley to A. J. Mason, 27 September and 22 November 1909, H. Boyd to Mason, 6 December 1909 and 11 February 1910, UCamA, CUR 39.37.
47 Hopkins to his mother, 4 December 1910, Hopkins Papers, ADD 7620 AA.
48 Langley to Mason, 15 February 1910, Langley, "Memorandum on a new physiology laboratory," 11 March 1910, T. G. Jackson to Mason, 17 May 1910, "Report of sites syndicate," 13 June 1909, UCamA, CUR 39.37.
49 *Reporter* (Cambridge), 1914, pp. 1019, 1082, 1210.
50 Langley to Mason, 1 February 1911, other correspondence, UCamA, CUR 39.37.
51 Fletcher to Lord Balfour, 6 May 1924, MRC, 1331A; Fletcher, "Professorial fellowships."
52 Fletcher, "Professorial fellowships," p. 3.
53 Hopkins, "Autobiography," p. 23.
54 J. Needham and D. M. Needham, "Sir F. G. Hopkins' personal influence and characteristics," in Needham and Baldwin, eds., *Hopkins and Biochemistry*, pp. 113–19.
55 Hopkins to M. Herrald, 16 January 1940, MRC, 2036.
56 Hopkins to H. H. Dale, 10 February 1914, MRC, PF 129.
57 "Report of the Council of the Senate on the proposed establishment of a professorship of bio-chemistry," 11 May 1914, *Reporter* (Cambridge), 1914, pp. 900–2, 1040; Fletcher to Hopkins, 29 April 1924 and Hopkins to Fletcher, 30 April 1924, MRC, PF 106; Vice Chancellor to Hopkins, 16 December 1914, Hopkins Papers, AD 7620 AAA.
58 Michael Sanderson, *The Universities and British Industry 1850–1970* (London: Routledge and Kegan Paul, 1972), ch. 4. Anon., *The University of Liverpool, 1903–1953* (at the University Press, 1953), pp. 10–24; Shimmin, *University of Leeds*, pp. 49–63.
59 Ernest Glynn, "Sir Rupert William Boyce...(1863–1911)," *J. Pathol. Bacteriol.* 16 (1911/2), 276–82; Hariette Chick letter, 10 September 1971, ULivA, D 139/2.
60 In Britain the term "biochemistry" apparently connoted a connection with microbiology. Plant physiologist F. F. Blackman defined biochemistry as "the study of the chemical physiology of lower organisms" (see Blackman to Mason, 22 February 1905, UCamA, CUR 39.44). Albert S. Grünbaum was at St. Thomas's Hospital with Sherrington in the 1890s and accompanied him to Liverpool. In 1904 he was appointed professor of pathology at Leeds. German-born, he changed his name to Leyden in 1914.
61 Glynn, "Boyce," p. 277; Johnston to Principal Dale, 1 February 1902, ULivA, 5/2. Johnston had pledged £5000 "for the university scheme" in 1901; after his daughter died in childbirth in 1902, he gave £25,000 for medical research, including £10,000 for biochemistry.
62 F. G. Hopkins, "Benjamin Moore (1867–1922)," *Biochem. J.* 22 (1928): 1–3; Anon., "Benjamin Moore," *Br. Med. J.* (1922 I): 417; Anon., *Lancet* (1923 I): 555–6; R. A. Morton, "Biochemistry at Liverpool, 1902–1971," *Med. Hist.* 16 (1972): 321–53; Benjamin Moore, *Dawn of the Health Age* (London: Churchill, 1911); Benjamin Moore, *The Origin and Nature of Life* (London: Williams & Northgate, 1911).
63 The Biochemical Club, "Minutes of committee meetings, 1911–1920," pp. 4–10, UCLonA.
64 Dean's annual report, 1912/13, 9 July 1913, in "Reports of the faculty of medicine," vol. 2, at p. 45, ULivA, S3094.
65 Sherrington to Sir John Brunner, 7 November 1907, ULivA, 5/3/9.
66 Report on the establishment of a lectureship in physiology, 1 June 1909 in "Reports of the medical faculty," vol. 1, at p. 29, ULivA, S3094; Anon., "Prof. H. E. Roaf," *Nature* 170 (1952): 910–1.
67 Sherrington to Monsarrat, 7 January 1914, ULivA, 5/3/9. Moore was, for a time, an associate professor of physiology at Yale.

68 Minute of the physiology subcommittee, 19 January 1914, in "Sub-Committees of the faculty of medicine minutes," ULivA, S3112. Moore was already teaching chemical physiology on an ad hoc basis.

69 Moore hoped to be put in charge of the Department of Biochemistry but was put under Hill in the Department of Applied Physiology; see Moore to Moulton, 2 February 2 and 18 March, 19 May, and 18 June 1914, Moulton to Moore, 16 March 1914, and correspondence between Moore and Fletcher, MRC, PF 178.

70 A meeting of the committee appointed to consider the applications for the chair of bio-chemistry, October 1914, in "Subcommittees of the faculty of medicine minutes," ULivA, S3112; Dean's reports for 1920/21 and 1921/22, in "Faculty minutes," vol. 2, pp. 151 and 168, ULivA; R. Peters, "Walter Ramsden (1865–1947)," *Biochem. J.* 42 (1948), 321–2.

71 H. S. Raper, "Julius Brerend Cohen 1859–1935," *Obit. Not. Fellows R. Soc.* 1 (1932–5): 503–13 (see p. 510). Cohen's biochemistry students included H. H. Dakin, Henry Raper, Percival Hartley, W. H. Dudley, Harold Raistrick, Arthur Wormall, J. H. Birkenshaw, P. W. Clutterbuck, and F. C. Happold – a formidable family; see H. H. Dale, "Percival Hartley," *Biogr. Mem. Fellows R. Soc.* 3 (1957): 81–100 (in particular, see pp. 81–2).

72 Harriette Chick, Margaret Hume, and Marjorie Macfarlane, *War on Disease: A History of the Lister Institute* (London: Andre Deutsch, 1971).

73 Arthur Landsborough Thompson, *Half a Century of Medical Research,* 2 vols.: *Origins and Policy of the Medical Research Council,* vol. I and *The Programme of the Medical Research Council,* vol. II (London: H.M. Stationery Office, 1973 and 1975).

74 Quoted in B. S. Platt, "Sir Edward Mellanby," *Annu. Rev. Biochem.* 25 (1956): 1–28. H. H. Dale, "Edward Mellanby," *Biogr. Mem. Fellows R. Soc.* 1 (1955): 193–222.

75 Richard B. Pilcher, *The Institute of Chemistry of Great Britain and Ireland. History of the Institute: 1877–1914* (London: Institute of Chemistry 1914), pp. 150, 155, 162.

76 F. G. Hopkins, "The analyst and the medical man," *Analyst* 31 (1906): 385 [reprinted in Needham and Baldwin, eds., *Hopkins and Biochemistry,* pp. 123–35 (quotation is from pp. 134–5)].

77 F. G. Hopkins, "The dynamic side of biochemistry," *Rep. Br. Assoc. Adv. Sci.* (1913): 652–68 [reprinted in Needham and Baldwin, eds. *Hopkins and Biochemistry* (quotation is from pp. 136–7)].

78 Ibid., p. 138.

79 Hopkins to Fletcher, 6 July and 4 August 1921, MRC, PF 106.

80 W. M. Fletcher, "The aims and boundaries of physiology," *Rep. Br. Assoc. Adv. Sci.* (1921): p. 125–53 (quotation is from p. 139).

81 Forster, "The laboratory of the living cell," *Rep. Br. Assoc. Adv. Sci.* (1921): 36–55.

82 W. M. Fletcher, Untitled draft for Arthur Balfour, 6 May 1924, MRC, 1331A.

83 In 1927 a visitor from Johns Hopkins got the same message from Fletcher, C. J. Martin, Dudley, Robert Robinson, Arthur Boycott, and Charles Harington: the best biochemist was one trained first in organic chemistry and then in biology; see W. G. MacCallum to L. H. Weed, 14 April 1927, Dean's files, JHMedA. T. R. Elliott made the same point to Richard Pearce; see Elliott to Pearce, 21 March 1920, RF, 401, box 30.

84 Fletcher to Robinson, 28 October 1931, Robinson to Fletcher, 23 October 1931, MRC, PF 55.

85 Robinson to Fletcher, 30 October 1931, Fletcher to Robinson, 2 November 1931, Robinson to Fletcher, 29 November 1932, MRC, PF 55. As the leading natural products chemist in Britain, Robinson was keenly interested in theories of biosynthesis and supported work on the border between chemistry and biology.

86 University College *Calendar* (1908/9, 1909/10, 1911/2). Plimmer advertised his course as preparation for the Royal Institute of Chemistry examination in biological chemistry.

87 "Faculty of medical science minutes," 1 July 1910, vol. I, pp. 3–4, 35–6, 64, 79, UCLonRO.

88 "Faculty of medical science minutes," 1 July 1910, vol. I, pp. 52–5, UCLonRO. A readership in physiological chemistry was created for Plimmer in 1912.

89 "Faculty of medical science minutes," 26 July 1917 and 31 May 1918, vol. I, pp. 116–17, 127, UCLonRO.

90 Drummond to L. B. Mendel, 26 August 1919, Mendel Papers. Drummond was then employed as a research chemist in the Cancer Hospital; see F. G. Young, "Jack C. Drummond," *Obit. Not. Fellows R. Soc.* 1 (1935): 595–606.

91 "Proposed plan for aid in developing a center for medical education and research," 14 May 1920, RF, 401, box 29; "Annual report, 1920," Rockefeller Foundation, pp. 17–26; Starling to Pearce, 9 January 1920, RF, 401, box 30.

92 Starling to Pearce, 9 January 1920, Dale to Pearce, 12 April 1920, and Elliott to Pearce, 11 February and 2 March 1920, RF, 401, box 30.

93 Elliott to Pearce, 16 September and 6 December 1921, RF, 401, box 30.

94 "Faculty of medical science minutes," 6 December 1922, 28 September 1923, and 30 January 1924, vol. 2, pp. 36–8, 51–2, 56–8, 67, UCLonRO.

95 George Barger, "The relation of chemistry to medicine," *Edinburgh Med. J.* 23 (II) (1919): 350–7; J. Waler, "The teaching of chemistry to students of medicine," *Edinburgh Med. J.* 20 (I) (1918): 48–60; J. Kendall, "Sir James Walker," *Obit. Not. Fellows R. Soc.* 1 (1935): 537–49; H. H. Dakin, "George Barger," *Obit. Not. Fellows R. Soc.* 3 (1940): 63–85; C. R. Harington, "George Barger," *J. Chem. Soc.* 142 (1939): 715–21.

96 Walker, "Teaching of chemistry," p. 50.

97 Faculty of science minutes, 13 January 1914 and 1 February 1917, in "College minutes," vol. 1 pp. 504–5, 543, UEdinA.

98 A. E. Schäfer, "Memorandum of 30 October 1918," p. 5, Dean D. H. Beare to Schäfer, 24 October 1918, UEdinA, Gen 2077/S.

99 "College minutes," 16 January and 6 March 1919, vol. 2, pp. 193–4, 223, 227, 245; "Medical faculty minutes," 10 and 24 June 1919 and Draft report, 18 November 1919, vol. 2, pp. 32–33, UEdinA. One of Barger's first acts as professor was to make general chemistry a prerequisite to admission.

100 R. Pearce, "Notes of RMP on Medical School University of Edinburgh, 14–22 February 1923," *Medical Education in Scotland*, pp. 89–90, RF, 405A, Pea-1; Pearce to Alan Gregg, 5 October 1923, RF, 405, box 2.

101 Report of Board of Studies, 14 January 1926, in "College minutes," vol. 4, p. 257, UEdinA.

102 J. A. H., "William D. Halliburton (1860–1931)," *Biochem. J.* 26 (1932): 269–71. William Robison, a chemist from Barger's group, was appointed in 1927. However, he was a poor entrepreneur, and an independent department was not established until 1957.

103 R. C. Garry, "Physiology and biochemistry," in Anon., *Fortuna Domus* (Glasgow: at the University Press, 1952), pp. 235–47; G. Wisehart, "Edward P. Cathcart (1877–1954)," *Obit. Not. Fellows R. Soc.* 9 (1954): 35–53.

104 E. P. Cathcart, "Dynamic biochemistry," *Edinburgh Med. J.* 35 (1928): 21–9 (quotation is from p. 22).

105 A. Neuberger, "James Norman Davidson," *Biogr. Mem. Fellows R. Soc.* 19 (1973): 281–303. Davidson accepted the chair on condition that he be free of interference by Cathcart.

106 Charlton, *Portrait of a University*, p. 179. A. V. Hill succeeded William Stirling as professor of physiology in 1920. His first reform was to establish a lectureship in chemical physiology; see Manchester University *Calendar* (1920/1).

107 H. S. Raper, "The synthetic activities of the cell," *Rep. Br. Assoc. Adv. Sci.* 1930: 160–75 (see p. 175).

108 Shimmin, *University of Leeds*, pp. 36–69; Report of Special Committee on Physiology, 11 February 1919, in "Senate minutes," ULeedsA; Undated memorandum from the Department of Physiology, circa May 1919, ULeedsA; B. A. McSweeney to Cyril Long, 1 February 1929, Long Papers.

109 Chapman, *Story of a Modern University* pp. 319–25; Diary of W. E. Tisdale, 12 November 1935, 5 February 1938, Hans Krebs to Tisdale, 16 November 1935,

other correspondence, and Warren Weaver to Krebs, 25 April 1945, RF, 401, box 204.

CHAPTER 4 *General biochemistry: the Cambridge School*

1 F. G. Hopkins, "Four lectures on the significance of variations in the constituents of urine," *Guy's Hosp. Gaz.* 21 (1907): 327–32, 383–8, 403–9, 423–8; F. G. Hopkins, "The utilization of proteins in the animal," *Sci. Progr.* (London) 1 (1906): 159–76; F. G. Hopkins, "Dr. Pavy and diabetes," *Sci. Progr.* (London) 7 (1912): 13–47.

2 F. G. Hopkins, "Biochemistry," in *Facilities for Study and Research* (Cambridge University Press, 1918), pp. 16–17.

3 N. Mutch, "A short quantitative study of histozyme, a tissue ferment," *J. Physiol. (London)* 44 (1912): 176–90; Harold Ackroyd and F. G. Hopkins, "Feeding experiments with deficiencies in the amino-acid supply: arginine and histidine as possible precursors of purines," *Biochem.* 10 (1916): 551–76; F. G. Hopkins, "Some oxidation mechanisms of the cell," *Bull. Johns Hopkins Hosp.* 32 (1921): 321–8.

4 Allbutt and Langley to Vice Chancellor, 22 February 1905, UCamA, CUR 39.44.

5 Hopkins, "Biochemistry," pp. 16–17; F. G. Hopkins, "Physiological chemistry," *Annu. Rep. Progr. Chem.* 11 (1914): 188–212.

6 F. G. Hopkins, "On current views concerning the mechanisms of biological oxidation," *Skand. Arch. Physiol.* 49 (1926): 33–59.

7 George Haines IV, *Essays on German Influence upon English Education and Science 1850–1914* (Hamden, Conn.: Archon Books, 1969); D. S. L. Cardwell, *The Organisation of Science in England* (London: Heinemann, 1957); Richard Glazebrook, *Science and Industry: The Place of Cambridge in Any Scheme for Their Combination* (Cambridge University Press, 1917); A. C. Seward, ed., *Science and the Nation, Essays by Cambridge Graduates* (Cambridge University Press, 1917).

8 Arthur Landsborough Thomson, *Half a Century of Medical Research*, 2 vols.: *Origins and Policy of the Medical Research Council*, vol. I; *The Programme of the Medical Research Council*, vol. II (London: H.M. Stationery Office, 1973 and 1975); T. R. Elliott, "Walter Morley Fletcher (1873–1933)," *Obit. Not. Fellows R. Soc.* 1 (1934): 153–63.

9 Elliott, "Fletcher," pp. 162–3.

10 Hopkins to Mellanby, August 1913, cited in B. S. Platt, "Sir Edward Mellanby," *Annu. Rev. Biochem.* 25 (1956): 1–28.

11 Fletcher to Hopkins, 23 June 1915, MRC, PF 106; F. G. Hopkins, "Feeding experiments illustrating the importance of accessory factors in normal dietaries," *J. Physiol. (London)* 44 (1912): 425–60.

12 Fletcher to Hopkins, 31 December 1917, MRC, PF 106; F. G. Hopkins, "Report on the Present State of Knowledge Concerning Accessory Food Factors (Vitamins)", (London: Special Report Series no. 38, Medical Research Council, 1919); Fletcher to Hopkins, 2 May and 8 August 1918, and 6 June 1919, Hopkins to Fletcher, 30 April 1918 and 9 June 1919, MRC, PF 106; F. G. Hopkins, "The present position of vitamins in clinical medicine," *Br. Med. J.* (1920 II): 147–60.

13 Hopkins to Fletcher, 4 July 1915, Hopkins to Fletcher, 30 April 1918 and 5 July 1917, MRC, PF 106.

14 Hopkins to Fletcher, 22 February 1917, Fletcher to Hopkins, 9 and 26 February 1917, MRC, PF 106.

15 Robert E. Kohler, "Walter Fletcher, F. G. Hopkins and the Dunn Institute of Biochemistry: a case study in the patronage of science," *Isis* 69 (1978): 331–5; F. G. Hopkins, "William Bate Hardy (1864–1933)," *Obit. Not. Fellows R. Soc.* 1 (1934): 327–33.

16 David Owen, *British Philanthropy 1660–1960* (Cambridge, Mass.: Harvard University Press, 1964).

17 Jeremiah Coleman, *Bequests of Sir William Dunn Baronet* (London: privately printed, 1930), MRC, 1331/A.

18 W. B. Hardy, "The Dunn estate," undated (circa September 1918), MRC, 1331A; Hardy to Hopkins, 19 June 1921, UCamA, BChem 3/5.
19 W. M. Fletcher, "Endowment of medical research," 11 November 1918, MRC, 1331A.
20 W. M. Fletcher, "Dunn estate," 30 August 1919, MRC, 1131A.
21 Hopkins to Fletcher, 9 June 1919, MRC, PF 106.
22 Hopkins to Fletcher, 9 June 1919, Fletcher to Hopkins, 9 and 11 June 1919, MRC, PF 106.
23 Fletcher memorandum to Balfour, 6 May 1924, MRC, 1331A.
24 Fletcher to Hopkins, 8 February 1921, MRC, PF 106.
25 Fletcher to A. Holland Hibbert, 29 December 1921, MRC, 1331A. Data on Hopkins's research associates are from J. Needham and E. Baldwin, eds., *Hopkins and Biochemistry* (Cambridge: Heffer, 1949), pp. 335–53.
26 Fletcher to Seligman, 24 January 1922, Seligman to Hibbert, 30 March 1922, MRC, 1331A.
27 Norman W. Pirie, "J. B. S. Haldane (1892–1964)," *Biogr. Mem. Fellows R. Soc.* 12 (1966): 219–49; Haldane to Hopkins, 19 June 1921, UCamA, BChem 3/5. Haldane was a polymath and an *enfant terrible*, cultivating a deliberately outrageous style. Selig Hecht observed in 1925 that Hopkins praised Haldane effusively in public; Fletcher, however, intimated that Haldane was a thorn in Hopkins's side. In 1927, Haldane was named in a divorce case and was ejected (temporarily) from his readership. He resigned in 1927; see Hecht to Crozier, 10 November, 6 and 14 December 1925, Crozier Papers; Fletcher to Hopkins, 29 July 1927, MRC, 1331A.
28 Marjorie Stephenson, "Muriel Wheldale Onslow (1880–1932)," *Biochem. J.* 26 (1932): 915–16; Muriel Wheldale, *The Principles of Plant Biochemistry*, (Cambridge University Press, 1931), part I.
29 Diary of H. M. Miller, 6 November 1939, Keilin to H. M. Miller, 2 January 1940, and "Outline of research on intracellular catalytic systems," Diary of H. M. Miller, 25 May 1939, RF, 401D, box 42.
30 A. C. Chibnall, "Postwar needs of the Department of Biochemistry," undated (circa 1943), UCamA, BChem 1/2; Chibnall to E. Mellanby, 25 October 1945, Malcolm Dixon, "Enzyme research at Cambridge," 25 and 30 October and 5 November 1945, Mellanby to Chibnall, 30 October 1945, 5 November 1946, MRC, 628.
31 F. G. Hopkins, "The dynamic side of biochemistry," *Rep. Br. Assoc. Adv. Sci.* (1913): 652–68 (reprinted in Needham and Baldwin, eds., *Hopkins and Biochemistry*, see pp. 150–2).
32 Mikulas Teich, "From 'enchyme' to 'cyto-skeleton': the development of ideas on the chemical organization of living matter," in M. Teich and Robert Young, eds., *Changing Perspectives in the History of Science* (London: Heinemann, 1973), pp. 439–72; R. A. Peters, "Co-ordinative biochemistry of the cell and tissues," *J. State Med.* 37 (1929): 683–709; J. Needham, "Frederick Gowland Hopkins," *Notes Rec. R. Soc. (London)* 17 (1962): 117–62 (see p. 119).
33 Dorothy Needham, *Machina Carnis: the Biochemistry of Muscular Contraction in Its Historical Development* (Cambridge University Press, 1971).
34 Baldwin had worked with Joseph Needham, who urged him to write the book on comparative biochemistry that Needham himself had once hoped to do; see Needham to Tisdale, 4 June 1935, RF, 401D, box 42; Anon., "Ernest F. Baldwin (1909–1969)," *Nature* 225 (1970): 569–70; Ernest Baldwin, *An Introduction to Comparative Biochemistry* (Cambridge University Press, 1937).
35 Hopkins, "Current views," p. 36.
36 R. Hill, D. Needham, and M. Stephenson, "Advantages of the present scheme," in Biochemistry Department Staff Minutes, April 1935, at p. 26, UCamA, BChem 1/1.
37 J. N. Pirie, "Topics omitted in this syllabus," Biochemistry Department Staff Minutes, April 1935, at p. 24, UCamA, BChem 1/1.
38 E. Holmes, "Memorandum on proposed Part II courses," Biochemistry Department Staff Minutes, April 1935, at p. 27, UCamA, BChem 1/1.

39 Hill et al., "Advantages,".
40 Biochemistry Department Staff Minutes, 30 April, 27 May and 10 July 1936, pp. 24, 31, UCamA, BChem 1/1.
41 "Memorandum on university relations," 20 May 1933, UCamA, BChem 4/2; *Reporter* (Cambridge), 14 June and 7 November 1932.
42 Holmes to Mellanby, 20 March 1935 and other correspondence, MRC, 1913; Elsie Watchorn, "Reports for 1933/34 and 1935/36," MRC, 2036.
43 In 1918 Hopkins complained of his inability to compete with "Harden and company" (Arthur Harden and Harriette Chick's group at the Lister Institute); see Hopkins to Fletcher, 30 April 1918, Fletcher to Hopkins, 8 August 1918, MRC, PF 106.
44 Fletcher to Coleman, 9 July 1928 and 5 January 1929, Hopkins to Fletcher, 19 July 1929 and other correspondence, MRC, 1331/A.
45 Fletcher to Hill, 20 January 1927, MRC, 1349; E. Mellanby, "Recommendations for better control of Nutritional Laboratory Cambridge," 3 July 1934 and other correspondence, MRC, 2037.
46 Hopkins to Fletcher, 4 July 1915, MRC, PF 106; F. G. Hopkins, "Biochemistry: its present position and outlook," *Lancet* (21 June 1924): 1247–52 (see p. 1251); Hopkins, "Physiological chemistry," *Annu. Rep. Progr. Chem.* 14 (1917): 190–4.
47 M. Stephenson, *Bacterial Metabolism* (London: Longmans Green, 1930), pp. vii, 8–16.
48 M. Robertson, "Marjory Stephenson, 1885–1948," *Obit. Not. Fellows R. Soc.* 6 (1949): 563–77; Hopkins to Fletcher, 14 March 1922, Hopkins to Thomson, 29 April 1922, Thomson to Hopkins, 13 May 1922, MRC, 2036.
49 Fletcher to Stephenson, 18 March 1929, Stephenson to Fletcher, 19 March 1929, MRC, PF 216. E. Mellanby, "Memorandum," 26 July 1946 and other correspondence, MRC, 2036.
50 C. Zobel, "Report on fellowship," 25 January 1948, RF, 401D, box 43.
51 Needham, "Hopkins," pp. 133, 162; J. Needham, *Biochemistry and Morphogenesis* (Cambridge University Press, 1942); J. Needham, "Memorandum to the vice-chancellor. . .on the question of the extension of the biochemical laboratory," Summer 1936, UCamA, BChem 4/6.
52 Needham, "Hopkins," p. 150; Needham "Memorandum," pp. 1–2.
53 Needham, "Memorandum," p. 2.
54 Needham to Tisdale, 22 January 1935, T. R. Hogness, "Fellowship report," 16 August 1937, RF, 401D, box 42.
55 Tisdale to Weaver, 12 June 1937 and 1 September 1937, diary of W. Weaver, 7 May 1935, RF, 401D, box 42.
56 Needham to Tisdale, 4 and 16 June 1935, J. Needham, "Memorandum for members of the proposed Institute of Physico-chemical Morphology," in the diary of W. Weaver, 7 May 1935, RF, 401D, box 42.
57 R. E. Kohler, "Warren Weaver and the Rockefeller Foundation program in molecular biology: a case study in the management of science," in Nathan Reingold, ed., *The Sciences in the American Context: New Perspectives* (Washington, D.C.: Smithsonian Institution Press, 1979), pp. 249–93.
58 Tisdale to Weaver, 12 June and 8 January 1937, Diary of H. M. Miller 27 October 1937, Diary of W. Weaver, 7 May 1935, RF, 401D, box 42.
59 Tisdale to Weaver, 8 January and 1 September 1937, Waddington to Miller, 26 October 1936, RF, 401D, box 42.
60 Diary of W. Weaver, 13–14 June 1936, Tisdale to Weaver, 8 January 12 July and 1 September 1937, Diary of Tisdale, 28 April 1938, Tisdale to Miller, 27 June 1939, RF, 401D, box 42.
61 Hopkins to Fletcher, 17 and 24 August 1924, MRC, PF 106; Fletcher to Hopkins, 5 October 1925, 28 July 1927, 28 July 1928, and 3 December 1928, Coleman to Fletcher, 17 November 1924 and 1 July 1925, Fletcher to Coleman, 16 February and 14 July 1925, Hopkins to Fletcher, 29 November and 9 December 1928, MRC, 1331/A.

62 Diary of W. Weaver, 31 May 1938, Diary of W. E. Tisdale, 28 April 1938, Diary of H. M. Miller, 6 November 1939, RF, 401D, box 42; Stephenson to Mellanby, 10 July 1934, 8 July 1935, 10 October 1935, and 13 and 24 July 1936, MRC, 2036.

63 J. Needham, "Sir F. G. Hopkins' personal influence and character," in Needham and Baldwin, eds. *Hopkins and Biochemistry* pp. 114–5.

64 Tisdale to Weaver, 22 December 1936 and 2–3 July 1937, RF, 401D, box 42. Francis Roughton was rumored to have also been considered.

65 Chibnall, "Postwar needs," undated (circa 1943), UCamA, BChem 1/2; Chibnall to Weaver, 11 October 1945, Diary of W. Weaver, 31 May 1948, RF, 401D, box 43.

66 Anon., "Edward Whitely, 1879–1945," ULivA, D139/2.

67 H. A. Krebs, "Sir Archibald Garrod," in Kenneth Dewhurst, ed., *Oxford Medicine* (Oxford: Sandford, 1970), pp. 127–35.

68 See Benjamin Moore's chapters in Leonard Hill, ed., *Recent Advances in Physiology and Biochemistry* (London: Arnold, 1906); B. Moore, *Biochemistry: A Study of the Origins, Reactions and Equilibrium of Living Matter* (London: Arnold, 1921), p. v.

69 R. E. Kohler, "A policy for the advancement of science: the Rockefeller foundation, 1924–1929," *Minerva* 16 (1978): 480–515.

70 R. M. Pearce, "Memorandum", 3 February 1923, Pearce to George Vincent, 7 February 1923, Pearce, "Medical Education in England," pp. 74–75, A. E. Garrod, "Note by the Regius Professor of Medicine," January 1923, RF, 401OUB.

71 Peters to Garrod, 16 February 1923, RF, 401OUB.

72 Pearce to Gregg, 23 September 1923, Pearce to Garrod, 6 December 1923, RF, 401OUB.

73 R. A. Peters, "Department of Biochemistry, Oxford," *Methods Probl. Med. Ed.* 18 (1930): 109–18 (see p. 115); R. A. Peters, "Forty-five years of biochemistry," *Annu. Rev. Biochem.* 26 (1957) (reprinted in *Excitement and Fascination in Science* (Palo Alto: Annual Reviews, 1965), pp. 363–80).

74 P. Fildes to E. Mellanby, 25 April 1944, Woods to A. L. Thomson, 8 March 1945, MRC, PF 254; R. A. Peters, "Ernest Walker (1900–1942)," *Biochem. J.* 37 (1943): 449–50.

75 M. Stephenson, "Sir F. G. Hopkins' teaching and scientific influence," in Needham and Baldwin, eds., *Hopkins and Biochemistry* pp. 29–38, (see p. 36).

CHAPTER 5 *European ideals and American realities, 1870–1900*

1 Jones to Abel, 16 July 1899, Abel Papers.

2 Thomas N. Bonner, *American Doctors and German Universities* (Lincoln: University of Nebraska Press, 1963).

3 Charles E. Rosenberg, *No Other Gods* (Baltimore, Md.: Johns Hopkins University Press, 1976), ch. 8; Margaret W. Rossiter, *The Emergence of Agricultural Science* (New Haven, Conn.: Yale University Press, 1975).

4 Richard Shryock, *The Unique Influence of the Johns Hopkins University on American Medicine* (Copenhagen: Munksgaard, 1954); Simon Flexner and J. T. Flexner, *William Henry Welch and the Heroic Age of American Medicine* (New York: Viking, 1941).

5 Rosenberg, *No Other Gods*, pp. 135–52.

6 Earl P. Ross, *Democracy's College: The Land Grant Movement in the Formative State* (Ames: Iowa State University Press, 1942).

7 Russell H. Chittenden, *History of the Sheffield Scientific School* 2 vols. (New Haven, Conn.: Yale University Press, 1928); Howard S. Miller, *Dollars for Research* (Seattle: University of Washington Press, 1970), ch. 4. Scientific schools were also established at Dartmouth, Princeton, Rutgers, Harvard, and Pennsylvania; Columbia's School of Mines belongs in the same category.

8 Hugh Hawkins, *Pioneer: A History of the Johns Hopkins University, 1874–1889* (Ithaca, N.Y.: Cornell University Press, 1960), p. 37.

9 Owen Hannaway, "The German model of chemical education in America: Ira Remsen at Johns Hopkins (1876–1913)," *Ambix* 23 (1976): 145–64.

10 Hugh Hawkins, "Transatlantic discipleship: two American biologists and their German mentor," *Isis* 71 (1980): 197–210.

11 Joseph Ben-David, *The Scientist's Role in Society* (Engelwood Cliffs, N.J.: Prentice-Hall, 1970), ch. 8.

12 Chittenden, *Sheffield School*, vol. I, ch. 4.

13 Ibid., vol. I, pp. 164–5, 239–40, vol. II, pp. 426–7; Chittenden to A. T. Hadley, 7 December 1909, Hadley Papers, box 17, f. 322; R. H. Chittenden, "Sixty Years of Service in Science: An Autobiography," 1936, Chittenden Papers, pp. 25–7. Physicist George F. Barker was professor of physiological chemistry and toxicology at the Yale Medical School from 1867 to 1874; see Chittenden to Lewis, 15 September 1924, Lewis Papers, box 3. Johnson's initiative in physiological chemistry was very likely a response to Barker's resignation.

14 Chittenden, "Autobiography," pp. 29–31. R. H. Chittenden, *The Development of Physiological Chemistry in the United States* (New York: Chemical Catalogue, 1928), pp. 34–6.

15 Chittenden, *Physiological Chemistry*, pp. 29–31.

16 Chittenden, "Autobiography," pp. 41–6.

17 A large correspondence with Kühne is preserved in the Chittenden Papers.

18 Thomas to Mendel, 22 December 1929, Mendel Papers.

19 Leslie B. Arey, *Northwestern University Medical School, 1859–1959* (Evanston, Ill.: Northwestern University Press, 1959), p. 92.

20 Chittenden to Hadley, 17 January 1906, Hadley Papers, box 17, f. 322. Chittenden, *Sheffield School*, vol. I, pp. 244–8, vol. II, p. 429; Chittenden, "Autobiography," pp. 62–5.

21 Chittenden to Welch, 2 October 1901, Welch Papers.

22 Chittenden to Hadley, 17 January 1906, Howell and Welch to Chittenden, 20 and 26 December 1905, Hadley Papers, box 17, f. 322.

23 Chittenden, *Sheffield School*, vol. II, pp. 430–2; Chittenden to Hadley, 17 January 1906, Hadley Papers, box 17, f. 322. The list is incomplete. Data after 1900 are not significant because recent graduates had not yet entered professional careers.

24 W. F. Norwood, "Medical education in the United States before 1900," in Charles D. O'Malley, ed., *The History of Medical Education* (Berkeley: University of California Press, 1970), pp. 463–500.

25 Wilfred B. Shaw, *The University of Michigan: An Encyclopedic Survey*, part V, *The Medical School, the University Hospital, the Law School, 1850–1940* (Ann Arbor: University of Michigan Press, 1951), vol. III, pp. 773–1034.

26 Ibid., vol. I, pp. 39–53 and vol. II, pp. 512–32; see also Edward C. Campbell, *History of the Chemistry Laboratory of the University of Michigan, 1856–1910* (Ann Arbor: University of Michigan Press, 1916).

27 Shaw, *University of Michigan*, vol. I, pp. 208–9; F. G. Novy, "MS on the History of the Medical School Laboratories," undated (circa 1947), UMichA, box 72; V. C. Vaughan, *A Doctor's Memories* (Indianapolis, Ind.: Bobbs Merrill, 1926), p. 195; V. C. Vaughan, *Albert Benjamin Prescott*, (Ann Arbor, Mich.: privately printed, 1906).

28 Vaughan, *Doctor's Memories*, pp. 101–2; Novy, "History."

29 Shaw, *University of Michigan*, vol. II, pp. 823–27; Novy, "History"; W. T. Vaughan, "Victor Clarence Vaughan," *J. Lab. Clin. Med.* 15 (1930): 817–21.

30 Medical faculty minutes, 8 October 1887, 11 February 1890, and 30 March 1896, U MichA; V. C., Vaughan, "Doctor's memories," *J. Lab. clin. Med.* 15 (1930): 902–27. (These are chapters not included in the published book.)

31 E. R. Long, "Frederick G. Novy," *Biogr. Mem. Nat. Acad. Sci.* 33 (1959): 326–50 (see p. 329); Ruth Good, "Dr. Frederick G. Novy: biographical sketch," *Univ. Mich. Med. Bull.* 16 (1950): 257–68 (see pp. 260–1.)

32 Vaughan to M. L. Burton, 18 April 1921, Burton Papers, box 3, f. 15.

33 University of Michigan *Calendar* (1903–4), pp. 180–1. By 1903 only 3 of 12 courses
    were in physiological chemistry; see Lyon to Burton, 2 April 1921, Burton Papers,
    box 3, f. 15.
34 Lewis to Hugh Cabot, 9 May 1922, Cabot to Lewis, 31 May 1922, 25 January
    1923, and 14 March 1923, Lewis to Cabot, 29 June 1922, Lewis Papers, box 4.
35 Alan Chesney, *The Johns Hopkins Hospital and the Johns Hopkins Medical School*
    (Baltimore, Md.: Johns Hopkins University Press, 1943), vol. I, pp. 206–12.
36 Welch to G. H. F. Nuttall, 20 and 23 February 1894, Welch Papers.
37 William Osler to Abel, 2 March 1893, Abel to Osler, 7 March 1893, Abel Papers;
    W. DeB. MacNeider, "John Jacob Abel, 1857–1938," *Biogr. Mem. Natl. Acad. Sci.*
    24 (1946): 231–57; Paul D. Lamson, "J.J. Abel – a portrait," *Bull. Johns Hopkins
    Hosp.* 68 (1941): 119–87.
38 J. J. Abel to Mary Abel, 22 July 1884, 14 October 1889, Abel Papers.
39 J. J. Abel to Mary Abel, 3 September 1889, Abel Papers.
40 J. J. Abel to Mary Abel, 31 October 1889, Abel Papers. "Nencki grasped my idea at
    once, and said, 'aha, I[ch] sehe, sie wollen es so machen dass sie sich später selbst
    helfen können.' I replied, 'Ja wohl, Herr Professor,' and thanked him."
41 J. J. Abel to Mary Abel, 14 October 1889, Abel Papers. "This is the great thread I
    find that has run through all my education since I first began at Vaughan's....I
    now recall conversations with Sewall expressing my ambition to do what I am
    now perhaps going to attain after all."
42 Ibid. and subsequent correspondence, Abel Papers.
43 J. J. Abel to Mary Abel, 23 June and July 1892 and other correspondence, Abel
    Papers.
44 Drechsel to Abel, 11 March 1894, see also 30 July 1894 and other correspondence,
    Abel Papers. "How strange that we find ourselves in analogous situations. You, a
    pharmacologist, must also teach physiological chemistry while I, a physiological
    chemist, teach pharmacology."
45 J. J. Abel to Mary Abel, 23 June 1892, Abel Papers. "The fact that I am not a
    systematically educated and drilled chemist is always popping out and annoying
    me."
46 Medical faculty minutes, 3 October 1895, 6 October 1896, 10 June 1897, 20 and 26
    February 1898, 31 March 1898, vol. A., pp. 133–4, 149–50, 190, 257–61, 306–13;
    JHUMedA; Abel to Chittenden, 28 May and 6 June 1897, Chittenden to Abel, 19
    May and 7 June 1898, Abel to Mathews, 19 November 1908, Welch to Abel, 3
    March 1898, Chittenden to Welch, 1 March 1898, Folin to Abel, 4 July and 5
    August 1898, Folin to W. H. Howell, 22 February 1898, Julius Stieglitz to Abel,
    15 November 1898, Abel Papers.
47 Medical faculty minutes, 5 March and 3 October 1896, June 1898, vol. A. pp. 170,
    206, 324, JHUMedA; W. M. Clark, "Walter Jennings Jones, 1865–1935," *Biogr.
    Mem. Natl. Acad. Sci.* 20 (1939): 79–139.
48 Clark, "Jones," p. 96; W. A. Noyes and J. F. Norris, "Ira Remsen, 1846–1927,"
    Biogr. Mem. Natl. Acad. Sci. 14 (1931): 207–57.
49 Clark, "Jones," pp. 93–4.
50 Ibid., p. 90.
51 George W. Corner, *Two Centuries of Medicine: A History of the School of Medicine,
    University of Pennsylvania* (Philadelphia: Lippincott, 1965), pp. 163–4; Hawkins,
    Pioneer, pp. 146, 243.
52 See Gerald Geison, "Divided we stand: physiologists and clinicians in the Ameri-
    can context," in Charles Rosenberg and Morris Vogel, eds., *The Therapeutic
    Revolution* (Philadelphia: University of Pennsylvania Press, 1979), pp. 67–90.
53 W. M. Fletcher and Wilmot Herringham, "Memorandum to the university
    grants committee" (London: H.M. Stationery Office, 1921), pp. 3–4.
54 Whitman to Harper, 13 March 1896, UChicPP, box 70, f. 22. On Loeb's appoint-
    ment, see Whitman to Harper, 15 January, 14 March, 17 and 30 August 1892,
    Harper Papers, box 15, f. 17; Loeb to Harper, 30 June 1891, 5 May 1892,

UChicPP, box 17, f. 13; C. O. Whitman, "General physiology and its relation to morphology," *Am. Nat.* 27 (1893): 202–7.

55 Whitman to Harper, 15 January 1892, UChicPP, box 15, f. 17; E. S. Monesh, "Charles Otis Whitman," *Biogr. Mem. Natl. Acad. Sci.* 7 (1913): 269–88.

56 Whitman to Harper, 14 February 1896 (Harper's letter to Whitman of 12 February 1896 is not present.), UChicPP, box 70, f. 22. Harper had a strong personal interest in neurophysiology, growing out of his concern with scientific theories of mind. Harper and Loeb had, of course, very different beliefs in the matter; see Herrick to Harper, undated (circa April 1891, 29 October 1891 and 12 November 1891), Harper memorandum, 9 May 1892, UChicPP, box 15, f. 2.

57 W. H. Howell et al., *History of the American Physiological Society Semicentennial, 1887–1937* (Baltimore, Md.: The Society, 1938); Chittenden, *Physiological Chemistry*, pp. 45–6.

58 Tait to E. A. Schäfer, 27 July 1921, UEdinA, Gen 2007/5, f. letters re laboratory.

59 W. J. V. Osterhout, "Jacques Loeb," *Biogr. Mem. Natl. Acad. Sci.* 13 (1930): 318–410.

60 Loeb to Benjamin I. Wheeler, 15 September 1906, UCalPP, box 23; see also J. Loeb, "Recent developments of biology," *Congr. Arts Sci. Univ. Expo.* 5 (1906): 13–24 (see p. 24).

61 Loeb to Wheeler, 15 September 1906, UCalPP, box 23.

62 Charles Rosenberg, *No Other Gods*, pp. 123–32.

63 Whitman's master plan included a position for a biological chemist, but it was set aside in 1892 along with agricultural and marine experiment stations; see Whitman to Harper, 15 January 1892, Harper Papers, box 15, f. 17.

64 University of Chicago *Register* (1897/98), pp. 315–16 and *1901/2*, pp. 315–17. Loeb lectured on chemical physiology in his course on general physiology.

65 Loeb to Harper, 16 July 1902, UChicPP, box 17, f. 13; Lewellys F. Barker to Harper, 25 August 1902, Loeb to Harper, 11, 22, 23, and 26 January, 11 July, and 11 November 1902, Harper to Loeb, 11 July 1902, UChicPP, box 45, f. 6.

66 Loeb to C. A. Herter, 4 April 1905, Abel Papers.

67 Loeb to B. I. Wheeler, 31 October 1908, UCalPP, box 23.

68 Loeb to Flexner, 1910, quoted by Osterhout, "Loeb," pp. 326–8.

69 See, for example, J. Loeb, "Recent developments of biology," *Science* 20 (1904): 777–86; J. Loeb, "Recent developments of biology," *Congr. Arts Sci. Univ. Expo.* 5 (1906): 13–24; J. Loeb "The biological problems of today: physiology," *Science* 7 (1898): 154–6; J. Loeb "Einige Bermerkungen über den Begriff, die Geschichte und Literatur der allgemeine Physiologie," *Arch. gesammte Physiol.* 69 (1898): 249–67.

70 Shaw, *University of Michigan*, vol. II, pp. 781, 845–55, 919–23; Corner, *Two Centuries*, pp. 178–84; J. A. Myers, "Richard Olding Beard, M.D., Minnesota pioneer in physiology...," *Lancet* 85 (1965): 302–8.

71 F. C. Waite, *Western Reserve University Centennial History of the School of Medicine* (Cleveland, Ohio: Western Reserve University Press, 1946), pp. 346–50.

72 Sherrington to Brunner, 7 November 1907, ULivA, 5/3.9.

73 John Field, "Medical education in the United States," in O'Malley, ed. *History of Medical Education*, pp. 501–30; Martin Kaufman, *American Medical Education: The Formative Years, 1765–1910* (Westport, Conn.: Greenwood Press, 1976).

74 Rosemary Stevens, *American Medicine and the Public Interest* (New Haven, Conn.: Yale University Press, 1971), ch. 2.

75 Arey, *Northwestern University*, pp. 140, 171.

76 Corner, *Two Centuries*, pp. 178–80, 187–94.

77 During the reform movement, a great deal was made of the "commercial" character of proprietary medical colleges. Many were indeed organized solely as profit-making companies, especially in the South and West, and a few made handsome profits on a small capital investment. By the 1890s, however, faculties were more likely to be dunned for contributions than to receive dividends. The benefits were more professional intangibles than cash. "Commercialism" was

simply a useful political stick with which Flexner and others beat good and bad alike.

78 Medical faculty minutes, 29 January 1894, vol. 7, pp. 305–23, UColA.
79 Shaw, *University of Michigan*, vol. III, pp. 915–1020.
80 Quoted by Corner, *Two Centuries*, pp. 205–7.
81 George Corner, *A History of the Rockefeller Institute 1901–1953* (New York: Rockefeller Institute Press, 1954), p. 44.

CHAPTER 6 *The reform of medical education in America*

1 "Medical education in the U.S. Annual presentation of education data for 1926..." *Am. Med. Assoc.* 87 (1926): 565–73; Willard C. Rappeleye, ed., *Final Report of the Commission on Medical Education* (New York: for the Commission, 1932), table 104.
2 A. D. Bevan et al., "Annual congress on medical education," *J. Am. Med. Assoc.* 74 (1920): 758; Medical council minutes, 13 November 1911, vol. 1, pp. 412–17, UPennA; Abraham Flexner, *Medical Education in the United States and Canada* (New York: Carnegie Foundation, 1910), p. 28.
3 Robert P. Hudson, "Abraham Flexner in perspective: American medical education, 1865–1910," *Bull. Hist. Med.* 46 (1972): 545–61; James G. Burrow, *Organized Medicine in the Progressive Era* (Baltimore, Md.: Johns Hopkins University Press, 1976); Richard Shryock, *The Unique Influence of the Johns Hopkins University on American Medicine* (Copenhagen: Munksgaard, 1954); Donald Fleming, *William H. Welch and the Rise of Modern Medicine* (Boston: Little, Brown, 1954); Richard Shryock, *Medical Licensing in America, 1650–1965* (Baltimore, Md.: Johns Hopkins University Press, 1967); John Field, "Medical education in the United States: late 19th and 20th centuries," in Charles O'Malley, ed., *The History of Medical Education* (Berkeley: University of California Press, 1970), pp. 501–30; Thomas N. Bonner, *American Doctors and German Universities* (Lincoln: University of Nebraska Press, 1963).
4 "Standards of medical education adopted by the AMA, July 1905," *J. Am. Med. Assoc.* (1906): 627, 632–3; "Report of the Council on Medical Education," *J. Am. Med. Assoc.* 53 (1909): 544–5, 54 (1910): 1974–5.
5 "Report of the meeting of the Council on Medical Education," 4 March 1912, Medical council minutes, vol. 1, pp. 450–1, UPennA; William Pepper to N. P. Colewell, 16 November 1914, C. A. Dabney to Colewell, 25 November 1914; Colewell to Pepper, 30 June 1916, Medical council minutes, vol. 2, pp. 108–11, 220–1, UPennA.
6 Bevan to George Dock, 27 October 1913, Faculty minutes, 5 November 1913, WashUMedA.
7 "Report of reference committee on medical education," *J. Am. Med. Assoc.* 66 (1916): 2083–4.
8 Ingals to W. R. Harper, 29 January 1900, UChicPP, box 57, f. 13.
9 Fred C. Zapffe to Allen Smith, 13 December 1909, Bevan to Smith, 18 January 1911, Smith to Allen, 20 January 1911, George Piersol, "Report on AAMC meeting of 13 November 1911," Medical council minutes, vol. 2, pp. 262, 357–58, 363, 418, UPennA.
10 Eugene Opie, "Report of delegate at meetings on medical education, February 24 and 25, 1914," Faculty minutes, 5 November 1913, WashUMedA. Representatives of the 15 or so better schools agreed to meet informally as a minority caucus so as not to disrupt the AAMC.
11 Laurence S. Veysey, *The Emergence of the American University* (University of Chicago Press, 1965); Frederick Rudolph, *The American College and University* (New York: Random House, 1962). See Guido H. Marx, "Some trends in higher education," *Science* 29 (1909): 759–87; Marx saw the increase of college attendance as a sign of "a rapid breaking down of...caste, class and privilege – a great social

upheaval signalling the imminence of a new social order...a great wave of awakening to a higher sense of social obligation and civic righteousness" (p. 763).

12 Edward A. Krug, *The Shaping of the American High School, 1880–1920* (Madison: University of Wisconsin Press, 1969); J. McKeen Cattell, "The American College," *Science* 26 (1907): 368–73.

13 Philip Hawk, "The physiological chemist: his training and profession," *The Jeffersonian* 15 (12) (1914): 1–3.

14 C. Judson Herrick, "What medical subjects can be taught efficiently in the literary college?" *Proc. Assoc. Am. Med. Coll.* 16 (1906): 34–8.

15 A. Flexner, "Adjusting the college to American life," *Science* 29 (1909): 361–72; Flexner, *Medical Education*, pp. 22–5; Raymond Fosdick, *Adventure in Giving, The Story of the General Education Board* (New York: Harper, 1952).

16 Wendy Jacobsen, "American medicine in transition: the case of the Yale Medical School, 1900–1920" (B.A. honors thesis, Wesleyan, 1976), YaUA, misc. mss 69; *Report of the president of Yale University* (New Haven, Conn.: Yale University Press, 1905/6, 1906/7); Yandell Henderson to F. P. Underhill, 15 February 1916, Underhill Papers.

17 Jerome Greene to H. A. Christian, 25 February 1909 and other correspondence, "Vote of faculty of medicine, 5 February 1909," Eliot Papers, box 207, f. Christian; Medical faculty minutes, 3 October 1908, 5 February 1909, vol. 7, pp. 35–6, 57, 115–19, HarvUMedA.

18 "Further report of the committee on university education in medicine," 4 January 1904, Medical faculty minutes, vol. 6, at p. 230 (see p. 13), HarvUMedA.

19 Frederick C. Waite, *Western Reserve University Centennial History of the School of Medicine* (Cleveland: Western Reserve University Press, 1946).

20 J.B. Mathews et al., *A History of Columbia University, 1754–1904* (New York: Columbia University Press, 1904); Edward C. Elliot, ed., *The Rise of a University* (New York: Columbia University Press, 1937); John Shrady, *The College of Physicians and Surgeons, New York,...A History* (New York: Lewis, n. d.).

21 "Report of Dean James W. McLane," 16 January 1899, "Report of the Committee on Curriculum," 18 November 1901, in Medical faculty minutes, vol. 8, p. 325, . vol. 9, pp. 271–4, UColA.

22 Between 1894 and 1897, 31 ± 3% of the freshman class dropped out; between 1898 and 1902, 20 ± 4% did so; in 1903 and 1904, the rate dropped to 12 to 15%. Figures are compiled from the Medical faculty minutes, vol. 9, pp. 272, vol. 10, pp. 191, 326, 459, vol. 14, p. 19, UColA.

23 "Report of the committee on curriculum," 25 April 1901, John G. Curtiss, "Memorandum to medical faculty," 21 October 1901, in Medical faculty minutes, vol. 9, pp. 177–8, 232–41, UColA.

24 Morris Bishop, *A History of Cornell* (Ithaca, N.Y.: Cornell University Press, 1952).

25 "Report of Dean McLane," 16 January 1899, pp. 2–3.

26 "Report on entrance examinations," 20 January 1902, "Report on entrance examinations," 18 February 1902, "Preliminary report of the committee on curriculum," 15 December 1902, in Medical faculty minutes, vol. 9, pp. 283–90, 304–8, vol. 10, pp. 35–8, UColA.

27 "Report of 20 January 1902", vol. 9, pp. 283–90, UColA.

28 Medical faculty minutes, 19 December 1904, 16 October 1905, vol. 10, pp. 352, 448, UColA.

29 Albert R. Lamb, *The Presbyterian Hospital and the Columbia-Presbyterian Medical Center* (New York: Columbia University Press, 1955), pp. 73–86.

30 George Corner, *Two Centuries of Medicine, A History of the University of Pennsylvania School of Medicine* (Philadelphia: Lippincott, 1965), pp. 189–90, 197.

31 Flexner to Welch, 1902, quoted by Corner, Ibid., pp. 205–7.

32 Corner, *Two Centuries*, p. 215; Medical council minutes, 18 November 1902, UPennA.

33 Medical council minutes, 15 October 1906, N. P. Colewell to Charles Frazier, 12 October 1906, vol. 1, pp. 84–6, 92, UPennA. This decision may have been influenced by the belief that the AMA was about to endorse a college requirement.

34 Medical council minutes, 20 September 1910, vol. 1, pp. 319–21, UPennA. Central High School graduates had only to take a summer course in laboratory science to be admitted.

35 Corner, Two Centuries, pp. 219–29; Joseph C. Aub and Ruth K. Hapgood, Pioneer in Modern Medicine, David Linn Edsall of Harvard (Boston: Harvard Medical Alumni Assoc., 1970), ch. 7.

36 Corner, Two Centuries, pp. 287–9; "Report of the Committee on the Reorganization of the Council," 5 February 1912, Medical council minutes, vol. 1, pp. 441–6, UPennA.

37 Edsall to Flexner, 3 February 1910, Flexner Papers, quoted by Aub and Hapgood, Edsall, pp. 86–7.

38 Aub and Hapgood, Edsall, pp. 98–101, 191; Correspondence with David Edsall, 1910–2, Flexner Papers.

39 Howell to Eugene Opie, 6 December 1910, Opie Papers, quoted by Aub and Hapgood, Edsall, p. 94.

40 Lusk to Shaffer, 17 January 1911, Shaffer Papers, box 12, f. 145.

41 Edsall to Flexner, 18 June 1912, Flexner Papers, quoted by Aub and Hapgood, Edsall, p. 102.

42 Corner, Two Centuries, pp. 234–6.

43 "Draft of annual report of board of overseers, 1899–1900," St. Louis Medical Collge Minutes, 1891–1905, WashUMedA.

44 G. Baumgarten, "Report to board of directors, Washington University," 4 June 1901, WashUMedA.

45 Marjory Fox, "History of the Washington University School of Medicine," unpublished manuscript, 1949–52, WashUMedA.

46 Ibid., ch. 3; D. B. Munger, "Robert Brookings and the Flexner Report, a case study of the reorganization of medical education," J. Hist. Med.23 (1968): 356–71.

47 G. Canby Robinson, Adventures in Medical Education (Cambridge, Mass.: Harvard University Press, 1952), pp. 111–2; see also Flexner, Medical Education, pp. 258–9.

48 Dock to Opie, 31 March 1910, Opie Papers.

49 P. Shaffer to Howland and Edsall, 6 October 1912, Medical faculty minutes, WashUMedA.

50 Fox, "Washington University Medical School," ch. 4, p. 28; Eugene Opie, "Adoption of standards of the best medical schools of Western Europe by those of the United States," Perspect. Biol. Med. 13 (1970): 309–42.

51 Opie to Howland, 10 August 1910, Opie Papers. One newspaper published a wholly fictitious "interview" with Opie.

52 Shaffer et al. to David Houston, 16 April 1912, Shaffer to Graham Lusk, 24 May 1912, Shaffer Papers, box 12, f. 146.

53 Shaffer to R. A. Hatcher, 23 April 1912, Shaffer to Lusk, 24 May 1912, Shaffer Papers, box 12, f. 146.

54 Richard Beard, "Memorandum of meeting of American Hospital Association, 20 September 1910," in Medical faculty minutes, 16 November 1910, vol. 14, pp. 12–23, UMinnA.

55 J. A. Myers, Masters of Medicine: An Historical Sketch of the College of Medical Sciences, University of Minnesota, 1881–1966 (St. Louis: Green, circa 1966), pp. 90–1; Medical faculty minutes, vol. 10, pp. 25–31, vol. 11, pp. 131–3, vol. 12, pp. 123–7, vol. 13, p. 115, vol. 18, p. 11, UMinnA.

56 Various authors, The University of Texas Medical Branch Galveston (Austin: University of Texas Press, 1967).

57 Ernest E. Irons, The Story of Rush Medical College (Chicago: Rush College, 1953); John M. Dodson, "The affiliation of Rush Medical College with the University of Chicago – a historical sketch," Rush Alumni Bull. 12–17 (1917–23).

58 Klebs to L. Hektoen, 18 January 1899, UChicPP, box 57, f. 9; Loeb to Harper, 8 March and 7 July 1900, Harper to Loeb, 9 August 1900, UChicPP, box 17, f. 13.

59 Ingals to Harper, 3 August 1896, 27 January 1898, 9 February 1899, 3 May 1902, UChicPP, box 57, f. 11,12, 14.

60 Alonzo Taylor to Wheeler, 25 July 1901, UCalPP, box 8.

61 Ingals to Harper, 14 November 1899, UChicPP, box 57, f. 12.

62 Ingals to Harper, 8 February 1901, UChicPP, box 57, f. 14.

63 Ingals to Harper, 30 March 1901, UChicPP, box 57, f. 14.

64 "Statement prepared by the Committee on Rush Medical College to be sent to New York," undated (circa February 1904), UChicPP, box 58, f. 5.

65 Ingals to Harper, 29 September and 1 October 1903, UChicPP, box 57, f. 14.

66 Ingals to Harper, 13 December 1906, UChicPP, box 58, f. 12.

67 Ingals to Harper, 4 February 1907, Ingals to "Dear Doctor," 9 February 1907, UChicPP, box 57, f. 14.

68 "Statement prepared by the committee on Rush...to be sent to New York," undated (circa 1904), "Statement made October 5th 1903 by the president to the trustees concerning the proposed union of Rush...and the university," UChicPP, box 58, f. 5; John D. Rockefeller to M. A. Ryerson, 26 September 1902, UChicPP, box 58 f. 11; Ingals to Harper, 29 September 1903, UChicPP, box 57, f. 14.

69 F. T. Gates to Harper, 18 December 1895, Harper Papers, box 8, f. 22; Harper to Gates, 20 December 1895, Gates Papers, box 1, f. 12.

70 Ingals to Harper, 3 October 1904, UChicPP,.box 57, f. 14.

71 Ingals to Judson, 25 June 1907, 16 January 1908, UChicPP, box 57, f. 14.

72 "A brief sketch of the relations of the University of Illinois to medical schools," undated (circa 1912), Edmund James Papers, box 25, f. medical school memoranda 1911–12; see also Edmund James Papers, box 22, f. P&S campaign 1905.

73 Ingals to J. S. Dickerson, 2 March 1914, UChicPP, box 58, f. 13.; Edmund James to Judson, 22 November and 1 December 1913, Frank Billings to Judson, 25 May 1913, Judson to James, 5 February 1914, Ingals to James, 2 March 1914, Memorandum of meeting of Rush faculty, 28 April 1914, UChicPP, box 19, f. 11.

74 Correspondence in the Edmund James Papers, box 22, f. Medical school reorganization...1911 and box 25, f. Medical school.

75 "A plan for establishing departments of medicine and surgery in the University of Chicago," 21 November 1916, UChicPP, box 20, f. 1.

76 B. I. Wheeler and J. B. Reinstein, "Report of the Committee on Relations of Medical Department of University of California," undated (circa 1902), UCalPP, box 7. Toland had been legally part of the university since 1873, but the regents had repeatedly refused to take financial responsibility for it.

77 Verne A. Stadtman, *The University of California, 1868–1968* (Berkeley: University of California Press, 1970); Wheeler and Reinstein, "Report," pp. 5–6; D'Ancona to Wheeler, 29 September 1903, UCalPP, box 14.

78 "Plan for a university hospital..." undated (circa 1902), p.15, UCalPP, box 9, f. Flint; "Report of the Committee on Medical Status in Reference to the Chair of Anatomy," undated (circa 1901), B. I. Wheeler to Joseph Flint, 6 March 1901, other correspondence, UCalPP, boxes 6 and 8, f. Taylor; Flint to Wheeler, 14 April 1902, 3 June and 17 September 1902, Wheeler to Flint 25 April 1902, UCalPP, box 9; Correspondence with Loeb and Taylor, UCalPP, boxes 8 and 10. (Only 3 of the 14 regents opposed Wheeler's medical plans; 2 of these were physicians.) For hints of medical and other politics, see Flint to Wheeler, 3 June 1902, UCalPP, box 9; John E. Budd to Wheeler, 19 September 1902, Wheeler to Budd, 20 September 1902, UCalPP, box 10, f. Loeb.

79 Taylor to Wheeler, 11 May 1905, Wheeler to Taylor, 12 May 1905, UCalPP, box 25.

80 Taylor to Wheeler, 27 February 1901, UCalPP, box 16.

81 Wheeler to Taylor, 28 February 1901, UCalPP, box 16.

82 "Plans for a university hospital," p. 15; Flint to Wheeler, 14 April 1902, UCalPP, box 9.

83 Flint to Wheeler, 14 June 1902, UCalPP, box 9; Correspondence regarding Stanford President David Starr Jordan's eagerness to attach Cooper Medical College, UCalPP, box 40, f. Carnegie.

84 Taylor to Wheeler, 25 July 1901, UCalPP, box 8.

85 D'Ancona to Wheeler, 29 September 1903, Wheeler, "Report to the regents," 6 October 1903, UCalPP, box 14.

86 Jacques Loeb, "Memorandum," undated (circa 1902), Wheeler to Loeb, 30 September, 15 November 1902, Loeb to Wheeler, 11 October, 26 November 1902, UCalPP, box 10.

87 Wheeler to Committee of regents, 6 October 1903, UCalPP, box 10. Enrollment dropped from 166 in 1900 to 112 in 1902.

88 Taylor to Wheeler, undated (circa June 1903), UCalPP, box 8.

89 Wheeler to regents, 6 October 1903, UCalPP, box 14; "Report of the Committee on Medical Status," 12 April 1904, UCalPP, box 19; Taylor to Wheeler, 29 May 1905, UCalPP, box 25; Wheeler to Flint, 18 July and 10 December 1906, UCalPP, box 29.

90 Wheeler to Henry Pritchett, 28 May 1909, UCalPP, box 40, f. Carnegie; Wheeler to Taylor, 9 January 1909, UCalPP, box 25.

91 Wheeler to Pritchett, 28 May 1909, 11 May 1910, UCalPP, box 40, f. Carnegie.

92 Loeb to Wheeler, 29 October 1908, UCalPP, box 23; Taylor to Wheeler, 18 December 1908, UCalPP, box 25.

93 Loeb to Wheeler, 31 October 1908, UCalPP, box 23.

94 D'Ancona's letter is not extant, but the gist of it is clear from Taylor and Loeb's replies; see Loeb to Wheeler, 31 October and 18 December 1908, Loeb to the medical faculty, 28 December 1908, UCalPP, box 25. Relations between D'Ancona and Loeb were chilly; see Loeb to Wheeler, 25 January 1909, 10 October 1908, Wheeler "Memorandum," 24 October 1908, UCalPP, box 23.

95 Loeb to Wheeler, 29 and 30 October 1908, UCalPP, box 23. Taylor to Wheeler, 18 December 1908, UCalPP, box 25.

96 Loeb to Wheeler, 29 October 1908, UCalPP, box 25. Zoologist Oliver P. Jenkins had taught college biology and was interested in ichthyology.

97 Loeb to Wheeler, 31 October 1908, UCalPP, box 23. Loeb characterized Moody as "...a kind of fanatic, who seems to be working with the zeal of a paranoiac towards 'crushing' the physiological and pathological departments, which have roused his wrath by requesting to cut down the amount of teaching in his course in Osteology."

98 Wheeler to Taylor, 9 January 1909, UCalPP, box 40.

99 Pritchett to Wheeler, 7 June 1909, UCalPP, box 40.

100 Wheeler to Pritchett, 11 May 1910, UCalPP, box 40.

101 Wheeler to Pritchett, 27 April 1911, Pritchett to Wheeler, 4 May and 6 September 1911, UCalPP, box 40.

102 Colewell to Allen Smith, 27 November 1918, Medical council minutes, vol. 2, pp. 328–9, UPennA.

103 Walter Fletcher and Wilmot Herringham, "Memorandum presented to the University Grants Committee," May 1921 (London: H.M. Stationery Office, 1921).

104 For example, "Report of the special committee," 18 October 1915, Medical faculty minutes, vol. 13, pp. 365–70, UColA.

CHAPTER 7 *From medical chemistry to biochemistry*

1 "A model medical curriculum," Report of the Committee of 100...Council on Medical Education of the AMA, *Am. Med. Assoc. Bull.* 5 (15 September 1909): 54–5.

2 Bowditch to Charles W. Eliot, 5 January 1905, Eliot Papers, box 203.

3 Aub to Abel, 14 May 1910, Abel Papers

4 R. E. Kohler, "The enzyme theory and the origins of biochemistry," *Isis* 64 (1973): 181–96.

5 Alsberg to Eliot, 20 August 1908, Eliot Papers, box 200.

6 R. H. Chittenden, *The Development of Physiological Chemistry in the United States* (New York: Chemical Catalogue, 1928), pp. 34–6, 40–3.

7 Various authors, *The University of Texas Medical Branch at Galveston* (Galveston: University of Texas Press, 1967), p. 432.

8 Medical faculty minutes, 6 June 1911, vol. 3, pp. 171–2, CornMedA; see also Medical faculty minutes, vol. 4, pp. 88–9, CornMedA.

9 Data on faculty and courses are conveniently assembled in Anon., "American medical colleges," *Bull. Am. Acad. Med.*, 4 (1900): 5–6. My count excludes two-year programs in the preclinical sciences only.

10 A. L. Muirhead to Abel, 16 September, 7 November 1898, Abel Papers.

11 Marston T. Bogert, "Charles F. Chandler," *Biogr. Mem. Natl. Acad. Sci.* 14 (1931): 125–81; Robert L. Larson, "Charles Frederick Chandler: his life and work," (Ph.D. diss., Columbia University, 1950).

12 Charles E. Pellew, *Manual of Practical Medical and Physiological Chemistry* (New York: Appleton, 1892).

13 University of California *Register* (1905/6–1908/9).

14 L. B. Rey, *Northwestern University Medical School 1859–1959* (Evanston, Ill.: Northwestern University Press, 1959), pp. 470–4.

15 W. S. Carter to Abel, 20 April 1908, Abel Papers. A one-year college requirement was planned for 1910.

16 Hollis to Abel, 26 September and 28 December 1908, Abel Papers.

17 L. J. Henderson to Eliot, 24 October 1908, Eliot Papers, box 219; see also Otto Folin to Eliot, 20 October 1908, Eliot Papers, box 215.

18 Mandel to Welch, 15 April 1894, Abel Papers; W. C. McTavish, "Professor John A. Mandel," *Science* 70 (1929): 29–30.

19 George Corner, *Two Centuries of Medicine, A History of the University of Pennsylvania School of Medicine* (Philadelphia: Lippincott, 1965), pp. 189–90, 197; John H. Long, "The relation of modern chemistry to modern medicine," *Science* 20 (1904): 1–14.

20 W. H. Warren, "The study of chemistry in medical schools," *St. Louis Med. Rev.* 58 (1909): 235–40.

21 Henry Mattill to P. A. Shaffer, 24 August 1936, Shaffer Papers, box 8, f. 81; University of Iowa *Calendar* 1900/1, pp. 386–7.

22 Harvard University *Catalogue* (1895/6), p. 430, (1896/7 p. 450.

23 Various authors, *Texas Medical Branch*, p. 42.

24 Hills to Eliot, 29 February and 4 March 1904, Eliot Papers, box 220.

25 Otto Folin, Untitled memorandum, "Folin Mins," undated (circa 1920), Shaffer Papers, box 6, f. 60.

26 Philip Shaffer, Untitled address on the 50th anniversary of the ABSC, 18 April 1956, pp. 5–6, Shaffer Papers, box 2, f. 18.

27 R. H. Chittenden, "Some of the present-day problems of biological chemistry," *Science* 27 (1908): 241–54 (quotation is from pp. 253–4).

28 "Model medical curriculum," p. 60.

29 Various authors, discussion, *Proc. Am. Assoc. Med. Coll.* 16 (1906): pp. 40–2, 45.

30 F. S. Lee, "What medical subjects can be taught efficiently in the literary school?" *Proc. Am. Assoc. Med. Coll.* 16 (1906): 19–25, (quotation is from pp. 21–22).

31 Ibid., various authors' discussion, pp. 23, 47–8.

32 C. Judson Herrick, "What medical subjects can be taught eficiently in the literary college?" *Proc. Am. Assoc. Med. Coll.* 16 (1906): 34–8. Herrick put physiological chemistry at 13 in a list of 14 subjects likely to be taught satisfactorily in literary colleges: only toxicology, human anatomy, and pathology ranked lower.

33 F. C. Waite, "What medical subjects can be taught efficiently in the college of liberal arts?" *Proc. Am. Assoc. Med. Coll.* 16 (1906): 25–33.

34 Ibid., p. 29. Waite felt that 100 to 200 of the 300 hours devoted to general, organic, and physiological chemistry in medical courses could be done in colleges. See also George M. Kober, "The past and present status of medical education in this country," *Proc. Am. Assoc. Med. Coll.* 17 (1907): 26–30.

35 "Model medical curriculum," pp. 55–6. The committee representing organic and physiological chemistry and physiology consisted of seven physiologists and only two biochemists (Otto Folin and A. P. Mathews).

36 Medical faculty minutes, 16 November 1896, 18 January 1897, 15 February 1897, vol. 8, pp. 185–6, 190–2, UColA. Chandler's critics had long felt that he was making himself rich by spreading himself thin.

37 Curtis to Seth Low, 2 February 1897, UColCF. The committee consisted of Low, Dean James McLean, Curtis, and Prudden.

39 Ibid.

40 Curtis to Low, 6 February 1897, UColCF.

41 Curtis to Low, 2 February 1897, Curtis to Low, 21 December 1896, Low to Curtis, 22 December 1896, UColCF.

42 Curtis to Low, 14 February 1897, UColCF.

43 Low to Curtis, 10 February 1897, Curtis to Low, 11 February 1897, UColCF.

44 Curtis to Low, 20 March 1897, UColCF.

45 "Report of committee," 19 April 1897, Medical faculty minutes, vol. 8, p. 196, UColA: Curtis to Low, 14 and 15 February 1897, UColCF.

47 "Report of Dean James W. McLane," 16 January 1899, Medical faculty minutes, vol. 8, pp. 325, UColA.

48 Butler to Chittenden, 14 December 1901, Chittenden to Butler, 2 December 1901, UColCF.

49 Medical faculty minutes, 21 March and 18 April 1898, vol. 9, p. 76, UColA; "Report of Committee on Curriculum on Entrance Examinations," 20 January 1902, Medical faculty minutes vol. 9, pp. 283, 290, UColA; Gies to Low, 11 October 1900, UColCF.

50 "Report of the Committee on Curriculum on Entrance Examinations," 20 January 1902, Medical faculty minutes, vol. 9, pp. 283–90, UColA; Gies to Butler, 19 January 1904, UColCF.

51 Medical faculty minutes, 18 January 1904, vol. 10, pp. 196–7, UColA; Gies to Butler, 11, 16, and 19 January 1904, UColCF.

52 Medical faculty minutes, 19 December 1904, 20 February 1905, vol. 10, pp. 325, 362–3, UColA.

53 Alfred C. Redfield, "The laboratories of physiology of the Harvard Medical School," *Methods Probl. Med. Educ.* 3 (1925): 19–34.

54 Harvard University *Catalogue* (1898/9), 535, (1899/1900), 560; Undated memorandum, "Department salaries," circa 1903, Eliot Papers, box 119, f. 304. On Pfaff, see Harry Trimble Papers, f. Pharmacology History, and A. S. Loevenhart to Abel, 17 January 1909, Abel Papers.

55 Medical faculty minutes, 5 May 1900, 5 January, 2 February, and 6 April 1901, vol. 6, pp. 31, 78–9, 90, HarvUMedA.

56 Bowditch to Eliot, 13 August 1902, Eliot Papers, box 102, f. 26.

57 Medical faculty minutes, 15 November 1899, 7 April 1900, vol. 6 pp. 1–2, 27–8, HarvUMedA. Chemist T. W. Richards had suggested to Bowditch that they try to get Emil Fischer for the new chair.

58 Cannon to Eliot, 28 October 1904, Eliot Papers, box 205.

59 Bowditch to Eliot, 6 December 1905, Eliot papers, box 203.

60 Gies to Butler, 15 June 1905, Gies to F. Keppel, 11 July 1905, UColCF.

61 Jackson to Eliot, 9 June 1905, Eliot Papers, box 222. Jackson suggested Arthur A. Noyes, head of the physical chemistry laboratory at MIT, or James M. Crafts, emeritus president of MIT and a distinguished technical chemist.

62 L. J. Henderson, "Memories," pp. 121–2, Henderson Papers; Harvard University *Catalogue* (1905/6–1906/7). Henderson's appointment was undoubtedly due to Jackson and Richards; see Jackson to Eliot, 20 September 1905, Eliot Papers, box 222.

63 Henderson, "Memories," pp. 86, 121, Henderson Papers; W. B. Cannon, "Lawrence J. Henderson," *Biogr. Mem. Natl. Acad. Sci.* 23 (1943): 31–58.

64 C. W. Eliot, Memorandum, undated (circa 27 May 1907), Eliot Papers, box 222, f. Jackson.

65 D. Bruce Dill, "The Harvard Fatigue Laboratory. Its development, contributions, and demise," *Circ. Res.,* Suppl. vols. 20 and 21 (March 1967): 161–70; Henderson, "Memories," pp. 75–6, Henderson Papers.

66 Eliot, Memorandum undated; Eliot did not mention Folin's two 1905 papers on the theory of protein metabolism. P. A. Shaffer, "Otto Knut Folin," *Biogr. Mem. Natl. Acad. Sci.* 27 (1952): 47–82.

67 Henderson, "Memories," p. 48; Joseph S. Davis, ed., *Carl Alsbrg, Scientist at Large* (Palo Alto, Calif.: Stanford University Press, 1948); Carl Alsberg, "Mechanisms of cell activity," *Science* 34 (1911): 97–105. Like Franz Hofmeister, Alsberg was interested in the organization of chemical reactions in the cell.

68 Alfred Kroeber, "The Making of the Man," in Joseph S. Davis, ed., *Carl Alsberg, Scientist àt Large* (Palo Alto, Calif.: Stanford University Press, 1948), pp. 3–22.

69 Henderson, "Memories."

70 Loeb to Welch, 8 March 1898, Abel Papers; see also Welch to Abel, 16 March 1898, Abel Papers.

71 Folin to Eliot, 27 August, 23 September, and 24 October 1908, Eliot Papers, box 213; see also Henderson to Eliot, 14 November 1907, 7 January, 24 October and 2 November 1908, Eliot Papers, box 219.

72 Bloor to Shaffer, 6 June 1949, Shaffer Papers, box 6, f. 60. I know of no corroborating evidence for Bloor's assertion. However, Folin did mention to Abel that Faust had been mentioned for a chair of pharmaology (probably by Henderson); see Folin to Abel, 6 May 1909, Abel Papers.

73 Alsberg to Eliot, 20 August 1908; Eliot Papers, box 200.

74 Folin to Eliot, 27 August 1908, Eliot Papers, box 213.

75 Alsberg to Eliot, 8 and 12 September 1908, Folin to Eliot, 27 August and 23 September 1908, Eliot Papers, box 213.

76 Folin to Eliot, 23 September 1908, Eliot Papers, box 213; Henderson, "Memories," pp. 163–4.

77 Jackson to Eliot, 11 January 1908, Jackson to Eliot, 20 September 1905; Eliot Papers, box 222. Jackson's testimonial may in fact have moved Eliot to keep Henderson at Harvard in 1905; see Eliot to Jackson, 15 January 1908, Eliot Papers, box 222.

78 Jackson to Eliot, 11 January 1908, Richards to Eliot, 29 January 1908, Eliot Papers, box 243.

79 Shaffer to Trimble, 10 June 1954, Trimble Papers, box 2. Although Shaffer did half his dissertation work with Folin, the Harvard chemists did not invite Folin to his dissertation examination. Th representative of the medical school was a professor from the Department of Public Health.

80 Folin to Eliot, 24 October and 9 November 1908, Eliot Papers, box 213; Richards to Eliot, 30 October and 19 November 1908, Joseph Warren to Richards, November 1908, Eliot Papers, box 243.

81 Henderson, "Memories," pp. 163–4.

82 Hawk to Lewis, 24 May 1952, Lewis Papers, box 1. Demonstrator was a rank equivalent to assistant professor.

83 Budget figures were compiled from the Medical Council minutes for the period from 1905 to 1914, UPennA.

84 Harrison to Marshall, 23 March and 28 April 1910, Harrison to Charles Frazier, 31 December 1910, in Provost's Letterpress, vol. 8, pp. 494–5, vol. 9, pp. 37, 187–8, UPennA.

85 Washington University *Register* (1908/9), pp. 167, 177–8; (1910/11), p. 205.

86 Shaffer to Dean Allison, 14 February 1922, p. 4, Deans' files, box 6, WashUMedA.

87 Warren to Shaffer, 4 April 1912; Warren to Shaffer, 5 ovember 1911, Shaffer Papers, box 12, f. 146; see also Warren to Terry, 18 June 1911, Terry Papers, box 11, f. 78. From Richards to E. A. Alderman, 26 April 1906, Alderman Papers, box 17: "He is essentially an organic chemist still, with . . . technical and physiological interests superposed. . . . His many duties have prevented him from publishing, . . . but he is by no means deficient in originality or power of thought."

88 Warren, "Study of chemistry," p. 238.

89 Opie and Howland to Dock, 15 May 1910, Opie Papers.
90 Dock to Erlanger, 12 May 1910, Opie Papers; Erlanger to Dock, 10/11 May 1910, Opie and Howland to Dock, 9 and 12 May 1910; Dock to Opie, 6 and 10 May 1910, Opie Papers; Shaffer to E. S. West, 20 November 1954, Shaffer Papers, box 11, f. 124.
91 Opie and Howland to Dock, 15 May 1910, Opie Papers.
92 Ibid. They regarded Alsberg as a good chemist but unoriginal in research.
93 Medical faculty minutes, 28 February 1899, 15 March 1901, 26 Mach 1901, vol. 1, p. 177 and vol. 2, pp. 80–4, CornMedA; "Report of Committee on Entrance Requirements," 6 May 1901, minutes 15 November 1901, 25 April 1902, vol. 2, pp. 88–94, 99–104, CornMedA.
94 Medical faculty minutes, 20 November 1908, vol. 3, p. 61, CornMedA; Cornell University Register (1909/10), pp. 271–2. Hawk's *Manual* was the only text.
95 Wolf to Shaffer, 21 January 1910, Shaffer papers, box 12, f. 145.
96 Shaffer to West, 20 November 1954, Shaffer Papers, box 11, f. 124. Shaffer felt that Ewing and Lusk never quite forgave his leaving Cornell for the "wild and raw west."
97 Lusk to Shaffer, 5 April 1911, Hatcher to Shaffer, 21 and 26 February 1911, Shaffer to Hatcher, 22 February 1911, Shaffer to Lusk, 25 April 1911, Shaffer Papers, box 12, f. 145.
98 Medical faculty minutes, 3 May 1918 and December 1919, vol. 4, pp. 186, 259, CornMedA; E. V. McCollum, "Stanley Rossiter Benedict," *Biogr. Mem. Natl. Acad. Sci.* 27 (1952): 155–77.
99 Verne Stadtman, *The University of California 1868–1968* (New York: McGraw-Hill, 1970), p. 128; University of California *Register* (1900/1–1901/2).
100 Jacques Loeb memorandum to B. I. Wheeler, undated, (circa September 1902), Wheeler to Loeb, 30 September 1902, Wheeler to A. W. Foster, 17 September 1902, UCalPP, box 10.
101 Taylor to Wheeler, undated (circa 6 February 1903), UCalPP, box 16. Lachman subsequently set up a consulting practice in San Francisco in organic chemistry and chemical engineering.
102 Wheeler to Taylor, 9 February 1903, UCalPP, box 16.
103 University of California *Register* (1902/3), pp. 366–8, (1903/4), pp. 239–40, (1904/5), pp. 352–3; O'Neill to Wheeler, 3 September 1908, UCalPP, box 23.
104 Loeb to Wheeler, 10 April 1905, UCalPP, box 23. Taylor told Wheeler that Green was an excellent analyst but not qualified to teach physiological chemistry; see Taylor to Wheeler, 8 May 1905, UCalPP, box 25.
105 Taylor t Wheeler, 8 May 1905, UCalPP, box 25.
106 Taylor to Wheeler, 14 August 1904 and undated (circa August 1904), UCalPP, box 24; A. E. Taylor, "On Fermentation," *Univ. Cal. Pub. Pathol.* (1904).
107 Taylor to Wheeler, 26 December 1908, 31 May 1909, Taylor to the medical faculty, 28 December 1908, UCalPP, box 25; Taylor to Loeb, 9 October 1908, Loeb Papers.
108 Wheeler to Taylor, 9 January and 28 May 1909, UCalPP, box 25.
109 Taylor to Wheeler, 2 July 1909, UCalPP, box 25.
110 Wheeler to Taylor, 7 July 1909, UCalPP, box 25.
111 Taylor to Wheeler, 7 September 1909, UCalPP, box 25.
112 Taylor to Loeb, 14 February 1910, Loeb papers.
113 University of Cincinnati *Catalogue* (1905/6), p. 12, (1906/7), pp. 196–200, (1910/11), pp. 253–4. University of Cincinnati, *Record* (1910/1), pp. 12–13.
114 University of Minnesota *Catalogue* (1909/10) pp. 45–6; E. P. Lyon, "Richard Olding Beard, 1865–1936," *Minn. Med.19 (1936): 683. Beard was himself interested in chemical aspects of physiology.*
115 *Medical faculty minutes, 1 March 1913, vol. 19, UMinnA; J. A. Myers, Masters of Medicine: An Historical Sketch of the College of Medical Sciences, University of Minnesota, 1881–1966* (St. Louis: Green, circa 1968); J. A. Myers, "Elias Potter Lyon, M. D.," *Lancet 85* (1965); 404–10.
116 Lyon to Shaffer, 4 June 1919, Shaffer Papers, box 9, f. 92.

117 "Minutes of the conference regarding the dean of the medical school," 30 September 1930, especially pp. 44–5; "Minutes of a meeting," 15 October 1930, UMinPP.
118 Orndorff to Abel, 28 February 1903, Abel Papers; Cornell University *Catalogue* (1897/8–1904/5).
119 Orndorff to Abel, 19 October 1908, Abel Papers. Orndorff was a student of Ira Remsen (Ph.D., 1887); see Cornell University *Catalogue* (1908/9–1909/10).
120 L. A. Maynard, "James B. Sumner," *Biogr. Mem. Natl. Acad. Sci.* 31(1958): 376–96.
121 F. C. Waite, *Western Reserve University Centennial History of the School of Medicine* (Cleveland: Western Reserve University Press, 1946), pp. 375–6, 390–2. Western Reserve *Catalogue* (1903/4), pp. 161–2, 173. Fiske was at Cleveland from 1915 to 1918 as successor to Howard Haskins, a professor of chemistry in the School of Pharmacy. Haskins had taught organic and biochemistry.
122 University of Virginia *Catalogues* (1905/6–1918/19); Kastle to Edwin A. Alderman, 17 December 1909 and other documents in the Alderman Papers, box 17. I owe thanks to Jeffrey Sturchio for this reference.
123 Paul F. Clark, *The University of Wisconsin Medical School, A Chronicle, 1848–1948* (Madison: University of Wisconsin Press, 1967), pp. 15–16; Harold C. Bradley to Joseph Erlanger, 5 September 1906, correspondence with Loevenhart 1908, Erlanger Papers, box 13, f. 136.
124 "Model medical curriculum," *Am. Med. Assoc. Bull.* 5 (15 September 199): 51–2.
125 Medical council minutes, 13 February 1911, vol. 1, pp. 361–3, UPennA. The 23 medical schools were: Harvard, Columbia, Johns Hopkins, Wisconsin, Michigan, Chicago/Rush, Minnesota, Western Reserve, Cornell, Yale, Washington University, California, Stanford, Syracuse, Virginia, Missouri, North and South Dakota, Utah, Northwestern, Toronto, McGill, Southern California, and Indiana.

CHAPTER 8 *Unity in diversity: the American Society of Biological Chemists*

1 Shaffer, "To the members of the executive faculty," December 1915, Shaffer Papers, box 5, f. 37; Shaffer to Flexner, 16 March 1920, GEB, B19, box 701; Shaffer to Flexner, 16 March 1921, Shaffer Papers, box 6, f. 37.
2 Taylor to A. Flexner, 1 June 1921, GEB, B19, box 701.
3 Simon Flexner to Abraham Flexner, 5 March 1920, GEB, B19, box 701.
4 Folin to A. Flexner, 18 March 1920, GEB, B19, box 701.
5 Folin to A. Flexner, 9 March 1920, GEB, B19, box 701; Memorandum, "Department of Biochemistry, Schools of Medicine," GEB, B19, box 701.
6 Shaffer to A. Flexner, 20 December 1921, Shaffer papers, box 6, f. 57.
7 Long to Abel, 23 October 1907, Richards to Abel, 18 December 1908, Abel Papers.
8 "Report of the Committee on the Rearrangement of Studies of the First and Second Years," Medical faculty minutes, vol. 14, pp. 67–70, UColA.
9 Untitled manuscript, "Folin Mins," undated (circa 1920), Shaffer Papers, box 60, f. 60. O. Folin, "Teaching of biological chemistry," *J. Am. Med. Assoc.* 74 (1920): 823–6.
10 A. P. Mathews, *Physiological Chemistry, A Text-Book and Manual for Students* (New York: Wood, 1915). The sixth and last edition appeared in 1939. Also see A. B. Macallum to Loeb, 1 March 1922; Loeb to Macallum, 8 March 1922, Loeb Papers; Arthur Cushny to Abel, 31 December 1907; Christian Herter to Abel, 15 October 1905, Abel Papers. E. N. Harvey, "Albert Prescott Mathews, Biochemist," *Science* 127 (1958): 743–4. Harvey writes that Mathews's book "...appeared at just the right time to inspire many a student to decide on a career in this rapidly growing...subject."
11 Gies to Shaffer, 3 January 1917, 4 December 1916, Shaffer Papers, box 7, f. 65. Idiosyncratically, Gies classified Philip Hawk, Walter Jones, A. P. Mathews, L. B. Mendel, and T. B. Robertson as "physiological chemists;" Otto Folin, W. B.

Macallum, and Philip Shaffer as "biological chemists;" Andrew Hunter, Victor Myers, and Frank Underhill as "pathological chemists;" Stanly Benedict, John Mandel, John Marshall, and Elbert Rockwood as "chemists."

12 R. E. Kohler, "The enzyme theory and the origin of biochemistry," *Isis* 64 (1973): 181–96.

13 "The Biochemical Club, minutes of committee meetings, 1911–1920," 8 July 1911, pp. 4–10, UCLonA; Herter to Abel, 24 May 1902, 30 October 1904, subsequent correspondence, Abel Papers.

14 Herter to Abel, 25 April 1907, Herter to Abel, 11 October 1906, Abel Papers. Herter took no role in organizing the ASBC.

15 Lewis to J. S. Fruton, 3 November 1952, Lewis Papers. Lewis noted that the organic chemists objected to his using the name "biochemistry" because they felt it might be construed as including bioorganic chemistry. They had no such objection to "biological chemistry."

16 Fruton to Lewis, 29 October 1952, Lewis Papers. Fruton adopted the name "biological chemistry" to signify a new emphasis on connections with the basic sciences and on graduate training.

17 R. H. A. Plimmer, *The History of the Biochemical Society 1911–1949* (Cambridge University Press, 1949); R. A. Morton, *The Biochemical Society. Its History and Activities 1911–1969* (London: Biochemical Society, 1969).

18 Alsberg to W. D. Bancroft, 3 November 1910, Wilder Bancroft Papers. I owe thanks to John W. Servos for this reference.

19 O. T. Williams, "Christian A. Herter," *Biochem. J.* 5 (1911): xxi–xxxi. R. M. Hawthorne, "Christian A. Herter," *Perspect. Biol. Med.* 18 (1974): 24–39.

20 Abel to Edmund James, undated (circa fall 1906); Harry Grindley to Abel, 3 January 1906, Abel Papers; see also correspondence in the James and Underhill Papers.

21 Abel to James, 29 May 1907, James to Abel, 2 January 1907, Abel Papers.

22 Gies, "American Society of Biological Chemists," *Science* 25 (1907): 139–42.

23 Gies to Abel, 8 January 1906, Abel Papers.

24 Gies to Abel, 13 November and 23 December 1906, Abel Papers.

25 Herter to Abel, 24 May 1903, Abel to Chittenden, 13 December 1906, Abel Papers.

26 Ibid. Also see Gies to Abel, undated (circa 10 December 1906), 12 December 1906, Abel Papers.

27 Abel to Mendel, 15 December 1906, Abel Papers.

28 Gies to Abel, 17 and 23 December 1906, Abel Papers.

29 Gies to Abel, 17 December 1906, Abel Papers.

30 Gies to Abel, 13 November 1906, Gies to Abel, 17 and 23 December 1906, Abel Papers.

31 Herter to Abel, 17 January 1908, Abel Papers.

32 Gies to Abel, 2 and 12 January, 22 March 1907, Grindley to Abel, 3 January 1907, Herter to Abel, 17 January 1908, Abel Papers.

33 Gies to Abel, 13 November 1906, Abel Papers.

34 Abel to Mendel, 15 December 1906, Abel Papers.

35 R. H. Chittenden, *The First Twenty-Five Years of the American Society of Biological Chemists* (New Haven, Conn.: at the Society, 1945), pp. 6–7. Two of the 81 founders could not be identified.

36 Gies to Abel, 12 December 1906, Abel Papers.

37 Benedict to Shaffer, 26 January 1915, Shaffer Papers, box 4, f. 28.

38 F. E. Breithut, "The status and compensation of the chemist in public service," *J. Ind. Eng. Chem.* 9 (1917): 64–79.

39 A. H. Dupree, *Science in the Federal Government* (Cambridge, Mass.: Harvard University Press, 1959); Stephen P. Strickland, *Politics, Science, and Dread Disease* (Cambridge, Mass.: Harvard University Press, 1972), ch. 1.

40 Alsberg to Abel, 18 December 1908, Abel Papers. Joseph S. Davis, ed., *Carl Alsberg, Scientist at Large* (Palo Alto, Calif.: Stanford University Press, 1948).

41 Clark to Joseph Ames, 25 May 1927, JHUMedA, f. Clark. Clark's team in 1926 consisted of five experienced assistants with Ph.D. degrees, three half-time assistants, two technicians, and a secretary. His research budget was $56,000 per annum. Few university departments could offer such amenities.

42 George W. Corner, *A History of the Rockefeller Institute 1901–1953* (New York: Rockefeller Institute Press, 1964); H. H. Donaldson, "Research foundations in their relation to medicine," *Science* 36 (1912): 65–74.

43 Nathan Reingold, "The case of the disappearing laboratory," *Am. Quar.* 29 (1977): 79–101; Stanley Coben, "Foundation officers and fellowships: innovation in the patronage of science," *Minerva* 14 (1976): 225–40.

44 Gies to N. M. Butler, 15 June and 17 October 1905, Gies to F. Keppel, 11 July 1905, UColCF.

45 Gies to Butler, 25 March 1913, Gies to Fackenthal, 28 June 1912, 10 July 1914, Gies to S. Lambert, 9 July 1917, UColCF.

46 Mathews to Abel, 19 April 1898, Folin to Abel, 4 July and 5 August 1898, Folin to Chittenden, 21 January 1898, Chittenden to Welch, 1 March 1898, Welch to Abel, 16 March and 3 May 1898, Folin to Howell, 22 February 1898, Loeb to Welch, 8 March 1898, Abel Papers; Otto Folin, "My scientific work," Folin Papers.

47 Eliot, Memorandum, 27 May 1907, Eliot Papers, box 222, f. Jackson.

48 Folin to Abel, undated (circa 1909), Abel Papers.

49 A. Flexner, *Medical Education in the United States and Canada* (New York: Carnegie Foundation, 1910), p. 71.

50 Abel to T. H. Sollman, 16 January 1908, R. H. Whitehead to Abel, 19 January 1908, Abel Papers.

51 Gies to Butler, 28 September 1907, 29 February 1908, UColCF; Gies to Abel, 17 October 1907, Abel Papers.

52 See Chittenden's annual reports in "Reports of the President of Yale University," 1898–1914.

53 Mendel to Lewis, 9 September 1913, Lewis Papers, box 3; Mendel to A. J. Carlson, 10 March 1924, UChicPP, box 17, f. 13.

54 "Memorial from the Ogden School of Science to the acting president," 26 January 1907, Minutes of the Faculty of the College of Arts, Literature and Science, UChicA, box 1.

55 Gies to Butler, 27 January and 4 February 1911, Butler to S. W. Lambert, 16 January 1911, UColCF.

56 Benjamin Harrow, Manuscript recollections of Gies (1956), Clarke Papers, f. Gies: "Gies was of German descent and ruled like the traditional Prussian. The people in the lab feared him. But he had his good side. Though he gave everybody hell sooner or later – including his assistant professors – he was always ready to defend his boys from outside attack."

57 Gies to Abel, 23 December 1906, Herter to Abel, 24 September and 12 November 1907, 13 November 1908, subsequent correspondence, Abel Papers.

58 Mathews to Abel, 1 March 1909, Gies to Abel, 7 and 14 November 1908, Chittenden to Abel, 25 November and 10 December 1908, Abel Papers.

59 Herter to Abel, 12 November and 15 December 1908, Abel Papers.

60 Herter to Abel, 23 March 1907, Abel Papers.

61 Herter to Abel, 21 February 1910, Abel Papers.

CHAPTER 9 *The clinical connection: biochemistry as applied science*

1 R. E. Kohler, "Medical reform and biomedical science: biochemistry, a case study," in Morris J. Vogel and Charles E. Rosenberg, eds., *The Therapeutic Revolution* (Philadelphia: University of Pennsylvania Press, 1979), pp. 27–66.

2 Gerald L. Geison, "Divided we stand: physiologists and clinicians in the American context," in Vogel and Rosenberg, eds., *Therapeutic Revolution*, pp. 67–90.

3 Russell C. Maulitz, " 'Physician versus biochemist': the ideology of science in clinical medicine," in Vogel and Rosenberg, eds., *Therapeutic Revolution*, pp. 91–107.

4 Samuel J. Meltzer, "The science of clinical medicine, what it ought to be and the men to uphold it," *J. Am. Med. Assoc.* 53 (1909): 508–12.
5 Taylor to Wheeler, 18 December 1908, UCalPP, box 25. Taylor was referring to Richard C. Cabot and W. T. Councilman.
6 Loeb to Wheeler, 29 and 31 October 1908, UCalPP, box 23.
7 Gies to Dean Hallock, 9 June 1906, pp. 2–3, Gies to S. W. Lambert, 28 September 1911, Gies to Butler, 10 June 1915, UColCF.
8 Medical faculty minutes, 18 March and 2 April 1913, WashUMedA.
9 See correspondence in GEB, B19, box 701.
10 Hollis to Abel, 26 September 1908, Abel Papers.
11 Christian to Eliot, 1 February 1909, Eliot Papers, box 207; see also Christian to Eliot, 23 January 1909, Eliot Papers, box 207.
12 Folin, Untitled typescript, Shaffer Papers, box 6, f. 60.
13 J. R. Angell to Harry P. Judson, 12 January 1912, UChicPP, box 58, f. 5; E. F. Ingals to J. Spencer Dickerson, 2 March 1914, UChicPP, box 58, f. 13; "Excerpt from a report made to the president on a proposed plan for medical expansion," 1912, UChicPP, box 59, f. 3; J. R. Angell, "Report of a meeting of Rush medical college faculty..." 28 April 1914, other correspondence, UChicPP, box 19, f. 10, and box 20, f. 11.
14 Angell to Judson, 12 January 1912, Herrick to Angell, 11 January 1912, Preston Keyes to Angell, 18 January 1912, Carlson to Angell, 12 January 1912, UChicPP, box 58, f. 5.
15 Wells to Angell, 16 January 1912, UChicPP, box 58, f. 5; E. R. Long, "Harry Gideon Wells, 1875–1943," *Biogr. Mem. Natl. Acad. Sci.* 26 (1949): 233–261. Wells was a student of Chittenden's (Ph.D., 1895).
16 Mathews to Abel, 22 November and 9 December 1908, Abel Papers. Mathews felt that the new American Society for Pharmacology should limit the number of physician members, to keep it "out of the clutches of the clinical men."
17 Shaffer to A. Flexner, 20 December 1921, Shaffer Papers, box 6, f. 57.
18 Shaffer to Opie, 13 August 1910, Opie Papers, f. Erlanger. Shaffer located his laboratories so as to be close to those of Opie and John Howland.
19 Eliot, Memorandum, 27 May 1907, Eliot Papers, box 213.
20 Gies to Dean Hallock, 9 June 1906, Gies, "Memorandum on Department of Biological Chemistry," enclosed in Gies to Butler, 9 February 1911, UColCF.
21 Hollis to Abel, 19 June 1911, Abel Papers.
22 Hatcher to Shaffer, 26 February 1911, Shaffer Papers.
23 Cole to Underhill, 27 May and 10 June 1910, Underhill Papers.
24 S. J. Meltzer, "Science of clinical medicine," p. 509; S. J. Meltzer, "Headships and organization of clinical departments," *Science* 40 (1914): 620–8.
25 For example, Lewellys F. Barker, "Medicine and the university," *Am. Med.* 4 (1902): 143–7.
26 S. J. Meltzer, "Chairman's address," *Congr. Sci. Arts* 5 (1904): 395.
27 Meltzer, "Science of clinical medicine," p. 510; J. H. Pratt, "The method of science in clinical training," *Boston Med. Surg. J.* 166 (1912): 835–42.
28 L. F. Barker, "On the cultivation of the clinical sciences of diagnosis and therapy," *Science* 37 (1913): 731–8.
29 S. J. Meltzer, "Headships," p. 627; W. H. Warren, "The study of chemistry in medical schools," *St. Louis Med. Rev.* 58 (1909): 235–40 (quotation is from p. 237).
30 Douglas Symmers, "Defects in the teaching of pathology and the lay professor," *J. Am Med. Assoc.* 73 (1919): 1651–5; Graham Lusk, "On the proposed reorganization of departments of clinical medicine in the United States," *Science* 41 (1915): 531–4; A. P. Mathews, "Comments," *Proc. Am. Assoc. Med. Coll.* 13 (1920): 107–17.
31 David Edsall, "Scheme for correlation in medical teaching," 7 December 1907, Medical council minutes, vol. I, pp. 152–6, UPennA.
32 "Report of the committee on the scheme of correlation in teaching," 25 March 1908, 10 October 1910, Medical council minutes, vol. I, pp. 162–7, 326, UPennA.
33 Taylor to Wheeler, 18 December 1908, UCalPP, box 25.

34 Yandell Henderson, "Clinical physiology – an opportunity and a duty," *J. Am. Med. Assoc.* 57 (1911): 857–9; R. G. Hoslans, "The correlation of clinical teaching and physiology," *Lancet Clin.* 107 (1912): 351–3.

34 Hugh Cabot, A. C. Abbott, B. D. Myers, A. S. Begg, and R. L. Wilbur, "Report of committee on curriculum," *Proc. Am. Assoc. Med. Coll.* 32 (1922): 73–91.

36 Richard M. Pearce, "Report of committee on education," 16 January 1914, Richard M. Pearce, "Report of committee on education in regard to elective course," January 1914, Graham Lusk, "On optional courses for the Cornell University Medical College." Medical faculty minutes, vol. 4, pp. 15–20, 25–26, 27–30, CornMedA.

37 Abel to Mathews, 19 November 1908, Abel Papers.

38 Shaffer to Dean Allison, 14 February 1922, pp. 7–8, Medical Deans' Papers, box 6, f. biol. chem, WashUMedA.

39 Folin to A. Flexner, 9 March 1920, Jones to Flexner, 9 March 1920, Shaffer to A. Flexner, 16 March 1920, GEB, B19, box 701.

40 P. A. Shaffer, Untitled address, 18 April 1956, Shaffer Papers, box 2, f. 18; Lusk, "On the proposed reorganization," pp. 531–4.

41 Christian to Eliot, 29 May and 5 June 1908, 1 February 1909, Eliot Papers, box 207; Dock to A. Flexner, 23 December 1913, Shaffer to Flexner, 6 July 1916, GEB, 2495, box 688.

42 Howland to Shaffer, 16 November 1917, Shaffer Papers, box 2, f. 18; correspondence with W. McKim Marriott, Shaffer Papers, box 13, f. 156.

43 Maurice B. Visscher to Hastings, 2 May 1928; Hastings to Visscher, 19 May 1928, Hastings Papers. Visscher was professor of physiology at the University of Tennessee.

44 Paul Starr, "Medicine and the waning of professional sovereignty," *Daedalus* 107 (1978): 175–93.

45 Shaffer to Flexner, 10 March 1920, GEB, B19, box 701.

46 Folin to A. Flexner, 10 March 1920, GEB, B19, box 701.

47 Hugh Cabot et al., "Report of committee," p. 76. A. Flexner, "Memorandum for Mr. Rockefeller re College of P & S," 21 December 1920, Cannon to Flexner, 10 March 1920, GEB, B19, box 701; Lyon to Burton, 30 April 1921; Cabot to Burton, 3 April 1921, Burton Papers.

48 Joseph Erlanger, C. M. Jackson, G. Lusk, W. S. Thayer, V. C. Vaughan, "An investigation of the conditions in the departments of the preclinical sciences," *J. Am. Med. Assoc.* 74 (1920): 1117–22.

49 Hugh Cabot, "The development of organized clinical teaching," *Colo. Med.* 22 (1925): 130–8; Louis B. Wilson, "The present status of the preclinical branches," *Chicago Med. Rec.* (November 1920): 1–6; Hugh Cabot et al., "Report of committee," p. 76; J. A. Myers, "Bridging the chasm between the fundamental and clinical branches in medical schools," *J. Am. Med. Assoc.* 81 (1925): 599–601.

50 Douglas Symmer, "Defects in the teaching of pathology and the lay professor," *J. Am. Med. Assoc.* 73 (1919): 1651–5; C. R. Stockard, "The laboratory professor and the medical sciences in the U.S.," *J. Am. Med. Assoc.* 74 (1920): 229–35.

51 Charles P. Emerson, "Professors and clinical professors of clinical subjects," *Proc. Assoc. Am. Med. Coll.* 32 (1922): 41–9 (for quotation, see pp. 45–6).

52 Otto Folin, Untitled typescript, Shaffer Papers, box 6, f. 60; O. Folin, P. A. Shaffer, and A. P. Mathews, "Report on teaching of biochemistry," *Proc. Assoc. Am. Med. Coll.* 13 (1920): 107–17 (reprinted in *J. Am. Med. Assoc.* 74 (1920): 823–6).

53 Contemporary handbooks of urinalysis give a good picture of the state of the art; for example, see H. Sahli, *A Treatise on Diagnostic Methods*, 4th ed. (Philadelphia: Saunders, 1907).

54 William D. Foster, *A Short History of Clinical Pathology* (Edinburgh: Livingstone, 1961); Joel Stanley Reiser, *Medicine and the Reign of Technology* (Cambridge University Press, 1978).

55 P. A. Shaffer, Untitled address, 18 April 1956, pp. 4–5, Shaffer Papers, box 2, f. 18.

56 P. A. Shaffer, "Otto Folin," *Biogr. Mem. Natl. Acad. Sci.* 27 (1952): 47–82; Lewis A. Conner, "Relation of laboratory aids to the practice of medicine and surgery," *J. Am. Med. Assoc.* 81 (1923): 871–3; George Dock, "Clinical pathology in the eighties and nineties," *Am. J. Clin. Pathol.* 16 (1956): 671–80.

57 Richard C. Cabot, "The limitations of urinary diagnosis," *Johns Hopkins Hosp. Bull.* 15 (1904): 174–7.

58 Charles P. Emerson, "Some clinical aspects of chemistry," *J. Am. Med. Assoc.* (1902): 1359–62 (for quotation, see p. 1359).

59 John H. Long, "The chemistry of the medical school," *J. Am. Med. Assoc.* 14 (1904): 946–7; H. Leffman, "Some applications of physical chemistry to problems in medicine," *Boston Med. Surg. J.* 174 (1916): 688–90; R. C. Cabot, "The historical development and relative value of laboratory and clinical methods of diagnosis," *Boston Med. Surg. J.* 157 (1907): 150–3.

60 Lewellys F. Barker, "Medical laboratories: their relationship to medical practice and to medical discovery," *Science* 27 (1908): 601–11 (for quotation, see pp. 607–8).

61 A. Flexner, *Medical Education in the United States and Canada* (New York: Carnegie Foundation, 1910), pp. 91–2.

62 George Dock, "Correlation of laboratory and clinical teaching," *South. Med. J.* 10 (1917): 187–91.

63 Thomas A. Flood, "The hospital laboratory: a first aid station, or a court of last appeal?" *Hosp. Prog.* 6 (1925): 561–4; Edward H. L. Corwin, *The American Hospital* (New York: Commonwealth Foundation, 1946).

64 John A. Hornsby and R. E. Schmidt, *The Modern Hospital* (Philadelphia: Saunders, 1913), pp. 379–80; Edward F. Stevens, *The American Hospital of the 20th Century* (New York: Architectural Record, 1918), p. 139; Francis C. Wood, "The hospital laboratory," *Bull. Am. Coll. Surg.* 3 (1917): 20–4; Max Kahn, "The department of laboratories," *Mod. Hosp.* 11 (1918): 271–4, in which Kahn wrote: "The reputation of the whole hospital is enhanced by the publication of the scientific researches conducted in its laboratory, and the whole medical staff should insist that research problems be investigated there, for the lay board is not aware of its great importance." Kahn was director of laboratories at Beth Israel in New York. See also O. J. Walker, "Organizing a modern hospital laboratory," *Mod. Hosp.* 16 (1921): 502–6.

65 Presbyterian Hospital (New York), *Annu. Rep.* 43 (1910/1): 15–16.

66 L. F. Barker, "Organization of the laboratories in the medical clinic of the Johns Hopkins Hospital," *Bull. Johns Hopkins Hosp.* 18 (1907): 193–7.

67 Charles Camac, "Hospital and ward clinical laboratories," *J. Am. Med. Assoc.* (1900): 219–27; Henry M. Hurd, "Laboratories and hospital work," *Bull. Am. Acad. Med.* 2 (1896): 483–95.

68 *Bull. Ayer Clin. Lab. Pa. Hosp.* 1 (1903): 1–3; Francis R. Packard, *Some Account of the Pennsylvania Hospital* (Philadelphia: Engle Press, 1938), pp. 108–9; "The William Pepper Laboratory of Clinical Medicine," *Boston Med. Surg. J.* 133 (1895): 603–4.

69 Christian to Eliot, 11 November 1908; Eliot Papers, box 207.

70 Clarence F. Graham, "The clinical laboratory of Albany Hospital," *Mod. Hosp.* 9 (1917): 158–62; Walker, "Organizing," p. 504; E. Gradwohl, "The proper recognition of the laboratory technician," *J. Am. Med. Assoc.* 76 (1921): 127.

71 A. N. Richards and T. G. Miller, "Survey of medical affairs, University of Pennsylvania," typescript, 1931, pp. 97–103; College of Physicians Library.

72 Barker, "Medical laboratories," p. 606; Barker, "Organization of the laboratories," p. 194.

73 Frederick A. Washburn, *The Massachusetts General Hospital: Its Development, 1900–1935* (Boston: Houghton-Mifflin, 1939), pp. 279–84; G. Stanley Hall, "The laboratory of the McLean Hospital," *Am. J. Insanity* 51 (1899): 358–64; Edward Cowles, "Reports," *Annu. Rep. Mass. Gen. Hosp.* 87 (1900): 161–2; 88 (1901): 170–91, 89 (1902): 200–1, 211–17.

74 Edward Cowles, "Reports," *Annu. Rep. Mass. Gen. Hosp.* 88 (1901): 170–2, 189–91; 89 (1902): 205–7; 90 (1903): 207–11; 91 (1904): 206–7; 93 (1906): 209.

75 Otto Folin, "A theory of protein metabolism" *Am. J. Physiol.* 12 (1905): 117–38.

76 Otto Folin, "Chemical problems in hospital practice," *Harvey Lect.* 3 (1907–8): 187–98 (for quotation, see pp. 196–7).

77 "Studies from the Department of Physiological Chemistry, Pathological Institute of the New York State Hospital," 1902/3; Samuel Bookman, "Twenty-five years of physiological chemistry at the Mt. Sinai Hospital (1902–1907)," *J. Mt. Sinai Hosp. N.Y.* 12 (1945): 870–90; D. D. Van Slyke and W. A. Jacobs, "Phoebus Aaron Theodor Levene, 1869–1940," *Biogr. Mem. Natl. Acad. Sci.* 23 (1945): 75–126; Joseph Hirsch and Beka Doherty, *Mt. Sinai Hospital of New York* (New York: Random House, 1952), pp. 127–35, 195–6. E. C. Dodds, "American impressions," *Middlesex Hosp. J.* 32 (1932): 49–62.

78 Barker, "Organization of the laboratories," pp. 193–7.

79 Folin, "Chemical problems," p. 189.

80 Warren, "The study of chemistry," pp. 235–40; Flexner, *Medical Education*, p. 102, in which Flexner wrote that clinical chemistry was "quite underdeveloped in America."

81 See Figure 8.4.

82 *Annu. Rep. N. Y. Postgrad. Hosp.* (1910): 13–15, (1915): 15–16, (1932): 30, (1939): 39–40.

83 Edward C. Kendall, *Cortisone* (New York: Scribners, 1971), pp. 23–6.

84 Frederick A. Washburn, *The Massachusetts General Hospital*, pp. 108, 117–19, 123–35; Joseph Aub and Ruth Hapgood, *Pioneer in Modern Medicine, David Linn Edsall of Harvard* (Boston: Harvard Medical Alumni Assoc., 1970), pp. 133, 137–8, 161–70; *Annu. Rep. Mass. Gen. Hosp.* 89 (1902): 83; 94 (1907): 94–8; 99 (1912): 118; 100 (1913): 126.

85 Aub and Hapgood, *Pioneer*, pp. 178–81; James Howard Means, *Ward 4* (Cambridge, Mass.: Harvard University Press, 1958), pp. 10–20; Arlie Bock to Van Slyke, 29 June 1924, Flexner Papers.

86 George Corner, *A History of the Rockefeller Institute 1901–1953* (New York: Rockefeller Institute Press, 1964), chs. 4 and 5; Cole to S. Flexner, 7 September 1910, Flexner Papers.

87 Knoop to M. James, 10 June 1913, S. Flexner to Cole, 29 July 1913, Cole to Flexner, 7 August 1913, Flexner Papers; S. Flexner to Abel, 25 March 1913, Abel Papers.

88 S. Flexner to Cole, 29 July and 11 August 1913, Flexner to Levene, 30 June 1913, Van Slyke to Flexner, 28 June 1913, Flexner Papers; D. D. Van Slyke, Interview, 1971, pp. 68–70, National Library of Medicine.

89 Cole to S. Flexner, 7 August 1913, Flexner to Van slyke, 6 November 1913, Flexner Papers.

90 Cole to S. Flexner, 4 November 1913, Flexner Papers.

91 Van Slyke, Interview, p. 18; D. D. Van Slyke, "Remarks upon receiving the Kober Medal," *Trans. Assoc. Am. Physicians* 57 (1942): 42–3. Corner, *Rockefeller Institute*, pp. 274–80; A. B. Hastings, "Donald Dexter Van Slyke," *J. Biol. Chem.* 247 (1972): 1635–40; S. Flexner to Van Slyke, 22 July 1914, Van Slyke to Flexner, 22 June 1914, Flexner Papers.

92 George E. Hale to Henry Pritchett, 7 October 1920, Hale Papers, box 33.

93 P. A. Shaffer, Memorandum, 20 November 1954, p. 1, Shaffer Papers, box 11, f. 124.

94 Joseph C. Aub, "Eugene F. DuBois (1882–1959)," *Biogr. Mem. Natl. Acad. Sci.* 36 (1962): 125–45. DuBois directed a medical service at Bellevue Hospital. Also see Lusk to S. Flexner, 19 February 1913, Flexner Papers.

95 Lusk to S. Flexner, 2 and 4 June 1919, 14 April 1923, Flexner Papers.

96 S. Flexner to Lusk, 3 June 1919, Lusk to Flexner, 4 June 1919, 17 February and 28 May 1920, Flexner to Lusk, 15 December 1920, Lusk to Flexner, 16 December 1920, Flexner Papers.

97 Means, *Ward 4*, p. 16.

98 See sketches of Peabody by F. G. Blake, Rufus Cole, G. C. Robinson, and others, February 1928, Flexner Papers; *Annu. Rep. Peter Bent Brigham Hosp.* 1 (1913/14): 118–19; *Annu. Rep. Roosevelt Hosp.* 37 (1908): 20, 38 (1909): 19, 41 (1912): 19.

99 Paul Titus to S. Flexner, 30 December 1927, Flexner Papers, f. Van Slyke; Albert P. Lamb, *The Presbyterian Hospital and the Columbia–Presbyterian Medical Center, 1868–1943* (New York: Columbia University Press, 1955), p. 168.

100 Folin to A. Flexner, 18 March 1920, GEB, B19, box 701.

101 A. B. Hastings to Glenn Cullen, 2 February 1940. Hastings to C. Sidney Burwell, 24 January 1936, penciled notes dated " '36–'37," Hastings Papers.

102 Franklin C. McLean, "Physiology and medicine: a transition period," *The Excitement and Fascination of Science* (Palo Alto, Calif.: Annual Reviews, 1965), pp. 317–32 (in particular, see p. 324); Marshall Urist, "Phoenix of physiology and medicine: Franklin Chambers McLean," *Perspect. Biol. Med.* 19 (1975): 23–58; F. C. McLean and N. Gorgas, *Medicine in the Division of the Biological Sciences, University of Chicago, 1927–1952* (University of Chicago Press, 1952); C. W. Vermeulen, *For the Greatest Good to the Greatest Number. A History of the Medical Center of the University of Chicago, 1927–1977* (University of Chicago, 1972), pp. 49–50, 52–5. Rufus Cole, "Hospital and Laboratory," *Science* 66 (1927): 545–52.

103 Hastings to Burwell, 24 January 1936, Hastings Papers, f. departmental.

104 E. C. Dodds, "American impressions," *Middlesex Hosp. J.* 32 (1932): 48–62 (see pp. 54–5); Corner, *Rockefeller Institute*, pp. 106–7, 274–83.

105 e. C. Dodds, "American Impressions," p. 51.

106 Oliver Gaebler, "Comments on the origins and development of clinical chemistry," *Clin. Chem.* 4 (1958): 331–8.

107 P. A. Shaffer, "Otto Knut Folin (1876–1934)," *Biogr. Mem. Natl. Acad. Sci.* (1952): 47–82. An English translation of Hilding Berglund's memoir in *Papers of the IV Medical Service, St. Eric's Hospital Stockholm* (1937) is present in the Harry Trimble Papers. See also Laura Grant Folin to Shaffer, 15 November [1952?], Shaffer Papers, box 6, f. 60; R. M. Archibald, "Donald Dexter Van Slyke (1883–1971)," *Am. Phil. Soc. Yearbook* 1971: 194–200.

108 E. V. McCollum, "Stanley Rossiter Benedict (1884–1936)," *Biogr. Mem. Natl. Acad. Sci.* 27 (1952): 155–77. H. D. Dakin, "Stanley R. Benedict," *Science* 85 (1937): 65–6; V. C. Myers to Shaffer, 14 January 1936, Shaffer Papers, box 5, f. 33. There is no biographical material on Myers. Chittenden thought him "a bright man, although rather heavy in some respects." See Chittenden to Taylor, 16 November 1910, Chittenden Papers.

109 Bloor to Shaffer, 6 June 1949, Shaffer Papers, box 6, f. 60.

110 Folin to A. Flexner, 18 March 1920, GEB, B19, box 701.

111 Folin to Eliot, 20 August 1908, Eliot Papers, box 213; Folin to A. Flexner, 9 March 1920, GEB, B19, box 701.

112 Myers to Trimble, 29 October 1934, Otto Folin Papers; Folin to Shaffer, 21 October 1934, Shaffer Papers, box 6, f. 60; E. A. Doisey, "An autobiography," *Annu. Rev. Biochem.* 45 (1976): 1–9.

113 Hastings to James Neill, 5 February 1937, Hastings Papers, f. Dill; Hastings to Edsall, 30 January 1942, Hastings Papers, f. Van Slyke; Wendell T. Caraway, "The scientific development of clinical chemistry to 1948," *Clin. Chem.* 19 (1973): 373–83.

114 Mendel to Carlson, 10 March 1924, UChicPP, box 17, f. 13; Moses Gomberg to M. L. Burton, 20 March 1921, Burton Papers, box 3, f. 15.

115 D. D. Van Slyke, Interview, p. 18; D. D. Van Slyke, "Donald D. Van Slyke on his 80th Year," *Clin. Chem.* 9 (1963): 645–63 (includes a full bibliography).

116 Van Slyke, "Remarks," pp. 42–3; Hastings, "Van Slyke," p. 1639; Van Slyke to S. Flexner, 29 June 1925, Flexner Papers; Van Slyke to Flexner, 2 September 1914, Rufus Cole Papers.

117 Julius Sendroy, "In Appreciation of D. D. Van Slyke," *Clin. Chem.* 17 (1971): 670–72; Van Slyke to S. Flexner, 29 June 1925; Flexner Papers; J. P. Peters and

D. D. Van Slyke, *Quantitative Clinical Chemistry*, 2 vols. (Baltimore, Md.: Williams and Wilkins, 1931–1932). J. R. Paul and C. N. H. Long, "John Peters (1887–1955)," *Biogr. Mem. Natl. Acad. Sci.* 31 (1958): 347–75.

118 Otto Folin and Hsien Wu, "A system of blood analysis," *J. Biol. Chem.* 38 (1919): 81–110; Otto Folin, "The clinical applications of pathological chemistry," *Lancet* (1913 II): 468.

119 A. I. Kendall to Shaffer, 13 October 1911, Shaffer Papers, box 12, f. 145 (in 1912 Kendall became professor of bacteriology and director of the Patten Research Fund at Northwestern); Bloor to Shaffer, 6 June 1949, Shaffer Papers, box 6, f. 60.

120 *Proc. Assoc. Am. Med. Coll.* 30 (1920): 115–16.

121 Myers to Shaffer, 14 January 1936, Shaffer Papers, box 5, f. 33.

122 McCollum, "Benedict," p. 160.

123 Myers to Shaffer, 14 January 1936, Shaffer Papers, box 5, f. 33; Benedict to Shaffer, 19 November 1934, Shaffer Papers, box 6, f. 60.

124 Myers to Shaffer, 14 January 1936, Shaffer Papers, box 5, f. 33; Thomas P. Nash, Jr. to Shaffer, 20 January 1937, Shaffer Papers, box 5, f. 33.

125 Myers to Shaffer, 14 January 1936, Shaffer Papers, box 5, f. 33.

126 J. S. Routh, "Training of clinical chemists in the U.S., a brief history," *Clin. Chem.* 20 (1974): 1251–3 (see p. 1251). Gaebler, "Comments on the origins," pp. 331–8.

127 Doisy, "An autobiography," p. 6; Doisy to Shaffer, 17 May 1919, Shaffer Papers, box 6, f. 51.

128 Hastings to Cullen, 2 February 1940, Hastings Papers. Hastings to John Peters, 27 December 1935, Peters to Hastings, 8 January 1936, Hastings Papers. Peters did not share Hastings's enthusiasm for Cullen, regarding him as shallow and unimaginative, and lacking in knowledge of physiology.

129 Doisey to Shaffer, 10 June 1920, Shaffer Papers, box 6, f. 51; Moses Gomberg to Burton, 20 March 1921, Burton Papers, box 3, f. 15.

130 Caraway, "Scientific development of clinical chemistry," pp. 373–83; Routh, "Training of clinical chemists," pp. 1251–3. Editorials in *Clinical Chemistry* refer continually to problems of professionalization.

131 Gaebler, "Comments on the origins," pp. 336–7.

CHAPTER 10 *Chemical ideals and biochemical practice*

1 R. E. Kohler, "Medical reform and biomedical science: biochemistry, a case study," in Morris J. Vogel and Charles E. Rosenberg, eds., *The Therapeutic Revolution* (Philadelphia: University of Pennsylvania Press, 1979), pp. 27–66.

2 Faust to Abel, 17 July 1895, Abel Papers.

3 Shaffer to A. Flexner, 20 December 1921, Shaffer Papers, box 6, f. 57.

4 W. G. MacCallum to Lewis H. Weed, 14 April 1927, Medical deans' files, JHUMedA.

5 Hans T. Clarke, "Some experiences in the training of research chemists," 20 May 1954, Clarke Papers.

6 Marston T. Bogert, "The function of chemistry in the conservation of our natural resources," *Science* 31 (1909):125–54; Samuel F. Sadtler, "Conservation and the chemical engineer," *Trans. Am. Inst. Chem. Eng.* 2 (1909):105–14. Frederick E. Breithut, "The status and compensation of the chemist in public service," *J. Ind. Eng. Chem.* 9 (1917):64–79. University of Wisconsin *Catalogue* (1908/9), 259–60 (an example of chemical boosterism); Joseph Kastle, "Concerning...the relation of chemistry to the industrial development of the South," 17 December 1909, E. A. Alderman Papers, box 17 (I owe thanks to Jeffrey Sturchio for this reference).

7 Marston T. Bogert, "American chemical societies," *J. Am. Chem. Soc.* 30 (1908):163–82 (see pp. 172–3).

8 Ibid., pp. 174–5; *J. Am. Chem. Soc. Proc.* 24 (1902):11, 18–19, 59.

9   Charles A. Browne and Mary E. Weeks, *A History of the American Chemical Society* (Washington: American Chemical Society, 1952), pp. 72–5. *J. Am. Chem. Soc. Proc.* 25 (1903):56, 88.
10 Owen Hannaway, "The German model of chemical education in America: Ira Remsen at Johns Hopkins, 1876–1913," *Ambix* 23 (1976): 145–64.
11 John Servos, "Physical chemistry in America, 1890–1933: origins, growth and definition" (Ph.D. diss. Johns Hopkins University, 1979).
12 Browne and Weeks, *History*, chaps. 3 and 4.
13 Ibid., pp. 74–5.
14 Ibid., pp. 78–9. Albert C. Hale, "Report," *J. Am. Chem. Soc. Proc.* 25 (1904): 13; W. F. Hillebrand, "The present and future of the American Chemical Society," *J. Am. Chem Soc.* 29 (1907): 1–18; Gies to Abel, 8 January 1906, Abel Papers.
15 Bogert, "American chemical societies," 179; Hillebrand, "The present and future," pp. 85–6.
16 Bogert, "American chemical societies," pp. 180–1.
17 *J. Am. Chem. Soc. Proc.* 30 (1908): 25–31; 31 (1909): 25–31; 34 (1912): 31.
18 *J. Am. Chem. Soc. Proc.* 30 (1908): 102; Browne and Weeks, *History*, pp. 94–5.
19 Herter to Abel, 13 November 1908, Abel Papers.
20 *J. Amer. Chem. Soc. Proc.* 28 (1906): 8–10; 29 (1907): 68; 30 (1908): 10–11 and 80–81; 31 (1909): 12–13.
21 Frank Cameron to W. D. Bancroft, 22 January 1909, Wilder Bancroft Papers. I owe thanks to John Servos for this reference.
22 W. A. Noyes, "Samuel W. Parr," *J. Am. Chem. Soc. Proc.* 54 (1932): 1–2; Parr to S. A. Forbes, 20 December 1904, 11 January 1905, UIllCS, box 4.
23 Parr to E. J. Townsend, 16 November 1906, UIllCS, box 8.
24 Noyes to Forbes, 3 March 1904, UIllCS, box 1; Parr to Townsend, 5 and 6 January and 10 October 1906, subsequent correspondence, box 2; Townsend to Edmund James, "Information regarding application for the headship of the chemistry department," 16 November 1906, Noyes to James, 7 March and 28 October 1906, Stratton to Parr, 16 January 1906, other correspondence, Edmund James Papers, box 8.
25 Grindley to Forbes, 27 April 1904, Grindley to R. S. Woodward, 10 April 1905, other correspondence, UIllCS, box 8. T. W. Richards described Grindley as a diamond in the rough: "He came to us a number of years ago, a forceful but uncultivated youth of unusual promise, and has fulfilled this promise by doing exceptional work in his present position. Much of this work, however, has concerned the chemistry of food stuffs and other practical problems. His interest is not so much in the purely scientific or philosophical side of the subject. It is said that he has lost much of his uncouthness and that his speech is now grammatical and suggests cultivation. Mental power and energy he has always had; and he will certainly make his mark in his line of work"; see Richards to Alderman, 26 April 1906, Alderman Papers, box 17 (I owe thanks to Jeffrey Sturchio for this reference).
26 James to Noyes, 12 January 1907, Noyes to James, 22 January 1907, James Papers, box 8.
27 Kemp to Townsend, 24 April 1906, UIllCS, box 9.
28 Ibid.; Kemp to James, 7 September 1906, Kemp, "Annual report of the Department of Physiology," 22 April 1907, UIllCS, box 9.
29 In 1905 Davenport had refused Grindley's request to be transferred to agriculture, apparently to avoid the extra expense of his project; see Davenport to Grindley, 6 January 1905, UIllCS, box 8.
30 Parr to Townsend, 18 March 1907, James to Noyes, 10 March 1907, UIllCS, box 2; James to Noyes, 18 March 1907, James Papers, box 8.
31 Parr to Townsend, 18 March 1907, James Papers, box 8.
32 James to Noyes, 18 March 1907, UIllCS, box 2.
33 Noyes to Parr, 5 March 1907, UIllCS, box 8, Noyes to James, 22 March 1922, Noyes to G. N. Lewis, 4 and 11 April 1907, Lewis to W. A. Noyes, 10 April 1907,

Ira Remsen to Noyes, 1 May 1907, A. A. Noyes to W. A. Noyes, 1 May 1907, James Papers, box 8.
34 Parr to W. A. Noyes, 30 April 1907, UIIICS, box 2; Parr to Townsend, 16 November 1906, UIIICS, box 8.
35 W. A. Noyes to Townsend, 25 May 1907, James Papers, box 8; Parr to W. A. Noyes, 30 April 1907, UIIICS, box 2.
36 James to W. A. Noyes, 29 May 1907, James Papers, box 8; Parr to Townsend, "Annual report of department," 27 April 1907, UIIICS, box 8; Noyes to Townsend, 25 May 1907, James Papers, box 8.
37 Servos, "Physical chemistry," pp. 141–53, 251–2.
38 Parr to W. A. Noyes, 30 April 1907, UIIICS, box 2; Grindley to Marshall, 15 May 1907, Grindley to W. A. Noyes, "Report of laboratory of physiological chemistry," in Noyes to James, 27 November 1907, Hawk to Grindley, 25 May and 19 June 1907, Grindley to Hawk, 17 June and 3 and 9 July 1907, Marshall to Grindley, 29 May 1907, James Papers, box 26.
39 For opinions of Hawk, see Chittenden to Grindley, 29 May 1907, Mendel to Grindley, 10 June 1907, Gies to Grindley, 13 June 1907, Sherman to Grindley, 10 June 1902, James Papers, box 26. Mendel considered Hawk a competent and energetic analyst, lacking in imagination and breadth, but a good team worker. Chittenden wrote in a similar vein that Hawk was "...not a brilliant man, but a thoroughly good and reliable one."
40 Kemp to James, 14 February 1908, Kemp to Townsend, 19 November 1907, "Memorandum in re Prof. Kemp" (undated), attached to Kemp's letter of resignation to the trustees, 1 May 1908, Kemp to James, 7 September 1906, 5 March 1908, UIIICS, box 9.
41 Minutes of regents' meetings, 10 March, 3 April, and 2 May 1908, other correspondence, James Papers, box 19, f. James–Kemp Affair; R. A. Swanson, "Edmund J. James, 1855–1925: a conservative progressive in American higher education" (Ph.D. diss., University of Illinois 1966), pp. 175–7.
42 W. A. Noyes to Townsend, 21 May 1908, UIIICS, box 8.
43 W. A. Noyes to Townsend, 17 December 1908, 19 March 1909, Noyes to David Kinley, 3 December 1910, UIIICS, box 9.
44 Hawk to W. A. Noyes, 7 April 1911, UIIICS, box 9.
45 W. Swanson, "Edmund J. James," pp. 175–7.
46 W. A. Noyes to James, 22 November 1912, UIIICS, box 8.
47 W. A. Noyes to Mathews, 19 February 1914, Noyes to K. C. Babcock, 19 February 1914, C. G. MacArthur to Noyes, 17 February 1914, Noyes to Babcock, 17 February 1914, UIIICS, box 1. A professorship of physiological chemistry was established in the medical school's Department of Physiology in 1921; see University of Illinois *Announcements* (1908/9), p. 189, (1909/10), pp. 309–10, (1911/12), pp. 266, (1914/15), pp. 238–9.
48 Lewis to Herbert Carter, 5 May 1952, Lewis Papers, box 1; Rose to Lewis, 18 March 1947, Lewis Papers, box 2.
49 P. A. Leighton, "Swains of progress," *Ind. Eng. Chem. News Ed.* 19 (1941): 1145–6.
50 Orndorff to Abel, 28 February 1903, Abel Papers.
51 Merle Curti and Vernon Carstenson, *The University of Wisconsin* (Madison: University of Wisconsin Press, 1949), vol. II, pp. 347–52. The degree course resembled that of the Sheffield School; see University of Wisconsin *Catalogue* (1908/9), pp. 259–60.
52 University of Virginia *Calendars* (1909–21); Joseph Kastle to Abel, 20 April 1909, Abel Papers; Kastle to R. M. Bird, 25 April 1909, Kastle, "Agreement between Dr. Kastle and Dr. Hough regarding the use of the Laboratory for Physiological Chemistry," 1 June 1909, Kastle to Edwin A. Alderman, 30 April 1909, UVaA, 2636, box 17.
53 Mendel to A. J. Carlson, 10 March 1924, UChicPP, box 17, f. 13.

54 H. B. Vickery, "Treat B. Johnson," *Biogr. Mem. Natl. Acad. Sci.* 27 (1952): 83–119; H. B. Vickery, "Rudolph J. Anderson," *Biogr. Mem. Natl. Acad. Sci.* 36 (1962): 19–50; H. B. Vickery, "Thomas B. Osborne," *Biogr. Mem. Natl. Acad. Sci.* 14 (1931): 261–304.

55 Charles H. Warren to J. R. Angell, 3 April 1936, Medical deans' files, box 21, YaUA. Edwin Cohn, William Mansfield Clark, and Adolf Butenandt were considered.

56 Robert E. Kohler, "Rudolf Schoenheimer, isotopic tracers, and biochemistry in the 1930s," *Hist. Stud. Phys. Sci.* 8 (1977), 257–298.

57 D. D. Van Slyke and W. A. Jacobs, "Phoebus Aaron Levene (1869–1940)," *Biogr. Mem. Natl. Acad. Sci.* 23 (1945): 75–126; George Corner, *A History of the Rockefeller Institute* (New York: Rockefeller University Press, 1965), pp. 340–2. Most of Levene's co-workers went into industrial research.

58 P. Hartley, "Henry Drysdale Dakin (1880–1952)," *Obit Not. Fellows R. Soc.*, 8 (1952): 129–48; Herter to Abel, 10 October 1905, 21 February 1910, Abel Papers; Fletcher to Stephenson, 15 July 1931, Dakin to Fletcher, 5 August 1931, MRC, 2036.

59 B. Helfrich, "Max Bergmann, 1886–1944," *Ber. dtsch. chem. Ges.* 102 (1969): i–xxvi; Hans T. Clarke, "Max Bergmann," *Science* 102 (1945): 168–70; Corner, *Rockefeller Institute*, pp. 342–5.

60 Henry G. Gale to Robert M. Hutchins, 4 October 1935, Gale to Frederick Woodward, 29 June 1936, UChicPP, box 101.

61 Schlesinger to Hutchins, 9 October 1935, Schlesinger to Gale, 31 January 1935, Schlesinger to Hutchins, 3 October 1935, UChicPP, box 101.

62 Conant to Hutchins, 17 September 1935, Roger Adams to Gale, 17 September 1935, Gomberg to Stieglitz, 6 February 1936, Schlesinger to Gale, 19 October 1935, 26 June 1936, Gale to F. Woodward, 29 June 1936, Butenandt to Hutchins, 3 August 1936, W. D. Harkins to Hutchins, 8 February 1937, Schlesinger to Hutchins, 5 December 1938, 27 May 1939, Harold Urey to Hutchins, 23 November 1938, UChicPP, box 101.

63 Conant to Adams, 23 January 1934, E. P. Kohler to Adams, 23 January 1934, Adams Papers, box 64. I owe thanks to Stanley Tarbell and Leon Gortler for these references.

64 E. P. Kohler to Adams, 15 March 1934, Adams Papers, box 64.

65 Medical council minutes, 2 August 1921, vol. 2, pp. 533, 536, UPennA; William Pepper to W. M. Clark, 12 September 1921, A. N. Richards to Clark, 20 and 23 June 1921, D. Bayne Jones to Clark, 15 April 1923, George Whipple to Clark, 14 May 1923, Van Slyke to Clark, 21 April 1923, Clark Papers.

66 William Haynes, *American Chemical Industry*, 6 vols. (New York: Van Nostrand, 1945), vol. 3, pp. 270–1, vol. 4, pp. 245–52; "The Chemical Foundation Inc.," 2 vols., manuscript, Francis P. Garvan Papers, small file no. 13 (I owe thanks to P. Thomas Carroll for this reference); Jan T. Levine, "Red, white, and blue: the political campaign to protect the American dye industry" (Honors B.A. thesis, University of Pennsylvania, 1980), E. F. Smith Collection.

67 Johnson to Hadley, 17 October 1919, YaUA, box 3, Misc. MSS.

68 Haynes, *American Chemical Industry*, vol. 4, pp. 250–7, 275–91, vol. 5, pp. 245–7.

69 Stieglitz to H. P. Judson, 15 December 1919, 19 January 1920, UChicPP, box 16, f. 1.

70 Julius Stieglitz, ed., *Chemistry in Medicine* (New York: Chemical Foundation, 1928); J. Stieglitz, *Chemistry and Recent Progress in Medicine* (Baltimore: Williams and Wilkins, 1926); J. J. Abel, Ried Hunt, J. Stieglitz, *The Future Independence and Progress of American Medicine in the Age of Chemistry; A Report* (New York: Chemical Foundation, 1921). The Chemical Foundation distributed 200,000 copies of *Chemistry in Medicine;* see "Chemical Foundation," ch. 15. Stieglitz's concern for creating jobs for chemists in biochemistry was sharpened by the temporary glut of chemists in the mid-1920s; see Stieglitz to Harold Smith, 4 May 1925, UChicPP, box 16, f. 2.

71 Folin to A. Flexner, 18 March 1920, GEB, B19, box 701.

72 John T. Edsall, Personal communication; R. M. Pearce, Memorandum of interview with A. N. Richards, 15 April 1922; William Pepper to A. Flexner, 2 October 1924, 6 February 1925, GEB, 2498, box 690; Minutes of Rockefeller Foundation Board, 5 December 1923, Edwin Embree to Josiah Penniman, 7 December 1923, Penniman to G. E. Vincent, 25 May 1925, GEB, 2498, box 690.

73 A. N. Richards and T. G. Miller, "Survey of medical affairs, University of Pennsylvania," 5 March 1931, College of Physicians Library. Eric Ball and John Buchanan, "David Wright Wilson," *Biogr. Mem. Natl. Acad. Sci.* 43 (1973): 261–84.

74 Fred C. Koch, A. J. Carlson, and A. L. Tatum to J. H. Tufts, 17 March 1925, UChicPP, box 17, f. 13; F. R. Lillie to Stieglitz, 6 February 1922, Lillie Papers, box 8, f. 16.

75 F. C. Koch, "List of researches in progress in physiological chemistry..." undated (circa 1926–7), UChicPP, box 107, f. 6; J. Stieglitz, "Endowment for research work in colloid chemistry...," to Rowland Haynes, 4 November 1927, UChicPP, box 101, f. 5.

76 Lewis to Max S. Dunn, 10 March 1936, Lewis Papers, box 6. W. C. Rose and M. J. Coon, "Howard Bishop Lewis," *Biogr. Mem. Natl. Acad. Sci.* 44 (1974): 139–73.

77 W. M. Clark, "Walter Jennings Jones, 1865–1925," *Biogr. Mem. Natl. Acad. Sci.* 20 (1938): 79–139 (see pp. 98). Jones advised Eli K. Marshall, a brilliant young biochemist, to go into pharmacology because it was a safer career; see T. H. Maren, "Eli Kennerly Marshall 1889–1966," *Bull. Johns Hopkins Hosp.* 119 (1966): 247-54 (see p. 24); W. M. Clark, "Autobiography," p. 4–5, Clark Papers.

78 Medical faculty minutes, 22 March and 12 May 1927, vol. G. pp. 21, 33, JHUMedA; W. G. MacCallum to L. H. Weed, 14 April 1927, Medical deans' files, JHUMedA.

79 Clark to Ames, 25 May 1927, Ames to Clark, 13 May 1927, Clark to Weed, 16 May 1927, Clark to Ames, 25 May 1927, Weed to Clark, 31 May 1927, JHUMedA.

80 Clark to Ames, 25 May 1927, JHUMedA; Clark to Barnet Cohen, 28 March 1937, Clark Papers.

81 Clark to Weed, 18 July 1927, JHUMedA, f. Clark; W. M. Clark, "Barnet Cohen," *Bacteriol. Rev.* 16 (1925): 205–9.

82 Clark to Weed, 29 July 1927, Weed to Clark, 7 August 1927, Clark Papers. The Dean was delighted with Clark's plans for organized team research.

83 Eric G. Ball, "The development of our current concepts of biological oxidations," *Proceedings of the Conference on the History of Bioenergetics* (Boston: American Academy of Arts and Sciences, 1973), pp. 92–114.

84 Clark to Alan Chesney, 28 June 1952, JHUMedA; Clark to Cohen, 28 March 1937; Clark to E. A. Park, 18 June 1936, Clark Papers.

85 Cannan to Clark, 20 April 1931, also 23 March 1924, Clark Papers.

86 Cannan to Clark, 15 May 1924, Joseph Needham to Clark, 19 June 1925, Clark Papers.

87 Needham to Clark, 19 June 1925, Clark Papers.

88 Clark to Chesney, 28 June 1952, JHUMedA; W. M. Clark, "Memorandum to Committee on Instruction and Examination," 5 June 1929, Clark Papers.

89 Marshall to Clark, 10 June 1950, Clark to Marshall, 23 May 1950, Clark Papers; Richards to A. Flexner, 24 December 1924. GEB, 2498.1, box 690; Dock to A. Flexner, 12 and 28 March 1913, GEB, 2495, box 688.

90 A. Flexner, "Memorandum for Dr. Buttrick re College of P&S," 1 June 1920, "Memorandum on P&S prepared for Mr. Rockefeller," 24 November 1920, William Darrach to Wallace Buttrick, 13 April 1920, S. Flexner to A. Flexner, 5 March 1920 and attached documents, Buttrick to Parsons, 29 May 1929, Pearce to Buttrick and Flexner, 26 April 1920, "Memorandum of conference," 13 April 1925, GEB, B19, box 701.

91 Benjamin Harrow to Clarke, 2 October 1956, A. Kent Balls to Clarke, 28 September 1956, Karshan to Clarke, 1 October 1956, Clarke Papers.

92 Medical faculty minutes, 21 November 1927, 16 April 1928, vol. 16, pp. 3, 13–14, 184, UColA; Darrach to Butler, 20 December 1927, 24 May 1928, UColCF.

93 H. T. Clarke, "Impressions of an organic chemist," *Annu. Rev. Biochem.* 27 (1958): 1–14.
94 Conant to Clarke, 23 May 1928, Clarke Papers.
95 Dakin to Darrach, 1 June 1928, UColCF.
96 W. W. Buffum to Darrach, 5 September 1928, Darrach to Butler, 7 September 1928, UColCF; see also Francis P. Garvan Papers, files D-6-21, cabinet 29, drawer 2 (I owe thanks to P. Thomas Carroll for this reference); F. B. Hanson, memorandum 25 October 1935, RF, 200D, box 132.
97 Data are from the Clarke Papers.

Year	1929	1930	1931	1932	1933	1934	1935	1936	1937	1938	1939	1940	1941	1942
Graduates	1	0	1	2	4	2	2	1	2	5	9	4	2	0

98 Du Vigneaud to Weaver, 26 February 1935, RF, 210D, box 1; V. Du Vigneaud, "Some reminiscences of my graduate student days," manuscript, 1965, Clarke Papers.
99 F. B. Hanson, memoranda, 10 January 1935, 15 January 1936, 30 March 1937, "Appraisal," May 1939, RF, 210D, box 1.
100 Du Vigneaud to Weaver, 26 January 1938, RF, 210D, box 1. There was a similar continuity of purpose in the succession at New York University. John Mandell was devoted to colloidal chemistry, a fashion of the 1920s; R. K. Cannan was a disciple of William Mansfield Clark's; see New York University *Bulletin* (1925), p. 438, (1930), p. 53; "Endowment and requirements, medical school," 1928, p. 4; S. A. Browne to E. E. Brown undated (circa 1930), p. 7, NYUCP; Walter Fletcher to R. K. Cannan, 11 July 1930; Cannan to Fletcher, 10 and 16 July 1930, MRC, 1435.
101 Maurice B. Visscher to Hastings, 20 November 1939, Hastings Papers, f. Logan.
102 Cullen to Hastings, 31 January 1940, Hastings Papers.
103 Cullen to Hastings, 21 March 1940 and other correspondence, Hastings Papers, f. Logan. Hastings described King as "a meticulous unimaginative sort of person;" see Hastings to James Neill, 29 April 1937, Hastings Papers.
104 Hastings to Peters, 27 December 1935, Hastings Papers. Hastings felt he could not live up to Folin's standards as a chemist; see Hastings to Shaffer, 12 November 1935, Hastings to Stieglitz, 27 December 1935, Hastings Papers. Hastings to Dexter, 23 October 1944: "I am really only a physiologist at heart, and a pretty poor chemist by our departmental standards," Medical Deans' Files, HarvMedA, f. Biochemistry; Harry Trimble, "Memorandum prepared at request of Dean Berry, 9 April 1959," Trimble Papers, box 1.
105 Hastings to Peters, 27 December 1935, Hastings Papers.
106 Physiologist John Fulton took a leading role in seeing to it that Mendel's successor was not one of his own school but an outsider with broader medical interests. W. C. Rose, H. B. Lewis, and other Mendel loyalists made discreet efforts to influence the selection. See extensive materials in the Medical deans' files, YaUA, box 21 (1935–6); correspondence with A. V. Hill, S. Bayne Jones and J. R. Angell, Cyril Long Papers; correspondence with Rebecca Hubbell, W. C. Rose, H. C. Bradley, Arthur Smith, and others, H. B. Lewis Papers, boxes 5 and 6.
107 Hastings to Joseph C. Hinsey, 5 February 1937, Hastings Papers, f. Dill.
108 Hastings to Peters, 27 December 1935, Hastings Papers.
109 Lewis to Marshall, 27 June 1951, Marshall to Lewis, 27 June 1951, Lewis Papers, box 2.

CHAPTER 11 *Biological programs*

1 Russell H. Chittenden, "Some of the present-day problems of biological chemistry," *Science* 27 (1908): 241–54, (for quotation, see pp. 242–3).

2 Felix Hoppe-Seyler, *Quellen der Lebenskräfte* (Berlin: Carl Habel, 1871), pp. 22–4; Fritz Rehbock, "Huxley, Haeckel and the oceanographers: the case of Bathybius Haeckelii," *Isis* 66 (1975): 504–33; Gerald Geison, "The protoplasmic theory of life and the vitalist–mechanist debate," *Isis* 60 (1969): 273–92.

3 Felix Hoppe-Seyler, "Vorwort," *Z. physiol. Chem.* 1 (1877): i–iii.

4 Jacques Loeb, "The biological problems of today: physiology," *Science* 7 (1898): 154–6; Robert E. Kohler, "The enzyme theory of life and the origins of biochemistry," *Isis* 64 (1973): 181–96.

5 R. E. Kohler, "The background to Eduard Buchner's discovery of cell-free fermentation," *J. Hist. Biol.* 4 (1971): 35–61; R. E. Kohler, "The reception of Eduard Buchner's discovery of cell-free fermentation," *J. Hist. Biol.*, 5 (1972): 327–53.

6 Franz Hofmeister, *Die chemische Organisation der Zelle* (Brunswick: Vieweg, 1901).

7 Pauline Mazumdar, "The antigen–antibody reaction and the physics and chemistry of life," *Bull. Hist. Med.* 48 (1974): 1–21. Pauline Mazumdar, "Karl Landsteiner and the problem of species, 1838–1960" (Ph.D. diss. Johns Hopkins University, 1976); John Parascandola and Ronald Jasensky, "Origins of the receptor theory of drug action," *Bull. Hist. Med.* 48 (1974): 199–220.

8 F. G. Hopkins, "The dynamic side of biochemistry," *Rep. Brit. Assoc. Adv. Sci.* (1913): 652–68; Z. M. Bacq, *Chemical Transmission of Nerve Impulses. A Historical Sketch* (Oxford: Pergamon, 1975).

9 Jacques Loeb, *The Dynamics of Living Matter* (New York: Columbia University Press, 1913); Jacques Loeb, *The Mechanistic Conception of Life* (University of Chicago Press, 1912); W. J. V. Osterhout, "Jacques Loeb (1859–1924)," *Biogr. Mem. Natl. Acad. Sci.* 13 (1930): 318–401.

10 Chittenden, "Present-day problems," pp. 248–52.

11 R. H. Chittenden and L. B. Mendel, eds., *The Sheffield Laboratory of Physiological Chemistry Yale University. Collected Papers,* vols. I–IX. (New Haven, Conn.: Sheffield Scientific School: 1896–1919); L. B. Mendel and P. H. Mitchell, "Chemical studies of growth," *Am. J. Physiol.* 20 (1907): 81–116; L. B. Mendel, "Nutrition and growth," *Harvey Lectures* (1914/15): 101–31.

12 A. T. Hadley, "Report of the president of Yale University," 1904, pp. 108–90; 1905, pp. 4–6, 1906 pp. 11–13, Chittenden to Hadley, 7 December 1909, Hadley Papers, box 17 f. 332; R. H. Chittenden, *History of the Sheffield Scientific School* 2 vols. (New Haven, Conn. Yale University Press, 1928).

13 Hadley, "Report of the president," 1905 pp. 116–18, 1906, pp. 9–10.

14 Hadley, "Report of the president," 1905, pp. 116–18, 1897, pp. 430–44.

15 Hadley, "Report of the president," 1905, pp. 116–18.

16 Chittenden, *History,* vol. 2, pp. 440–48.

17 R. H. Chittenden in Hadley, "Report of the president of Yale University," 1912, pp. 196–8, 1913, pp. 194–5.

18 R. H. Chittenden, "The relation of chemistry to practical medicine," *N.Y. Med. J.* 68 (1898): 943–51.

19 Jones to Abel, undated (circa 1899), Abel Papers (Kutscher was Kossel's prickly and unapproachable assistant); John Parascandola, "Yandell Henderson," *Dict. Sci. Biogr.* VI: 264–5.

20 "Report of the committee on the Department of Physiology," 1917, Medical deans' files, box 21, YaUA.

21 Henderson to Hadley, 17 January 1906, Henderson to Chittenden, 17 January 1906, Hadley Papers, box 17, f. 322.

22 G. Blumer, "Relation of the medical school to the Department of Physiological Chemistry in the scientific school," 15 November 1915, pp. 1–2, Medical deans' files, box 21, YaUA.

23 Henderson to Underhill, 15 June 1911, 9 March 1915, Underhill to Henderson, 10 March 1915, Underhill Papers.

24 Henderson to Blumer, 17 November 1914, excerpted in Blumer to Underhill, 18 November 1914, Underhill Papers.

25 Blumer to Henderson, 17 November 1914, excerpted in Blumer to Underhill, 18 November 1914, Underhill Papers.

26 *The Past, Present, and Future of the Yale University School of Medicine*, (New Haven, Conn.: Yale University, 1922), pp. 22–4.

27 C. W. Warren to J. R. Angell, 3 April 1936, Mendel to M. C. Winternitz, 19 March 1930, with report for 1929–30, A. H. Smith to S. Bayne-Jones, 20 January 1936, other correspondence, Medical deans' files, box 21, f. Physiological sciences, YaUA.

28 Gies to Butler, 10 January 1903, Butler to Gies, 9 January 1903, UColCF.

29 Douglas Sloan, "Science in New York City, 1867–1907," *Isis* 71 (1980): 35–76.

30 Gies to Abel, 13 November 1906, Abel Papers.

31 Gies to Dean Hallock, 9 June 1906, p. 6, Gies to Seth Low, 9 November 1899, Low to Gies, 10 November 1899, Gies to Frederick Keppel, 24 October 1901, Gies to Butler, 19 January 1904, UColCF.

32 Gies to Seth Low, 1 October 1902, Gies to Hallock, 9 June 1906, pp. 4–6, Gies to Butler, 18 April and 19 October 1905, Gies to Keppel, 9 May 1905, UColCF.

33 Gies to Keppel, 9 May 1905, Gies to Butler, 17 October 1905, Gies to Hallock, 9 June 1906, UColCF; W. J. Gies, ed., *Biochemical Researches* (New York: Columbia University, 1903).

34 Gies to Butler, 29 December 1909, Butler to Gies, 5 April 1909, UColCF.

35 Gies to Butler, 29 December 1909, pp. 1–2.

36 E. C. Kendall, "Henry C. Sherman," *J. Chem. Educ.* 32 (1955): 510–13; P. L. Day, "Henry Clap Sherman (1875–1955)," *J. Nutr.* 61 (1975): 3–11.

37 R. H. Chittenden, *The Development of Physiological Chemistry in the United States* (New York: Chemical Catalogue, 1930): pp. 132–3, 215–16.

38 Raphael Kurzok to Hans T. Clarke, 25 September 1956, A. K. Balls to Clarke, 28 September 1956, Clarke Papers, f. Gies.

39 Names of graduates were obtained from Columbia University *Bulletin of Information* 26 (1911), Columbia *Bulletin* (1912, 1913), and a list (1913–54) in the Clarke Papers.

40 Maxwell Karshan to Clarke, 1 October 1956, Clarke Papers; Gies to Butler, 10 June 1915, 23 November 1916, Gies to S. W. Lambert, 9 January 1917, UColCF; H. T. Clarke, "William John Gies (1872–1956)," *Am. Phil. Soc. Yearbook* (1956): 111–15. Clarke apologized for the cool tone of his memoir: "only a dentist could have written a warm obituary"; see Clarke to Eisenhart, 12 October 1956, Benjamin Harrow, Biographical sketch of Gies (1956), Clarke Papers, f. Gies.

41 Gies to Shaffer, 27 January 1916, other correspondence, Shaffer Papers.

42 R. Kurzok to Clarke, 25 September 1956, Clarke Papers, f. Gies.

43 Mathews to Abel, 19 April 1898, Abel Papers; A. N. Harvey, "Albert Prescott Mathews, Biochemist," *Science* 27 (1958): 443–4.

44 Curtis to Low, 10 October 1898, UColCF.

45 Bowditch to Eliot, 25 January 1902, Eliot Papers, box 103, f. 26; Herter to Abel, 15 October 1905, Abel to Mathews, 19 October 1905, Abel Papers.

46 Loeb to W. R. Harper, 22 January 1902; see also Loeb to Harper, 23 and 26 January and 11 November 1902, UChicPP, box 45, f. 6.

47 University of Chicago *Register* (1906–7), pp. 265–6, (1909–1910), pp. 375–6, (1916–17), pp. 268–70.

48 A. P. Mathews, "The residual valency of anesthetics and its importance in anesthesia," *Int. Z. phys. chem. Biol.* 1 (1914): 433–49; Arthur Cushney to Abel, 31 December 1907, Abel Papers.

49 Loeb to A. B. Macallum, 8 March 1922, Macallum to Loeb, 1 March 1922, Loeb Papers.

50 University of Chicago *Register* (1916–17), pp. 268–9,

51 Hadley R. Marston, "Thorburn B. Robertson," *Aust. J. Exp. Biol. Med. Sci.* 9 (1932): 1–21; Loeb to Wheeler, 27 March 1905, 8 October and 2 November 1907, UCalPP, box 23; T. B. Robertson, "On the normal rate of growth of an individual and its biochemical significance," *Arch. entwicklungsmech. Org.* 25 (1908): 581–614.

J. Loeb, "On the chemical character of fertilization and its bearing upon the theory of life phenomena," *Science* 26 (1907): 425–37. T. B. Robertson, "A biochemical conception of the phenomena of memory and sensation," *The Monist* 19 (1909): 367–86.

52 T. B. Robertson, *Principles of Biochemistry for Students of Medicine, Agriculture and Related Sciences* (Philadelphia: Lea and Febiger, 1920).

53 Robertson to David P. Barrows, 11 February and 11 March 1915, UCalPP.

54 Robertson to Barrows, 11 March 1915, UCalPP. Robertson to Moffit, 15 January 1915, C. M. Torrey to Robertson, 2 November 1915, Robertson to Wheeler, 22 November 1915, Robertson to H. R. Hatfield, 24 May 1916, other correspondence, UCalPP, box 82.

55 Robertson to Barrows, 11 February and 11 March 1915, UCalPP.

56 Martin Hanke, "Fred Conrad Koch, 1876–1948," *Arch. Biochem.* 17 (1948): 207–9.

57 Bloor to Barrows, 23 August 1920, UCalPP, box 115; Bloor to Barrows, 18 and 23 February 1922, 30 June and 7 July 1922, Barrows to Bloor, 5 July 1922, UColPP, box 147. Bloor was appointed at Rochester on the advice of Van Slyke and Folin. Rush Rhees to A. Flexner, 3 October 1922, GEB, B23, box 708. Anon., "Dr. Walter Ray Bloor," *Genesee Valley Chemunications* (September 1950): 8–9, 20.

58 David Greenberg, "Carl Louis August Schmidt," *Science* 104 (1946): 387; D. Greenberg, "Recollections of the history of biochemistry at the University of California, 1900–970," Unpublished manuscript, pp. 9–11, 23–5, UCalA. Schmidt's group remained in Berkeley; he himself worked on the physical chemistry of proteins.

59 Loeb to Traube, 29 December 1913, Loeb to Taylor, 9 November 1912, Loeb Papers; Wolfgang Ostwald, "Martin Fischer zum 60 Geburtstag," *Kolloid Z.* 89 (1939): 1–12.

60 Loeb to Meyerhof, 3 October 1923, Loeb Papers.

61 Loeb to Robertson, 23 December 1914, Loeb to T. H. Morgan, 9 and 10 March 1922, Hardolph Wasteneys to Loeb, 24 March 1919, Loeb Papers.

62 Loeb to S. Flexner, 1 February, 1924, Flexner Papers. Flexner did not take Loeb seriously and calmed him down; see Flexner to Loeb, 7 February 1924, Loeb to Flexner, 4 August and 8 September 1923, Flexner Papers.

63 Loeb to Rudolph Höber, 10 November and 11 December 1923, Meyerhof to Loeb, 12 June 1923, Karl Neuberg to Loeb, 10 October and 28 December 1923, Loeb to Neuberg, 11 December 1923, Loeb to Warburg, 3 December 1920, 18 May 1923, Warburg to Loeb, 14 October 1923, Loeb Papers.

64 Warburg to Loeb, 20 December 1920, Loeb Papers.

65 A. Flexner to Rush Rhees, 10 April and 14 May 1923, Rhees to Flexner, 7 and 11 May 1923, Meyerhof to Flexner, 12 May 1923, GEB, B23, box 708. W. Pepper to Flexner, 26 February 1923, GEB, 2498, box 690; Flexner to E. D. Burton, 5 November 1923, Memorandum from dean of faculties to Burton, 16 November 1923, Mendel to Carlson, 10 March 1924, Carlson to Burton, 24 April 1924, UChicPP, box 17, f. 13.

66 A. Flexner to Rush Rhees, 14 May 1923, GEB, B23, box 708.

67 George H. Whipple to A. Flexner, 24 May 1923, GEB B23, box 708. "I have known a number of continental physiologists and have worked with some of them. I have a feeling that their point of view does not coincide with ours in contrast to that of the English physiologists who think much more like the Americans in medical research and general physiology. I also feel that it is very difficult for them to understand our students and for students and junior members of the staff to understand them.... I think that the transplantation of a continental physiologist to this country... would be quite a serious experiment."

68 Morse to Loeb, 5 April 1915, Loeb Papers.

69 Loeb to Morse, 8 April 1915, Loeb Papers. I owe thanks to Philip Pauly for these citations.

70 T. H. Morgan to H. J. Thorkelson, 2 February 1926, GEB, 2451, box 691; George Wald, "Selig Hecht, 1892–1947," *J. Gen. Physiol.* 32 (1949): 1–16; Hecht to Crozier, 14 February, 2 May, and 10 May 1921, Crozier Papers.

71 R. Gerard, "Ralph Staynard Lillie, 1875–1952," *Science* 116 (1952): 496–7.

72 Morgan to Thorkelson, 2 February 1926, GEB, 2451, box 691.

73 Loeb to Lillie, 12 November 1923, UChicPP, box 17, f. 13; Lillie to Morgan, 28 January 1926, GEB, 2451, box 691.

74 Morgan to Thorkelson, 2 February 1926, J. W. V. Osterhout to Thorkelson, 6 March 1926, Butler to W. W. Brierly, 30 March 1926, GEB, 2451, box 691. Hecht to Crozier, 11 and 29 March 1926, Crozier Papers.

75 Frank R. Johnson, "Edmund Newton Harvey," *Biogr. Mem. Natl. Acad. Sci.* 39 (1967): 193–6. Harvey wrote: "Jacques Loeb's *The Dynamics of Living Matter* had just appeared in 1906, and I now feel that Ralph Lillie and I were both greatly influenced by Loeb's materialistic view of biological problems. There was no doubt that I had found my proper approach to the great subject of biology . . . Loeb's definition of living organisms as 'chemical machines' appealed greatly to me" (pp. 206–7).

76 Harvey to E. G. Conklin, 26 October 1916, 17 August 1918, 5 June 1919, Conklin Papers, box 31.

77 H. J. Thorkelson, Memorandum of interview with H. B. Fine, E. G. Conklin, and Karl T. Compton, 22 May 1925; Fine, Conklin, and Compton, "Memorandum in support of the application to the General Education Board for its support of work in the fundamental sciences at Princeton University," 22 May 1925, pp. 5–6, GEB, 2431, box 675.

78 H. J. Thorkelson, Memorandum of visit to Princeton, 20 October 1925, GEB, 2431, box 675.

79 "Memorandum . . . to the GEB," appendix II, p. 1.

80 Thorkelson, Memorandum, President Hibben to General Education Board, 21 October, 1925, H. A. Smith to Thorkelson, 26 October 1925, GEB, 2431, box 675.

81 Compton to Thorkelson, 22 October 1925, GEB, 2431, box 675.

82 Thorkelson, Memorandum of visits to Princeton, 28 October and 5 November 1928, Thorkelson to Hibben, 20 November 1925, subsequent correspondence, GEB, 2431, box 675.

83 Harvey to Conklin, 15 December 1921, Harvey to C. F. W. McClure, 4 June 1926, Conklin Papers, box 31.

84 H. J. Thorkelson, Memorandum of meeting with R. L. Wilbur, 5 October 1926, GEB, 2301, box 653.

85 Swain to Wilbur, 26 September 1927, Swain Papers, box 2, f. 14; Swain to Wilbur, 27 April 1920, Swain Papers, box 1, f. 5; Swain to Wilbur, 19 December 1929, Swain Papers, box 2, f. 14; J. P. Baumberger, "A history of biology at Stanford University," *Bios* 25 (1954): 123–47.

86 Ray Lyman Wilbur, "Altering the medical curriculum," *J. Am. Med. Assoc.* 88 (1927): 723–5 (for quotation, see p. 724).

87 Swain to Wilbur, 18 May 1928, Wilbur Papers, box 66.

88 Ibid. The number of graduate students in the physical and biological sciences grew from 85 in 1920 to 235 in 1926. Wilbur to E. G. Martin, 23 January 1929, Wilbur Papers, box 69.

89 Wilbur to Taylor, 27 July 1928, Wilbur Papers, box 66.

90 Taylor to Wilbur, 6 December 1928, Martin to Wilbur, 7 December 1928, Wilbur Papers, box 69; Luck to Taylor, 14 January 1930, Wilbur papers, box 72.

91 E. G. Martin, "Report of Committee . . . Plan for the Establishment of a School of Biology," 2 February 1922, Swain Papers, box 1, f. 6; Wilbur to Martin, 23 January 1929, Wilbur Papers, box 69.

92 G. M. Smith et al. to the Faculty of biological sciences, May 1929, Wilbur Papers, box 69. Opinion was divided whether it was in the best interests of the preclinical departments to loosen their attachment to the medical school; see Reports of subcommittees, 17 April 1930, Wilbur papers, box 72.

93 Martin to the Executive Committee, 27 May 930, Wilbur Papers, box 72.

94 Taylor to Swain, 27 February 1931, Wilbur Papers, box 75.

95 Edsall to A. Lawrence Lowell, 29 January 1920, Edsall to Henry P. Walcott, 12 March 1920, David Edsall Papers, f. Physical chemistry.

96 J. T. Edsall, "Edwin Joseph Cohn, 1892–1953," *Biogr. Mem. Natl. Acad. Sci.* 35 (1961): 47–84.

97 Alexander Muralt to H. B. Hanson, 11 February 1938, RF, 200, box 141.

98 John to Cannon, 11 February 1937, David Edsall Papers; John T. Edsall and W. H. Stockmayer, "George Scatchard, 1892–1973," *Biogr. Mem. Natl. Acad. Sci.* 52 (1980); 335–77.

99 Muralt to Hanson, 11 February 1938, RF, 200, box 141.

100 Cohn to Morgan, 11 June 1928, Cohn to Edsall, 29 March 1929, David Edsall Papers; Cohn to Weaver, 20 April 1937, RF, 200, box 141.

101 Diary of W. Weaver, 1 November 1937, RF, 200, box 141. Pauling believed that his own work on the geometry of the peptide bond and hydrogen bonds gave more fundamental information on the structure and function of proteins.

102 Cohn to Weaver, 20 April 1937, RF, 200, box 141; Hastings to Stieglitz, 27 December 1935, Hastings Papers; Hecht to Crozier, 30 August 1925, Crozier Papers.

103 Trustees' minutes, 21 May 1937, 6 April 1938, other correspondence, RF, 200, box 141.

104 Diary of W. Weaver, 13 April 1937, RF, 200, box 141.

105 E. S. Ryerson, "Coordination of the courses as a means of increasing the efficiency of the medical curriculum, undated (circa 1922 or 1923), Edsall to Lyon, 29 January 1920, David Edsall Papers, f. Curriculum.

106 Edsall to Carl Binger, 5 December 1924, Edsall to A. Lawrence Lowell, 16 December 1924, Edsall, Memorandum, undated (circa December 1924), David Edsall Papers, f. Tutors.

107 Edsall fought a running battle with department heads, deans, and students who saw the biochemical sciences program as a preprofessional course; see Lewis to Edsall, 25 June 1925, Edsall to Lewis, 25 June 1925, Edsall to Davis, 12 January 1926, Edsall to Ward, 9 April 1926, R. M. Ferry to Dean C. H. Moore, 23 January 1929, David Edsall Papers, f. Tutors.

108 Samuel Eliot Morison, *Three Centuries of Harvard, 1636–1936* (Cambridge, Mass.: Harvard University Press, 1937); Abbott Lawrence Lowell, *At War with Academic Traditions in America* (Cambridge, Mass.: Harvard University Press, 1934).

109 Correspondence between David Edsall and G. B. Baxter, G. H. Parker, and Theodore Lyman, 1924, Crozier to Ronald Ferry, 18 February 1932, David Edsall Papers, f. Tutors.

110 There are hints that Henderson was active behind the scenes in setting up the Tutors Program; see correspondence between David Edsall and C. H. Moore, December 1926, Edsall to Ferry, 25 January 1926, Edsall to A. L. Lowell, 10 December 1924, 19 January 1925, and correspondence with Hallowell Davis, January 1925, David Edsall Papers, f. Tutors; John T. Edsall, Personal communication.

111 John T. Edsall, "Development of biochemistry at Harvard University," Unpublished essay, August 1975, Survey of Sources; D. Edsall to H. Davis, 12 January 1926, Davis to Edsall, 4 April 1928, David Edsall Papers, f. Tutors.

112 R. M. Ferry and J. T. Edsall, Undated memorandum (circa 1932), Ferry to Dean K. B. Murdock, 28 March 1932, Memorandum (probably by Ferry), February 1934, D. Edsall to Ferry, 25 January 1932, David Edsall Papers, f. Tutors.

113 Edsall to Ferry, 25 January 1932, David Edsall Papers, f. Tutors.

114 Robert A. Emerson to Crozier, 5 May 1931, Crozier to Emerson, 24 March and 11 May 1931, Crozier Papers; Crozier to Hecht, 2 January 1926, Hecht Papers: Crozier wrote, regarding some remarks of G. N. Lewis's: "The childish freedom wherewith chemists speculate about biological matters often gives me a cold fury."

115 Ferry to Murdock, 28 March 1932, David Edsall Papers, f. Tutors; J. T. Edsall, Personal communication, May 1979.
116 Crozier to Ferry, 18 February 1932, David Edsall Papers, f. Tutors. Crozier suggested that a new centralized laboratory be built specifically for the Tutors Program.
117 E. P. Kohler to Adams, 23 January and 15 March 1934, Conant to Adams, 23 January 1934, Roger Adams Papers. I owe thanks to Leon Gortler and D. Stanley Tarbell for these references.
118 Conant to Adams, 23 January 1934, Roger Adams Papers. John T. Edsall recalls that most biologists showed little interest in biochemistry, ignoring Jeffries Wyman's work on the physical biochemistry of proteins; see J. T. Edsall, "Development of biochemistry," August 1975, Survey of Sources.
119 Millikan to Morgan, 1 August 1929, Millikan Papers, box 18, f. 11; T. H. Morgan, "Biology 1930/31," memorandum, Morgan Papers, box 3.
120 John Servos, "The knowledge corporation: A. A. Noyes and chemistry at Caltech, 1915–1930," *Ambix* 23 (1976): 175–86; Robert Kargon, "Temple to science: cooperative research and the birth of the California Institute of Technology," *Hist. Stud. Phy. Sci.* 8 (1977): 3–32; Garland E. Allen, *Thomas Hunt Morgan* (Princeton University Press, 1978), ch. 9.
121 Wycliffe Rose, memorandum of telephone conversation with Arthur Fleming, 4 October 1923, Wycliffe Rose, Memorandum of interviews with G. E. Hale, 2 and 3 October 1923, GEB, 1103, box 611; Noyes to Hale, 17 August 1923, Hale Papers, box 23.
122 Noyes to Hale, 20 October and 22 December 1922, 18 February, 26 March, and 8 May 1923, Hale Papers, box 3.
123 Noyes to Hale, 2 February 1925, Hale Papers, box 33; Noyes to Abel, 31 May 1924, 1 December 1925, Abel to Noyes, 9 September 1925, other correspondence, Abel Papers.
124 "Application to the General Education Board..." 19 January 1925, pp. 7–8, GEB 1103.2, box 612.
125 Ibid., p. 17; A. A. Noyes, "Plans for the development of biology at the California Institute of Technology and its relation to a medical school in Los Angeles," undated (circa 20 March 1925), GEB, 1103.2, box 612.
126 Millikan to H. Pritchett, 13 January 1926, A. A. Noyes, "Outline of a possible plan for the cooperation of the California Institute in developing the proposed metabolic research laboratory," undated (circa 30 March 1925), Millikan to Pritchett, 13 January 1926, Noyes to Millikan, 13 January 1926, Millikan Papers, box 18, f. 7.
127 Hale to Rose, 24 April 1927, GEB, 1103.2, box 612; R. A. Millikan, Memorandum of talk with Morgan, University Club New York, 16 May 1927, Millikan Papers, box 18, f. 9; Morgan to Hale, 8 July, 10 September, 22 October, and 31 October 1927, Hale to Morgan, 22 July, 3 August, 6 September, and 18 October 1927, Morgan Papers, box 1; Millikan to Rose, 16 February 1928, Thorkelson, Memorandum, 23 March 1928, GEB, 1103.2, box 612.
128 Noyes to Millikan, 11 May 1927, Lorena Breed to Noyes, 6 and 18 May 1927, L. L. Snow to Breed, 23 April 1927, Noyes to Breed, 10 June 1927, Millikan Papers, box 18, f. 9.
129 Noyes to Millikan, 4 March 1927, Hale Papers, box 33; Conant to Noyes, 16 May 1927, Noyes Papers, box 49, f. 4, Thorkelson, Memorandum, 24 March 1927, GEB, 1103.2, box 612.
130 Noyes to Morgan, 31 August 1927, Morgan to Noyes, 3 July 1928, Morgan Papers, box 1; Morgan to Fleming, 19 January 1929, Millikan Papers, box 18, f. 11.
131 Millikan, Memorandum of talk with Morgan, 16 May 1927, Millikan Papers, box 18, f. 9. Morgan projected a staff of four or five for physiology and a budget of $25,000, apart from biochemistry and biophysics: see Morgan to Fleming,

1 August 1927, Millikan Papers, box 18, f. 9; Morgan to Hale, 8 July 1927, Morgan Papers, box 1.

132   Hale to Morgan, 3 and 8 August 1927, Morgan Papers, box 1; Rose to Flexner, 3 November 1927, GEB, 1103.2, box 612.

133   See Hale to Morgan, 24 August 1927, Morgan to Hale, 22 October 1927, Morgan Papers, box 1.

134   Morgan to Hale, 15 August 1927, Millikan Papers, box 18, f. 9.

135   Morgan, Memorandum, undated (circa April 1928), Millikan Papers, box 18, f. 10; Hecht to Crozier, undated (circa January 1928), Crozier to Hecht, undated (circa 20 January 1928), Hecht Papers.

136   Morgan to Millikan, 28 May 1928, Millikan Papers, box 18, f. 10. Morgan thought highly of Michaelis's work, but "On the other hand he is not young, and already has collected about himself a few young Jews. He himself is markedly Semitic. I have my doubts whether we should want to start under these conditions, and shall make no moves. Possibly next year we might invite him for a year, but this too is dubious."

137   Noyes to Hale, 2 January 1928, Hale Papers, box 33. In 1936 Raymond became director of research at Searle Laboratories.

138   Morgan to Mason, 13 May 1933, Morgan Papers, box 1; Morgan, Report for 1930/31, Morgan Papers, box 3; Noyes to Morgan, 22 July 1932, Noyes Papers, box 49, f. 4.

139   Emerson to Crozier, 24 March 1931, Crozier Papers.

140   Emerson to Crozier, 1 December 1931, Crozier Papers; Hecht to Jacinto Steinhardt, 7 November 1934, Hecht Papers.

141   A. A. Noyes, "Notes on the Kerckhoff Laboratories," undated (circa August 1933); see also Hale to S. Flexner, 21 August 1933, Noyes Papers, box 49, f. 4; Noyes to Morgan, 25 August 1933, Noyes, Confidential notes on the Kerckhoff situation, undated (circa August 1933), Millikan Papers, box 18, f. 14.

142   Extensive correspondence in the Noyes, Millikan, and Morgan Papers.

143   Borsook to S. Flexner, 30 April 1934, Flexner to Borsook, 8 May 1934, Flexner Papers; Morgan to Millikan, undated, Millikan to John Balderston, 6 December 1940, Millikan Papers, box 18, f. 6. Borsook's publications show the following shift from physical chemistry to metabolism and nutrition:

Period	Thermodynamics, enzymology	Nutrition	Nitrogen metabolism	Other
1930–4	7	2	2	4
1935–9	4	2	8	
1940–4	1	7	10	

CHAPTER 12   *Epilogue: Toward a molecular biology?*

1   R. E. Kohler, "Rudolf Schoenheimer, isotopic tracers, and biochemistry in the 1930s," *Hist. Stud. Phys. Sci.* 8 (1977): 257–98.

2   Stanley to S. Flexner, 7 April and 8 June 1936, November 1940; Flexner Papers.

3   Joseph S. Fruton, *Molecules and Life* (New York: Wiley, 1972); Horace F. Judson, *The Eighth Day of Creation* (New York: Simon and Schuster, 1979); Robert Olby, *The Path to the Double Helix* (Seattle: University of Washington Press, 1974).

4   There were a few noteworthy exceptions. Hans Krebs was one of the first outside Beadle's circle to do biochemical genetics, and he arranged for Hugh McIlwain to study bacterial genetics, with an eye to developing the field in Britain. See the Diary of G. R. Pomeranz, 2 May 1947, RF, 401D, box 43; Krebs to Beadle, 2 June 1949, Krebs to A. L. Thomson, 8 March 1947, MRC, 497.

5   Kohler, "Schoenheimer," pp. 257–98.

6 Alexander to Hastings, 1 March 1938, Hastings to Dean Burwell, 1 and 16 March 1938, correspondence with SubbaRow, Hastings, Memorandum on the responsibilities of a Department of biochemistry, 19 October 1942, Hastings Papers.

7 Hanke to Hastings, 8 November 1938, Vennesland to Hastings, 3 October 1939, Hastings, "To be discussed with Miss Vennesland," undated, Vennesland to Hastings, 29 October and 22 December 1941, Hastings Papers; Harry Trimble, "Notes on Fiske and Hastings," 9 April 1959, Trimble Papers.

8 Trimble, "Fiske and Hastings," 9 April 1959, Vennesland to Hastings, 23 December 1946, Eric Ball and Hastings to Dean Burwell, 6 November 1947, Hastings Papers, f. Anfinson; E. Ball, Memorandum, "Teaching of graduate students," Hastings to G. P. Berry, Hastings's department report, 8 September 1949, Hastings Papers, f. Departmental.

9 David Greenberg, "Recollections of the history of biochemistry at the University of California, 1900–1970," pp. 27, 61, UCalA; W. C. Pomeroy to R. G. Sproul, 25 April 1938, UCalPP, box 451; Archie Woods to Sproul, 27 April 1939, Carl Schmidt to Sproul, 27 April 1939, 2 May 1941, 26 December 1945, UCalPP, boxes 474, 544, 658.

10 Howard B. Lewis to A. C. Furstenberg, 7 October 1937, 21 September 1938, Lewis Papers, box 4.

11 Lewis to Mattill, 30 June 1948, Lewis Papers, box 1; Lewis to Max S. Dunn, 10 March 1936, Lewis Papers, box 5; Lewis to Rose, 30 March 1947, Lewis Papers, box 2.

12 Mattill to Lewis, 3 February 1948, 1 September and 30 October 1945, Lewis Papers, box 1.

13 Lewis to Mattill, 2 May 1946, Lewis Papers, box 1; Lewis to Minor J. Coon, 22 April 1947, Lewis to R. J. Gustavson, 22 April 1947, Lewis to Dean Furstenberg, 15 November 1954, H. B. Lewis, "Possible appropriations for support of medical research," and "Department of Biological Chemistry research progress," undated, Lewis Papers, box 2.

14 The leading texts in 1950 were Benjamin Harrow, *Biochemistry for Medical, Dental and College Students* (Philadelphia: Saunders, 1938), and Israel Kleiner, *Human Biochemistry* (St. Louis, Mo.: Mosby, 1945). Harrow, a biochemist, emphasized basic chemistry; Kleiner, a clinical chemist, emphasized human physiology and clinical applications. (Kleiner gave 20% of his text to clinical methods, 2% to recent topics. Harrow gave them 10% and 13%, respectively.) H. B. Lewis took the middle road: although his medical students preferred Kleiner, he assigned whichever text had been most recently revised: see H. B. Lewis to Kleiner, 3 November 1950, P. Hawk to Lewis, 24 May 1952, 21 January 1953, Lewis Papers, box 1. By 1955 Lewis had switched to a new generation of general biochemistry texts: see Edward S. West and Wilbur R. Todd, *Textbook of Biochemistry* (New York: Macmillan, 1951); Joseph S. Fruton and Sofia Simmonds, *General Biochemistry* (New York: Wiley, 1953); Abraham White, Philip Handler, and Emil Smith, *Principles of Biochemistry* (New York: McGraw-Hill, 1954); Lewis to W. A. Krehl, 4 April 1952, Lewis to Crossman, 14 January 1953, Lewis Papers, box 1.

15 Luck to Greenberg, 29 January 1954, Luck Papers.

16 Eleanor Darby to Clarke, 14 March 1963, Clarke Papers.

17 I. C. Gunsalus, "Biochemistry at a graduate level, relation of biochemistry to biology and new approaches to biochemistry," Address to the ASBC meeting, 16–20 April 1963, Clarke Papers.

18 Philip Handler, "The education of professional biochemists," Address to the ASBC meeting, 16–20 April 1963, Clarke Papers.

19 Erwin Chargaff, *Essays on Nucleic Acids* (Amsterdam: Elsevier, 1963), p. 176.

20 Morton is quoted by E. A. Dawes, "Place of biochemistry in the new universities," *Nature* 203 (1964): 131–2.

21 Ibid.

22 J. C. Kendrew et al., *Report of the working group on molecular biology* (London: H.M. Stationery Office, 1968), p. 2.

23 Hans Krebs, *Biochemistry, "Molecular Biology," and Biological Sciences* (London: Biochemical Society, 1969), p. 5.

24 Hill to Cyril Long, 2 June 1936, Long Papers.

25 Hubert [illeg.] to Shaffer, 26 October 1936, Shaffer Papers, box 13, f. 171.

26 R. E. Kohler, "Warren Weaver and the Rockefeller Foundation program in molecular biology: a case study in the management of science," in Nathan Reingold, ed., *The Sciences in the American Context: New Perspectives* (Washington: Smithsonian Institution Press, 1979), pp. 249–93.

Index

Cornell Medical School, (*cont.*)
  biochemistry at, 185–6, 281, 283
  clinical research in, 239–40
Cornell University
  biochemistry at, 190–1, 267
Cowles, Edward, 234
Crane, William H., 190
Crozier, William J., 317, 321, 384
  n114
Cullen, Glenn, 239, 374 n128
Curtiss, John G., 114, 134–5
  and biochemistry at P&S, 172–6

Dakin, Henry, 213, 269–70, 280
D'Ancona, A.A., 149, 151–3, 189
Danelli, William J., 267–8
Darrach, William, 280
Davenport, Eugene, 262, 264
Davis, Hallowell, 316
Debye, Peter, 314–15
Denis, Willey, 238, 244
Deyer, George, 266
diabetes, 227, 229, 245
diagnosis
  biochemistry in, 227–31
  clinicians and, 229–30
  see also laboratories, diagnostic
disciplinary programs, 213–14, 252,
  288, 295, 324–5
disciplines
  definition of, 1–3, 7
  history of, 1–3
Dixon, Malcolm, 83
Dock, George, 128, 142, 184–5, 225,
  231
Dodds, Edward C., 40, 242–3, 251
Doisey, Edward, 244, 248
Drechsel, Edmund, 24, 29, 30, 35,
  106–7, 343 n75
Drummond, Jack, 67–8
DuBois, Eugene, 238, 240, 372 n94
Du Bois-Reymond, Emil, 28–30
Dunn, Sir William
  bequests, 78–81
Du Vigneaud, Vincent, 281–3

ecology of knowledge, 8, 324–5
Edinburgh, University of, 45–6
  biochemistry at, 68–9
Edsall, David, 128, 223
  and clinical research, 237–8
  at Pennsylvania, 138–9

and Physical Chemistry Laboratory,
  313–14
and Tutors Program, 316
Edsall, John T., 316–17
Eicholz, Alfred, 48
Eliot, Charles W., 128–30, 177–80
Elliott, T.R., 48, 68
Embden, Gustav, 28, 37
embryology, biochemical, 48
  at Cambridge, 73, 83, 85–7
Emerson, Charles, 227, 229
Emerson, Robert, 318
Emerson, Robert L., 177
enzymes, 48–9, 56, 83, 287, 289
Erlangen, University of, 20
Erlanger, Joseph, 142, 184
Evans, Earl A., Jr., 281, 328
Ezrahi, Yaron, 5–6

Faust, Edwin, 107, 254
Ferry, Ronald M., 316–17
Fischer, Emil, 36
  students of, 267, 270
Fischer, Martin, 190, 230, 306
Fiske, Cyrus, 191, 225
Fletcher, Walter M., 48, 63–5, 156,
  254
  and Dunn Estate, 78–82
  and F.G. Hopkins, 52–4, 77–8,
  85, 87–8
  secretary of MRC, 76–7
Flexner, Abraham, 129, 138, 141–2,
  211, 230, 236, 280
Flexner, Simon, 119, 137, 232,
  238–9, 240, 269, 306
Flexner Report, 125
Flint, Joseph, 145, 149, 151–2
Flügge, Karl, 35
Folin, Otto K., 107, 194–5, 211, 225,
  226, 228–9
  background and character, 180–1
  at Harvard, 179–82, 219, 275
  and hospitals, 220, 235–6, 241
  at McLean Hospital, 234–5
  professional role, 244–8
Foster, Michael, 42, 47–59, 50, 75, 86
Frazier, Charles H., 138–9
Fribourg, University of, 18–19, 25
Fruton, Joseph, 270, 281
Fulton, John, 283, 379 n106

Gaebler, Oliver, 250
Gale, Ernest F., 86